Liver Transplantation: Update of Concepts and Practice

Editors

KALYAN RAM BHAMIDIMARRI
PAUL MARTIN

CLINICS IN LIVER DISEASE

www.liver.theclinics.com

Consulting Editor
NORMAN GITLIN

August 2014 • Volume 18 • Number 3

ELSEVIER

1600 John F. Kennedy Boulevard • Suite 1800 • Philadelphia, Pennsylvania, 19103-2899

http://www.theclinics.com

CLINICS IN LIVER DISEASE Volume 18, Number 3
August 2014 ISSN 1089-3261, ISBN-13: 978-0-323-32016-0

Editor: Kerry Holland
Developmental Editor: Casey Jackson

Clinics in Liver Disease (ISSN 1089-3261) is published quarterly by Elsevier Inc., 360 Park Avenue South, New York, NY 10010-1710. Months of issue are February, May, August, and November. Business and Editorial Offices: 1600 John F. Kennedy Blvd., Ste. 1800, Philadelphia, PA 19103-2899. Customer Service Office: 3251 Riverport Lane, Maryland Heights, MO 63043. Periodicals postage paid at New York, NY and additional mailing offices. Subscription prices are $295.00 per year (U.S. individuals), $145.00 per year (U.S. student/resident), $401.00 per year (U.S. institutions), $395.00 per year (foreign individuals), $200.00 per year (foreign student/ resident), $498.00 per year (foreign instituitions), $340.00 per year (Canadian individuals), $200.00 per year (Canadian student/resident), and $498.00 per year (Canadian institutions). Foreign air speed delivery is included in all *Clinics* subscription prices. All prices are subject to change without notice. **POSTMASTER:** Send address changes to *Clinics in Liver Disease*, Elsevier Health Sciences Division, Subscription Customer Service, 3251 Riverport Lane, Maryland Heights, MO 63043. **Customer Service: Telephone: 1-800-654-2452 (U.S. and Canada); 314-447-8871 (outside U.S. and Canada). Fax: 314-447-8029. E-mail: journalscustomer service-usa@elsevier.com (for print support); journalsonlinesupport-usa@elsevier.com (for online support).**

Reprints. For copies of 100 or more of articles in this publication, please contact the Commercial Reprints Department, Elsevier Inc., 360 Park Avenue South, New York, NY 10010-1710. Tel.: 212-633-3874; Fax: 212-633-3820; E-mail: reprints@elsevier.com.

Clinics in Liver Disease is covered in *MEDLINE/PubMed (Index Medicus)*, Science Citation Index Expanded, Journal Citation Reports/Science Edition, and Current Contents/Clinical Medicine.

Contributors

CONSULTING EDITOR

NORMAN GITLIN, MD, FRCP (LONDON), FRCPE (EDINBURGH), FACG, FACP
Formerly, Professor of Medicine, Chief of Hepatology, Emory University; Currently, Consultant, Atlanta Gastroenterology Associates, Atlanta, Georgia

EDITORS

KALYAN RAM BHAMIDIMARRI, MD, MPH
Assistant Professor of Clinical Medicine, Division of Hepatology, Miami Transplant Institute, University of Miami, Miami, Florida

PAUL MARTIN, MD, FRCP, FRCPI
Chief, Division of Hepatology, Miller School of Medicine, University of Miami, Miami, Florida

AUTHORS

SUMEET K. ASRANI, MD, MSc
Division of Hepatology, Baylor University Medical Center, Dallas, Texas

THIAGO BEDUSCHI, MD
Miami Transplant Institute, University of Miami, Miami, Florida

KALYAN RAM BHAMIDIMARRI, MD, MPH
Assistant Professor of Clinical Medicine, Division of Hepatology, Miami Transplant Institute, University of Miami, Miami, Florida

SUPHAMAI BUNNAPRADIST, MD
Division of Nephrology, Department of Medicine, Kidney and Pancreas Transplant Program, David Geffen School of Medicine at UCLA, Los Angeles, California

MICHAEL R. CHARLTON, MBBS, FRCP
Professor of Medicine, Director of Hepatology and Medical Director of Liver Transplantation, Intermountain Medical Center, Murray, Utah

SANDY FENG, MD, PhD
Professor, Division of Abdominal Transplantation, Department of Surgery, University of California, San Francisco, San Francisco, California

IVO W. GRAZIADEI, MD
Department of Internal Medicine II (Gastroenterology and Hepatology), Medical University of Innsbruck, Innsbruck; Department of Internal Medicine, District Hospital Hall, Hall in Tirol, Austria

SOHAIB K. HASHMI, BS
Harrison Surgical Scholar, Department of Surgery, The University of Pennsylvania, Philadelphia, Pennsylvania

PETER C. HAYES, MBChB, PhD
Department of Hepatology, Royal Infirmary of Edinburgh, Edinburgh, United Kingdom

DEIRDRE KELLY, FRCPCH, FRCP, FRCPI, MD
Professor of Paediatric Hepatology, The Liver Unit, Birmingham Children's Hospital, University of Birmingham, Birmingham, United Kingdom

WILLIAM H. KITCHENS, MD, PhD
Department of Surgery, Massachusetts General Hospital, Boston, Massachusetts

JENNIFER C. LAI, MD, MBA
Assistant Professor, Division of Gastroenterology/Hepatology, Department of Medicine, University of California, San Francisco, San Francisco, California

JAMES F. MARKMANN, MD, PhD
Chief of the Division of Transplantation, Department of Surgery, Massachusetts General Hospital; Claude E. Welch Professor of Surgery at Harvard Medical School, Boston, Massachusetts

PAUL MARTIN, MD, FRCP, FRCPI
Chief, Division of Hepatology, Miller School of Medicine, University of Miami, Miami, Florida

NORMA C. McAVOY, MBChB, MRCP
Consultant Gastroenterologist and Honorary Senior Lecturer, Department of Hepatology, Royal Infirmary of Edinburgh, Edinburgh, United Kingdom

JACQUELINE G. O'LEARY, MD, MPH
Medical Director, Hepatology Research; Medical Director, Liver and Transplant Unit, Division of Hepatology, Baylor University Medical Center, Dallas, Texas

PAIGE M. PORRETT, MD, PhD
Division of Liver Transplantation, Assistant Professor of Surgery, Department of Surgery, The University of Pennsylvania, Philadelphia, Pennsylvania

KAYVAN ROAYAIE, MD, PhD
Division of Abdominal Organ Transplantation, Department of Surgery, Oregon Health and Sciences University, Portland, Oregon

SASAN ROAYAIE, MD
Liver Cancer Program, Hofstra-North Shore LIJ School of Medicine, Lenox Hill Hospital, New York, New York

MARCELO S. SAMPAIO, MD, PhD
Division of Nephrology, Department of Medicine, Kidney and Pancreas Transplant Program, David Geffen School of Medicine at UCLA, Los Angeles, California

ABRAHAM SHAKED, MD, PhD
Division of Liver Transplantation, Eldrige L. Eliason Professor of Surgery, Department of Surgery; Director, Penn Transplant Institute, The University of Pennsylvania, Philadelphia, Pennsylvania

JAMES F. TROTTER, MD
Medical Director of Liver Transplantation, Baylor University Medical Center, Dallas, Texas

ELIZABETH C. VERNA, MD, MS
Assistant Professor of Medicine, Division of Digestive and Liver Diseases, Center for Liver Disease and Transplantation, Columbia University College of Physicians and Surgeons, New York, New York

RODRIGO VIANNA, MD
Director of Transplant Services; Professor of Clinical Surgery, Miami Transplant Institute, University of Miami, Miami, Florida

RUSSELL H. WIESNER, MD
Professor of Medicine, Mayo College of Medicine, Rochester, Minnesota

JO WRAY, PhD, C PSYCHOL
Health Psychologist, Critical Care and Cardiorespiratory Division, Great Ormond Street Hospital for Children NHS Foundation Trust, London, United Kingdom

HEIDI YEH, MD
Division of Transplantation, Department of Surgery, Massachusetts General Hospital, Boston, Massachusetts

Contents

Viral hepatitis is both a leading indication for liver transplant (LT) and an important cause of posttransplant graft loss and mortality. Treatment and prevention of hepatitis B virus in LT recipients, with the observed corresponding improvement in post-LT outcomes, is among the great success stories in transplantation. By comparison, treatment of hepatitis C virus with safe and effective regimens is only just becoming a reality. Chronic hepatitis E virus infection in LT recipients represents a newly described phenomenon that can also lead to graft loss; early diagnosis and treatment may be key in the management of these patients.

The role of liver transplant for treatment of early hepatocellular cancer (HCC) is no longer contested. However, its benefit relative to other therapies for patients with very early (<2 cm) HCC is still a matter of debate. Twenty years after the establishment of the Milan criteria, we are beginning to realize that the number and size of tumors may not be the best metric by which to prognosticate outcomes and allocate organs. A better assessment of tumor aggressiveness is clearly needed.

The rapid development of new diagnostic tests and improved therapy, especially the success of liver transplantation, has changed the outcome for children with liver disease, many of whom survive into adolescence without liver transplantation. The indications for transplantation in adolescence are similar to pediatric indications and reflect the medical advances made in this specialty that allow later transplantation. These young people need a different approach to management that involves consideration of their physical and psychological stage of development. A focused approach to their eventual transition to adult care is essential for long-term survival and quality of life.

The greatest challenge facing liver transplantation today is the shortage of donor livers. Demand far exceeds supply, and this deficit has driven expansion of what is considered an acceptable organ. The evolving standard has not come without costs, however, as each new frontier of expanded donor quality (i.e., advancing donor age, donation after cardiac death, and split liver) has possibly traded wait-list for post-transplant morbidity and mortality. This article delineates the nature and severity of risk associated with specific deceased donor liver characteristics and recommends strategies to maximally mitigate these risks.

James F. Trotter

Living donor liver transplantation is a procedure that has waned in its application over the past decade but remains a beneficial procedure for properly selected candidates. This review discusses some of the newer, relevant studies in the field, focusing on outcomes with hepatocellular carcinoma, ABO-incompatible transplant, and issues in donor complications and safety.

Kalyan Ram Bhamidimarri, Thiago Beduschi, and Rodrigo Vianna

Intestinal transplantation is the definitive therapy for patients with irreversible intestinal failure and can be combined with transplantation of other abdominal organs, such as stomach, spleen, and pancreas with or without liver. There is an increasing trend in the volume of intestinal and multivisceral transplantation in the past few decades and there is also increasing trend in patient and graft survival primarily due to improved patient selection, advances in immunosuppression, and improved perioperative management. This review summarizes the various key elements in patient selection, types of grafts, and updates in the perioperative management involved in multivisceral transplantation.

Ivo W. Graziadei

Many nonviral diseases that cause liver failure may recur after liver transplantation. Although most studies have shown that a recurrent disease does not negatively affect patient and graft survival in the intermediate postoperative course, there is growing evidence that, especially in patients with primary sclerosing cholangitis and in patients with recurrent abusive alcohol drinking, disease recurrence is a significant risk factor for graft dysfunction and graft loss. Therefore, the recurrence of nonviral diseases has become a clinically important and prognostically relevant issue in the long-term management of recipients of liver transplantation.

Paige M. Porrett, Sohaib K. Hashmi, and Abraham Shaked

Advances in pharmacologic immunosuppression are responsible for the excellent outcomes experienced by recipients of liver transplants. However, long-term follow up of these patients reveals an increasing burden of morbidity and mortality that is attributable to these drugs. The authors summarize the agents used in contemporary liver transplantation immunosuppression protocols and discuss the emerging trend within the community to minimize or eliminate these agents from use. The authors present recently published data that may provide the foundation for immunosuppression minimization or tolerance induction in the future and review studies that have focused on the utility of biomarkers in guiding immuno-suppression management.

Long-term survival following liver transplantation is profoundly affected by conditions unrelated to graft function. Many causes of mortality are contributed to by the metabolic syndrome. The approach to metabolic syndrome in liver transplant recipients requires consideration of transplant-specific factors, particularly immunosuppression. Enhancing long-term outcomes for liver transplant recipients necessitates minimizing the amount of immunosuppression required to prevent rejection. Studies to determine the optimal approach to minimize the impact of metabolic syndrome and complications of immunosuppression in transplant recipients are needed.

Hepatic retransplant is the sole option for survival in many patients suffering hepatic dysfunction after liver transplant, but it is associated with significantly increased hospital costs and inferior outcomes compared to primary transplants. In this review, the indications for both early and late liver retransplant are presented. The controversy regarding retransplant in patients infected with hepatitis C virus is discussed, and the recipient and donor graft characteristics impacting survival following hepatic retransplant are analyzed. With improved risk stratification models to match retransplant candidates with appropriate donor grafts, it is hoped that the clinical outcomes of retransplant will continue to improve.

CLINICS IN LIVER DISEASE

Preface

Liver Transplantation: Update of Concepts and Practice

 CrossMark

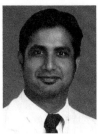
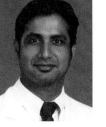

Kalyan Ram Bhamidimarri, MD, MPH   Paul Martin, MD, FRCP, FRCPI
Editors

Liver transplantation has remarkably changed the outlook for patients in whom advanced liver disease was once typically fatal. In the current issue of the *Clinics in Liver Disease*, we sought assistance from a distinguished group of experts to compile an update on concepts and practices in this ever-evolving field.

Organ allocation policies were profoundly changed after the adoption of the Model for End Stage Liver Disease (MELD) in 2002, and we now refer to the transplant periods as "pre- and post-MELD eras." Dr Wiesner discusses the current changing trends of organ allocation policies, including the recent "Share 35" policy in the first article. The articles by Professor Hayes on cardiopulmonary issues and Dr Bunnapradist on kidney disease address the workup and management of the transplant candidate in the peritransplant setting.

Dr O'Leary discusses acute chronic liver failure, which is now recognized as an important entity, and the management of viral hepatitis, especially hepatitis C, which is rapidly evolving, is discussed by Dr Verna. Dr Roayaie addresses the key role of liver transplant in the management of primary liver cancer, while Dr Feng discusses the current role and strategy in the transplantation of extended criteria or marginal liver grafts. Dr Kelly provides her expertise from a pediatric angle in dealing with the issues and challenges in an adolescent transplant patient.

Living donor liver transplantation, which is an important option for many potential recipients, is discussed by Dr Trotter, while intestinal and multivisceral transplantation is discussed by the group from the University of Miami, led by Dr Vianna. The remarkable improvement in long-term outcomes after liver transplantation is a reflection of the advancements in the immunosuppression, as discussed by Dr Shaked, and posttransplant care, as related by Dr Charlton. Long-term outcomes unfortunately are diminished by recurrence of primary liver disease in the graft, as reviewed by Dr Graziadei. Dr Markman discusses the difficult issue of retransplantation, making the current issue wholesome and complete.

Clin Liver Dis 18 (2014) xiii–xiv
http://dx.doi.org/10.1016/j.cld.2014.05.015
1089-3261/14/$ – see front matter © 2014 Elsevier Inc. All rights reserved.

liver.theclinics.com

We are extremely thankful to the authors who have contributed their time and effort to provide us with their expertise and insights in this issue on liver transplantation. We also thank Dr Norman Gitlin and the Elsevier editorial staff for providing us the opportunity to edit the issue.

Kalyan Ram Bhamidimarri, MD, MPH
Medicine/Hepatology
Miller School of Medicine Center For Liver Diseases
University of Miami
1500 NW 12th Avenue, Suite 1101
Miami, FL 33136, USA

Paul Martin, MD, FRCP, FRCPI
Division of Heaptology
University of Miami
1500 NW12th Avenue, 1101E
Miami, FL 33136, USA

E-mail addresses:
KBhamidimari@med.miami.edu (K.R. Bhamidimarri)
pmartin2@med.miami.edu (P. Martin)

Evolving Trends in Liver Transplantation

Listing and Liver Donor Allocation

Russell H. Wiesner, MD

KEYWORDS

- Liver transplantation • MELD • Liver donor allocation • Chronic liver disease

KEY POINTS

- The MELD-based allocation policy is excellent at prioritizing patients with chronic liver disease on the waiting list based on survival.
- Exception criteria are needed because of such conditions as hepatocellular cancer, with tumor progression being used as a surrogate for patient survival.
- MELD can be tweaked by adding serum sodium and other variables; but overall the impact would be minimal and reprograming is expensive and cumbersome.

INTRODUCTION

The success of liver transplantation in the past three decades as a life-saving procedure for patients with end-stage liver disease has led to the ever-increasing disparity between the demands for liver transplantation and the supply of donor liver organs. This demand has been fueled by an increasing prevalence of cirrhosis and hepatocellular cancer (HCC) related to the hepatitis C epidemic, and to the increase in obesity-related liver disease.[1] Today, nearly 1 in 10 patients waiting for a donor liver organ die on the waiting list.[2] Therefore, donor allocation and distribution remains a challenge and a moral issue as to how these organs can be equitably distributed. This article reviews the evolution of the liver allocation policy and discusses in detail the challenges we face today.

HISTORY

Donor liver allocation dates back to the Transplantation Act of 1983 when there were only a few liver transplant centers in the United States. However, with the increasing success of liver transplantation and expanded indications, the number of patients seeking this life-saving procedure continued to grow. At the same time, the number

Disclosure: None.
Mayo College of Medicine, Rochester, MN 55905, USA
E-mail address: rwiesner@mayo.edu

of institutions offering liver transplantation also increased. By the mid-1990s, livers were allocated based on blood type; time on the liver transplant waiting list; and whether a patient was in the intensive care unit (ICU), hospital, or an outpatient. There was no criterion to define which patients should be in the ICU or which patients should be hospitalized. Indeed, many centers admitted patients to the ICU solely to facilitate their placement at the top of the liver waiting list. In retrospect, it was noted in the model for end-stage liver disease (MELD) era that the number of patients proceeding to liver transplantation from the ICU dropped dramatically from 24% in the pre-MELD era to 13% in the post-MELD era.[3] There was also noted to be a strong relationship between the number of centers in an organ procurement unit, and the number of patients undergoing liver transplant directly from the ICU.

An attempt to rectify this problem was made in 1998 by implementation of a new system incorporating the Child-Turcotte-Pugh score (CTP) as an index for liver disease severity and prognosis. This scoring system was originally used to predict the outcome of portal-cava shunt surgery in patients with cirrhosis.[4] Adoption of the CTP-based allocation system was intended primarily to reflect waiting list mortality and severity of liver disease. However, the use of the CTP score for the prioritization of liver transplant candidates had several major drawbacks. First, ascites and encephalopathy were subjectively assessed and were influenced by such therapies as diuretics, albumin administration, and lactulose therapy. In addition, a score of three points was allocated for any serum bilirubin value higher than 3.0 mg/dL and any serum albumin level value of 2.8 mg/dL or less. This "ceiling and floor affect" for bilirubin and albumin, respectively, meant that many patients ended up with the same overall CTP score, even though they may have had vastly different values of these two variables. Indeed, a patient with a serum bilirubin of 25 mg/dL received the same CTP score as the patient who had a serum bilirubin of 3 mg/dL. As a result, time spent on the waiting list became the major selection factor of liver candidates having identical CTP scores. Finally, there was no parameter in the CTP score that reflected renal function, a key prognostic marker in patients with end-stage cirrhosis. Two studies found time spent on the waiting list was not associated with risk of death on the waiting list.[5,6] In the end, the revised allocation policy based on the CTP score ultimately proved unworkable and unfair to patients with the most severe liver disease. Because of considerable disagreement among transplant centers on how livers should be allocated, the United Network for Organ Sharing (UNOS) and the Department of Health and Human Services intervened in 1999 and challenged the transplant community with "The Final Rule."[7] Among the conditions of the Final Rule were that allocation policies should be based on objective and measurable medical criteria of patients or categories of patients who are medically suitable candidates for liver transplantation. In addition, it noted that patients should be rank-ordered according to severity of disease and predicted mortality on the liver waiting list. The Final Rule stipulated that waiting time should be deemphasized, that allocation should be designed to achieve equitable allocation of organs among patients, and that organs should be distributed over as broad a geographic area as feasible in order of decreasing medical urgency. Finally, the Final Rule noted that neither place of residence nor place of listing should be a major determinant of access to a liver transplant. This challenge was ultimately met by the adoption of the MELD score by UNOS in February 2002.

MELD

The MELD score was first used and published in 2000 by Malinchoc and colleagues[8] to predict survival in patients undergoing elective transjugular intrahepatic portal-cava systemic shunts. In 2001, the Mayo Clinic group modified the score to predict mortality in a wide range of liver disease etiologies and severities.[9] In the final model, cause of liver disease was eliminated from the model and three biochemical variables were used: (1) serum bilirubin, (2) international normalized ratio (INR), and (3) serum creatinine level. Retrospective studies demonstrated that the MELD score had a high degree of discriminative ability in prediction of 3-month survival in patients with cirrhosis, regardless of the cause of liver disease, and was independent of complications of liver disease, such as ascites, encephalopathy, variceal bleeding, and spontaneous bacterial peritonitis.[9] The final assessment of the MELD score was made using 3437 patients on the UNOS liver transplant waiting list. In this study the MELD score was found to be superior to the CTP score for predicting 3-month survival.[10] The C statistic for predicting 3-month survival on the waiting list was 0.83. This study led to the adoption of the MELD score for liver donor allocation in the United States in February 2002. Since that time, the MELD score has been validated around the world and is presently used in many countries today to allocate donor liver organs.[11–13] Indeed, there are more than 1000 papers published in the last decade on the MELD score. The MELD score has been thoroughly scrutinized and a decade later remains the standard by which to predict mortality in patients with end-stage liver disease.

ADVANTAGES OF THE MELD SCORE

Advantages of the MELD score are its statistical validation and the use of objective widely available laboratory tests (serum bilirubin, serum creatinine, and INR of prothrombin). Today several online calculators are available for calculating the MELD score. It initially was thought that the MELD score might prioritize sicker patients who were more likely to die following liver transplantation.

The impact of the MELD allocation policy resulted in a reduction in waiting list registration by 12%, a reduction in death on the waiting list by 5%, decreased median waiting times from 676 to 416 days, and patients transplanted within 30 days of listing increased from 23% in the pre-MELD era to 37% in the post-MELD era.[14] In the MELD era although sicker patients were transplanted posttransplant survival actually slightly improved, thus dispelling concerns that many had about reducing death on the waiting list, but increasing death posttransplant.[15,16] However, transplantation of sicker patients with higher MELD scores has led to an increase in the cost of liver transplantation and resource use.[17,18]

Finally, the MELD-based allocation system has allowed increasing transparency and allows evidence-based decision making to refine allocation and distribution policy to maximize outcomes using this scarce donor resource.

DISADVANTAGES OF THE MELD SCORE

The MELD allocation policy is an urgency-based system, which means that the risk of death on the waiting list is paramount, irrespective of the degree of survival benefit after liver transplantation. In reality, the MELD era has seen a small increase in overall patient survival despite increases in MELD score at the time of transplant. However, this increase in survival may be related to the increased number of patients with HCC with low MELD scores who are given exception points. In the final analysis, patients with the highest MELD score have reaped the most benefit.[19]

The second potential disadvantage is that there is considerable variation in MELD score known to occur based on laboratory methodology.[20–22] This is particularly true of INR and serum creatinine measurements. Differences in measurement can mean up to a seven MELD point variation depending on how these biochemical parameters are determined. Specifically, variability has been seen in the measurement of INR. However, major issues regarding serum creatinine have been raised, which can be influenced by extrarenal factors, such as total muscle mass, ethnicity, and gender. It has been noted that women tend to have lower median MELD scores compared with men at the time of transplantation. In addition, females are more likely to die on the waiting list in the post-MELD era compared with the pre-MELD era.[23,24] Women are not only disadvantaged because of smaller size, but are also disadvantaged in that their serum creatinine underestimates the degree of renal dysfunction.

A third disadvantage of the MELD system is that it has been shown that the quality of life does not correlate well with severity of liver disease as measured by the MELD score.[25]

Challenges that remain with regard to MELD allocation include that 15% of patients are prioritized incorrectly; the MELD exception scores are nonstandardized (discussed next), and HCC patients are overprioritized compared with non HCC patients (discussed next). In addition, there remains marked geographic disparity with regard to mean MELD scores at the time of transplant and regarding overall waiting time.[26] Finally, because serum creatinine is one of the three factors making up the MELD score, there has been a four-fold increase in the number of liver-kidney transplants since the start of the MELD allocation system.[27] Ongoing attempts are being made to further define which liver transplant patients need simultaneous liver-kidney transplant and which do not.

MELD EXCEPTIONS

One of the major requirements of fair organ allocation is equitable access and distribution of organs to candidates regardless of their underlying liver disease, race, or gender. However, there are several patients with diseases who are poorly served by using the pure MELD allocation system; patients with HCC constitutes such a group of patients. In the absence of MELD exception points, patients with HCC could have an increased risk of waiting list drop-out, generally because of tumor progression even though typically they have a relatively low risk of waiting list mortality caused by liver disease severity. Other conditions underserved by the MELD allocation policy are patients with cirrhosis and hepatopulmonary syndrome or portal pulmonary hypertension, familial amyloidosis, and primary oxaluria.

In HCC patients, MELD exception points were originally granted to patients whose tumor burden fell within the so-called Milan Criteria (stage 1–2) disease. Accordingly, it was determined that the risk of tumor progression, rather than 3-month death on the waiting list, should be used to adjust the MELD score for these patients. The adoption of a risk-based allocation system using MELD exception points has lowered waiting list mortality for HCC patients in the post-MELD era.[28,29] Originally in 2002, stage 1 tumors ($\leq$2 cm) were given a 15% risk of dying within 3 months, which equated to a MELD score of 24. Patients with stage 2 tumors (single tumor >2 cm but <5 cm or 2–3 tumors <3 cm) were given a 30% risk of becoming untransplantable, which equated to MELD score of 29. It was soon realized that HCC patients were overprioritized and on April 2003, the stage 1 tumors were reduced to a MELD exception of 20 or a risk of 8% mortality; the stage 2 tumors were reduced to a MELD of 24 or a mortality risk of 15% over the ensuing 3 months. In January 2004, it was decided that stage 1 tumors should not get MELD exception points because of the low risk of falling off the waiting list and because of the frequent misdiagnosis of small tumors. Stage 2 tumors remained at a MELD score of 24 or a 15% mortality risk. Finally, in 2005 because HCC patients were found to have continued prioritization over non-HCC patients with comparable MELD scores, the stage 2 tumors were decreased to a MELD exception score of 22, which stands today. Despite these efforts to reduce MELD allocation priority for HCC patients, HCC patients continue to have substantial lower waiting list drop-out rates and a higher transplantation rate compared with patients with chronic liver disease who have identical MELD scores (**Fig. 1**).[30] Indeed, today, HCC patients remain at a marked advantage when compared with non-HCC patients. A recent study has shown that liver transplant candidates with HCC have a high degree of variability with regard to waiting list drop-out rates depending on tumor size, number, serum α-fetoprotein level, and response to local-regional therapy.[30] The incidence of waiting list drop-out in HCC patients who have a single tumor of 2 to 3 cm, an α-fetoprotein of less than 20 ng/mL, and who have had a complete response to local-regional therapy have less than a 2% chance of becoming untransplantable in a 2-year period of time. In addition, transplant surgeons often showed favoritism in selecting HCC patients for transplant because of their low biologic MELD score, excellent 1-year survival, and low resource use.

In summary, the current allocation policy for HCC may need revision based on the individual patient's tumor characteristics. A prolonged waiting time before application of MELD exception points for HCC patients is currently being considered by UNOS.

EVIDENCE-BASED MODIFICATIONS TO THE MELD SCORE

With the advent of the MELD allocation system, free of physician and center bias, discrepancies were defined with regard to access to liver transplant, geographic variation in MELD score at the time of transplant, variation in waiting list mortality, and transplantation rates.[31,32] To address these differences, UNOS implemented a policy in 2005 called Share 15 to mandate offering donor livers over a larger distribution area for patients with MELD scores higher than 15. This was a result of a study reported by Merion and colleagues, which showed that patients transplanted with a MELD score of less than 15 had a higher risk of dying with the transplant than without the transplant.[19] Thus, the conclusion was that livers should be prioritized to those

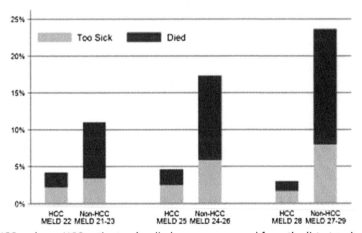

Fig. 1. HCC and non-HCC patients who died or were removed from the list at various MELD scores. (*From* Goldberg D, French B, Abt P, et al. Increasing disparity in waitlist mortality rates with increased model for end-stage liver disease scores for candidates with hepatocellular carcinoma vs candidates without hepatocellular carcinoma. Liver Transpl 2012;18:438; with permission.)

patients having a MELD score of greater than 15 before being offered to patients who had lower MELD scores (**Fig. 2**). The result was a decrease in waiting list death rate of patients; however, regional sharing of livers did not increase, which was the ultimate goal. Why did regional sharing not increase with the livers? Before Share 15 went into effect, applications for a MELD 15 exception numbered 5 between 2002 and 2005. Following the mandatory Share 15 policy, there were 452 applications for a MELD 15 exception, which allowed 81% of these patients to be transplanted with a MELD below 15 (median, 11).[33] The reasons for these exceptions included ascites (57%), encephalopathy (32%), and pruritus (3%). All these variables should be accountable for the MELD score itself. Fifty-three percent of these MELD 15 exceptions were from single-center organ procurement organizations. The conclusion of this study was that these exceptions were requested for the sole purpose to keep local organs and prevent sharing to sicker patients. It points to a continued need for a national review board to standardize criteria for MELD exceptions, which continues to be a challenge in the allocation system.[34,35]

CAN WE IMPROVE THE MELD ALLOCATION POLICY?

In **Fig. 3** we note several factors that enter into the liver allocation policy of which MELD is only a single component. MELD does not increase access to the liver transplant waiting list, it does not take into account the number of MELD exceptions that are given by review boards, it does not correct for geographic disparity, and it is very poor at predicting posttransplant survival with a C statistic of approximately 0.60. Finally, it does not deal with gender or racial disparity issues. MELD can be improved by adding several variables, such as ascites and encephalopathy, which would add to MELD's predictability; however, these variables are subjective and thus cannot reliably be used in an objective-based formula.

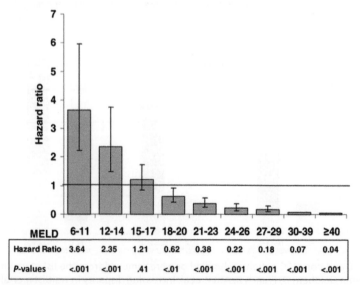

MELD	6-11	12-14	15-17	18-20	21-23	24-26	27-29	30-39	≥40
Hazard Ratio	3.64	2.35	1.21	0.62	0.38	0.22	0.18	0.07	0.04
P-values	<.001	<.001	.41	<.01	<.001	<.001	<.001	<.001	<.001

Fig. 2. Mortality risk of liver transplantation versus waiting based on MELD. (*From* Merion RM, Schaubel DE, Dykstra DM, et al. The survival benefit of liver transplantation. Am J Transplant 2005;5:310; with permission.)

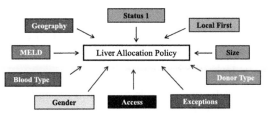

Fig. 3. Factors involved in allocation policy.

Hyponatremia has been shown to add to the MELD score's predictability, particularly in those patients having ascites; however, this would only apply to a small percentage of patients on the waiting list, and it would involve the high cost of reprograming the UNOS allocation system.[36] Finally, donor recipient age, race, and center effect are important factors that would add to MELD's predictability, but obviously cannot be used in a public allocation policy.[37] Even with adding the variables discussed previously, it is unlikely that the C statistic at predicting survival would be greater than 0.9 because of the random events that occur in patients on the waiting list. One of the major challenges that remain to improve the MELD allocation policy is to standardize the criteria for exceptions, which would be resolved by forming a national review board.

FUTURE CHANGES TO LIVER ALLOCATIONS

The most recent change to the liver allocation policy has been the Share 35 policy. With this policy, any person with a MELD score of 35 or greater goes to the top of the liver waiting list and, therefore, any liver procured in the region must be allocated to the person with a MELD score of 35 or greater before it can be offered locally to a patient with a MELD score of less than 35. Although this policy has been in place for only 6 months, it seems that the mean MELD score being transplanted is increasing and approaching the mid-30s in many regions. Indeed, the experience at Mayo Clinic, Rochester is that in the last 6 months we only transplanted one patient with a standard criteria donor with a MELD of less than 35. The result seems to be that we are transplanting extremely sick patients who frequently need prolonged rehabilitation care following transplantation. Death rate following transplantation may well increase, in addition to cost and resource use. Data are being collected to assess this change in policy.

SUMMARY

The MELD-based allocation policy is excellent at prioritizing patients with chronic liver disease on the waiting list based on survival. Exception criteria are needed because of such conditions as HCC, with tumor progression being used as a surrogate for patient survival. MELD can be tweaked by adding serum sodium and other variables; but overall the impact would be minimal and reprograming is expensive and cumbersome. MELD exceptions continue to be challenging, and a national review board to standardize exception criteria is needed. Broader data sharing has been advocated and is one solution to the geographic disparity that has been documented. However, with Share 35 we may well be transplanting patients who are too sick. Finally, the MELD allocation policy allows transparency, which permits a much more rigorous assessment of results and for highlighting areas for improvement.

REFERENCES

1. Charlton MR, Burns JM, Pedersen RA, et al. Frequency and outcomes of liver transplantation for nonalcoholic steatohepatitis in the United States. Gastroenterology 2011;141:1249–53.
2. Charlton MR. The lethal and enduring inequity of deceased donor liver allocation policy for hepatocellular carcinoma in the United States [editorial]. Am J Transplantation 2013;13:2794–6.
3. Snyder J. Gaming the liver transplant market. J Law Econ Organ 2010;26: 3546–68.
4. Pugh R, Murray-Lyon I, Dawson J. Transection of the oesophagus for bleeding oesophageal varices. Br J Surg 1973;60:646–9.
5. Freeman RB Jr, Wiesner RH, Harper A, et al. The new liver allocation system: moving toward evidence-based transplantation policy. Liver Transpl 2002;8:851–8.
6. Institute of Medicine Committee on Organ Procurement and Transplantation Policy. Organ procurement and transplantation: assessing current policies and the potential impact of the DHHS final rule, vol. 1. Washington, DC: National Academy Press; 1999. p. 1–38.
7. Hussong S. Administrative developments: DHHS issues organ allocation final rule. J Law Med Ethics 1999;27:380–2.
8. Malinchoc M, Kamath PS, Gordon FD, et al. A model to predict poor survival in patients undergoing transjugular intrahepatic portosystemic shunts [see comments]. Hepatology 2000;31:864–71.
9. Kamath PS, Wiesner RH, Malinchoc M, et al. A model to predict survival in patients with end-stage liver disease. Hepatology 2001;33:464–70.
10. Wiesner RW, Edwards E, Freeman R, et al. Model for end-stage liver disease (MELD) and allocation of donor livers. Gastroenterology 2003;124:91–6.
11. Cejas NG, Villamil FG, Lendoire JC, et al. Improved waiting-list outcomes in Argentina after the adoption of a model for end-stage liver disease-based liver allocation policy. Liver Transpl 2013;19(7):711–20.
12. Dubowski P, Oberkofler CE, Bechir M, et al. The model for end-stage liver disease allocation system for liver transplantation saves lives, but increased morbidity and cost: a prospective outcome analysis. Liver Transpl 2011;17:674–84.
13. Da Silva Machado AG, de Medeiros Fleck A Jr, Marroni C, et al. Impact of MELD score implementation on liver allocation: experience at a Brazilian center. Ann Hepatol 2013;12:440–7.
14. Freeman R, Wiesner R, Edwards E. Results of the first year of the new liver allocation plan. Liver Transpl 2004;10:7–15.
15. Wiesner RH. Patient selection in an era of donor liver shortage; current US policy. Nat Clin Pract Gastroenterol Hepatol 2005;2:24–30.
16. Freeman RB Jr. Model for End-Stage Liver Disease (MELD) for liver allocation: a 5-year score card. Hepatology 2008;47:1052–7.
17. Axelrod DA, Koffron AJ, Baker T, et al. The economic impact of MELD on liver transplant centers. Am J Transplant 2005;5:2297–301.
18. Axelrod DA, Dzebisashvili N, Lentine K, et al. Assessing variation in the costs of care among patients awaiting liver transplantation. Am J Transplant 2014;14:70–8.
19. Merion RM, Schaubel DE, Dykstra DM, et al. The survival benefit of liver transplantation. Am J Transplant 2005;5:307–13.
20. Trotter JF, Brimhall B, Arjal R, et al. Specific laboratory methodologies achieve higher model for endstage liver disease (MELD) scores for patients listed for liver transplantation. Liver Transpl 2004;10:995–1000.

21. Porte RJ, Lisman T, Tripodi A, et al. The International Normalized Ratio (INR) in the MELD score: problems and solutions. Am J Transpl 2010;10:1349–53.
22. Goulding C, Cholongitas E, Nair D, et al. Assessment of reproducibility of creatine measurement and MELD scoring in four liver transplant units in the UK. Nephrol Dial Transplant 2010;25:960–6.
23. Cholongitas E, Marelli L, Kerry A, et al. Female liver transplant recipients with the same GFR as male recipients have lower MELD scores—a systemic bias. Am J Transpl 2007;7:685–92.
24. Lai J, Terault NA, Vittinghoff E, et al. Height explains the gender difference in wait-list mortality under the MELD-based liver allocation system. Am J Transplant 2010;10(12):2658–64.
25. Saab S, Ibrahim AB, Shpaner A, et al. MELD fails to measure quality of life in liver transplant candidates. Liver Transpl 2005;11(2):218–23.
26. Yeh H, Smoot E, Schoenfeld DA, et al. Geographic inequity in access to livers for transplantation. Transplantation 2011;91(4):479–86.
27. Singal AK, Salameh H, Kuo YF, et al. Evolving frequency and outcomes of simultaneous liver-kidney transplants based on liver disease etiology. Transplantation, in press.
28. Freeman RB, Edwards EB, Harper A. Wait list removal rates among patients with chronic and malignant liver diseases. Am J Transpl 2006;6:1416–21.
29. Wiesner RW, Freeman RB, Mulligan DC. Liver transplantation for hepatocellular cancer: the impact of the MELD allocation policy. Gastroenterol 2004;127:261–7.
30. Goldberg D, French B, Abt P, et al. Increasing disparity in waitlist mortality rates with increased model for end-stage liver disease scores for candidates with hepatocellular carcinoma vs. candidates without hepatocellular carcinoma. Liver Transpl 2012;18:434–43.
31. Mehta N, Dodge JL, Goel A, et al. Identification of liver transplant candidates with hepatocellular carcinoma and a very low dropout risk: implications for the current organ allocation policy. Liver Transpl 2013;19:1343–53.
32. Freeman RB. A decade of model for end-stage liver disease: lessons learned and need for re-evaluation of allocation policies. Curr Opin Organ Transplant 2012;17: 211–5.
33. Bittermann T, Makar G, Goldberg D. Exception point applications for 15 points: an unintended consequence of the Share 15 Policy. Liver Transpl 2012;18: 1302–9.
34. Volk ML. Center differences in model for end-stage liver disease exceptions: fairness, local culture, and norms of practice. Liver Transpl 2013;19:1287–8.
35. Goldberg DS, Makar G, Bittermann T, et al. Center variation in the use of nonstandardized model for end-stage liver disease exception points. Liver Transpl 2013; 19:1330–42.
36. Kim WR, Biggins SW, Kremers WK, et al. Hyponatremia and mortality among patients on the liver-transplant waiting list. N Engl J Med 2008;359:1018–26.
37. Asrani SK, Kim WR, Edwards EB, et al. Impact of the center on graft failure after liver transplantation. Liver Transpl 2013;19:957–64.

Cardiac and Pulmonary Issues in LT Assessment Candidates

Norma C. McAvoy, MBChB, MRCP, Peter C. Hayes, MBChB, PhD*

KEYWORDS

- Liver transplant • Assessment • Cardiovascular complications
- Pulmonary disorders

KEY POINTS

- Liver disease and associated portal hypertension can result in dyspnea from a variety of mechanisms.
- Coronary artery disease (CAD) is common in liver transplant (LT) assessment patients, with cardiovascular (CV) complications now an increasing cause of long-term morbidity and mortality post-LT.
- Accurate CV risk assessment is a key issue as LT candidates are increasing in age with increased incidence of comorbid states at presentation. Risk assessment can be difficult with no clear consensus in all transplant centers.
- Pulmonary vascular disorders are uncommon but are a serious complication of liver disease with their presence having the potential to greatly affect prognosis. Hepatopulmonary syndrome (HPS) and portopulmonary hypertension (PPH) should therefore be routinely sought in all LT assessment candidates.
- LT is the key treatment option for HPS, but is contraindicated in patients with PPH with mean pulmonary artery pressure (mPAP) greater than 40 mm Hg.

INTRODUCTION

With the incidence of liver disease increasing worldwide, a growing number of patients are being referred for assessment for LT. Unfortunately, the donor pool is not expanding at the same rate, which consequentially results in increasing demand on a finite resource. It is therefore imperative that the candidate who undergoes an LT gets maximal benefit with a resultant maximal increase in life expectancy. This article addresses some of the main cardiac and pulmonary issues that may occur in LT assessment candidates.

Disclosure: None.
Department of Hepatology, Royal Infirmary of Edinburgh, 51 Little France Crescent, Edinburgh EH16 4SA, Great Britain
* Corresponding author.
E-mail address: P.Hayes@ed.ac.uk

Clin Liver Dis 18 (2014) 529–541
http://dx.doi.org/10.1016/j.cld.2014.05.001   liver.theclinics.com

CARDIAC ISSUES

Patients with end-stage liver disease exhibit a hyperdynamic state that is characterized by a low systemic vascular resistance and high arterial compliance. The associated increase in cardiac output and demand may contribute to the wide range of CV abnormalities and events seen in patients with cirrhosis.

With the optimization of donor grafts, advancements in surgical techniques, and closer management of immunosuppressant regimes, patient outcomes post–orthotopic liver transplant (OLT) have greatly improved. CV complications have therefore become a major cause of morbidity and mortality post-OLT, including a leading cause of non–graft-related death in the longer term.[1] **Box 1** lists common cardiac issues that can arise in LT candidates.

Preexisting Coronary Artery Disease

- The aging worldwide population has naturally resulted in a change in demographics of current LT assessment patients. Candidates are older and therefore have significant comorbid states, such as diabetes mellitus, hypertension, and CAD, at the time of assessment.
- Prevalence of CAD has been estimated to be 6% to 26% in LT candidates, with silent moderate or severe CAD detected in 13.3%.[2]
- In general, the initiation and progression of atherosclerotic CV disease seems to involve factors such as vascular inflammation, a prothrombotic state, endothelial dysfunction, and plaque instability. It is unknown whether these factors are common to patients with liver disease or if novel, as yet unknown, factors have a role. Several novel biomarkers have been postulated, but no clear consensus exists.
- Evaluation of cardiac risk and cardiac function can be difficult in LT candidates due to limited exercise tolerance or concurrent pharmacotherapy that limits heart

---

Box 1
Cardiac issues commonly seen in LT candidates

Preoperative Factors

Accurate preoperative cardiac risk assessment

Preexisting coronary artery disease

Cirrhotic cardiomyopathy

Alcohol-related cardiomyopathy

Hypertrophic cardiomyopathy

Prolonged QT interval/cardiac arrhythmias

Pericardial effusion

Portopulmonary syndrome/hepatopulmonary syndrome

Liver disease with known association with cardiac disease, eg, hemochromatosis, nonalcoholic fatty liver disease

Postoperative factors

Pulmonary edema

Cardiac arrhythmias

Immunosuppression-related cardiac toxicity

Development of metabolic syndrome post-LT

Table 1
Methods used in the assessment of LT candidates

Assessment Method	Comment
EKG	Examine for prolonged QT interval, LVH, any arrhythmia
Echocardiography	Examine for assessment of diastolic and systolic function, valvular abnormalities, and PAP Bubble study should be performed if evidence of hypoxia Dobutamine stress testing may be of limited value
Computed tomography (CT)	Coronary artery calcification scores CT coronary angiography
Exercise stress test	May be of limited value due to patients having a poor functional and exercise capacity (unable to achieve target heart rates)
Cardiopulmonary exercise testing	Examine for reduced aerobic capacity
Cardiac catheterization	Right heart catheterization studies mandatory if pulmonary hypertension suspected Coronary angiography

Abbreviations: EKG, electrocardiography; LVH, left ventricular hypertrophy; PAP, pulmonary artery pressure.

rate or blood pressure response. **Table 1** lists methods of cardiac assessment but protocols vary from unit to unit.

Cirrhotic Cardiomyopathy

Definition
- Cardiac dysfunction characterized by reduced contractile ventricular responsiveness to stress, systolic and diastolic impairment, and electrophysiology abnormalities, in the absence of other known causes of cardiac disease (**Box 2**).

Pathophysiology
- Mechanism is complex and not completely understood.
- Reduced density of beta receptors on cardiomyocytes with altered β-adrenergic signaling has been proposed.[3,4]
- Additional factors are thought to include adjustments of ion channels with activation of cellular signaling pathways by vasoactive cytokines, nitric oxide, and endocannabinoids.

Clinical features
- It affects up to 50% of patients with end-stage liver disease,[5] independently of liver etiology, with changes also reported in children with cirrhosis.[6]
- Diagnosis is difficult, as patients have near-normal cardiac function at rest.
- Most patients are diagnosed during phases of clinical decompensation of cirrhosis, in which they present with features of diastolic heart failure and/or high-output heart failure. Development of high output in the postoperative period (after LT or transjugular intrahepatic portosystemic shunting [TIPSS] insertion) is highly suggestive.

Investigation
- Electrophysiological abnormalities
     Prolonged QT and serum norepinephine levels correlate with severity of liver disease (Child-Pugh score)[7]
- Evidence of autonomic dysfunction: alteration of circadian heart rate variability
- Echocardiography (features described in **Box 2**)

Box 2
Cirrhotic cardiomyopathy: 2005 World Congress of Gastroenterology proposed diagnostic criteria

Diagnostic criteria

Systolic dysfunction

- Blunted increase in CO with exercise, volume challenge, or pharmacologic stimuli
- Resting LVEF less than 55%

Diastolic dysfunction

- Prolonged deceleration time (>200 ms)
- Prolonged isovolumetric relaxation time (>80 ms)
- E/A ratio less than 1.0 (age corrected)

Supportive criteria

- Electrophysiological abnormalities
- Abnormal chronotropic response
- Electromechanical uncoupling
- Prolonged QTc interval
- Enlarged left atrium
- Increased myocardial mass
- Increased BNP and proBNP levels
- Increased troponin I levels

Abbreviations: BNP, brain natriuretic peptide; CO, cardiac output; E/A, early diastolic/atrial filling ratio; LVEF, left ventricular ejection fraction.

Management

- There is no specific pharmacologic treatment. Medical therapy should be optimized for heart failure in the setting of left ventricular (LV) systolic dysfunction.
- Drugs that affect ventricular repolarization should be used with caution, as these prolong the QT interval, which has been linked with increased risk of sudden death in cirrhosis irrespective of cause.[8]
- Presence of pre-LT heart failure may resolve post-LT,[9] so presence of cirrhotic cardiomyopathy does not prohibit LT.
- Autonomic dysfunction is also reversed in some cases post-OLT.[10]

Alcohol-Related Cardiomyopathy

Definition

- A form of dilated cardiomyopathy, which is a result of chronic alcohol excess.

Pathophysiology

- Complex but thought to be due to the direct toxic effects of alcohol on heart muscle, which results in cell death and alteration of myocyte function.

Clinical features

- Symptoms same as those seen in other forms of cardiomyopathy and in the late stages may include peripheral edema, loss of appetite, exertional dyspnea, orthopnea, fatigue, and productive cough (frothy white or pink sputum).

Investigations

- Abnormal results in cardiac examination: loud heart sounds and presence of mitral regurgitation or tricuspid regurgitation with or without signs of heart failure.
- Cardiomegaly on chest radiograph (CXR).
- Electrocardiogram abnormalities.
- Echocardiogram abnormalities: findings in alcohol-related cardiomyopathy (ACM) are similar to those in persons with idiopathic dilated cardiomyopathy (DC).
  4-Chamber dilatation
  Globally decreased ventricular function (changes in ventricular function may depend on the stage, in that asymptomatic ACM is associated with diastolic dysfunction, whereas systolic dysfunction is a common finding in patients with symptomatic ACM)
  Mitral and tricuspid regurgitation
  Pulmonary hypertension
  LV hypertrophy
- Cardiac catheterization or angiogram can confirm the diagnosis.

Management

- There should be complete abstinence from alcohol.
- A low-sodium diet and fluid restriction is followed in addition to administration of ACE inhibitors, β-blockers, and nitrates.
- Patients with congestive heart failure may be considered for surgical insertion of a pacemaker, which can improve heart function.
- Heart transplant may be considered when heart failure is deemed irreversible and worsening.

Posttransplant Metabolic Syndrome

- With increasing long-term survival post-LT, metabolic syndrome and its individual components (diabetes mellitus, hypertension, dyslipidemia, and obesity), are increasingly being identified to be key factors contributing to late morbidity and mortality.[11]
- The development of non-alcoholic fatty liver disease (NAFLD) after LT for non-NAFLD cirrhosis is also being increasingly recognized,[12] with NAFLD itself thought to be a risk factor of CV event.[13]
- Potential risk factors for posttransplant metabolic syndrome have been identified (**Table 2**).
- Classical cardiac risk factors such as diabetes, hypertension, and hyperlipidemia should be closely monitored post-LT. CV risk assessment should be performed at regular intervals, with immunosuppression regimens closely monitored and need reevaluated.

Regardless of OLT, this increased cardiac risk remains[14] and may rise further particularly in those with preexisting heart disease.[15]

PULMONARY ISSUES

Concerns regarding pulmonary function in any operative candidate have to be fully investigated, as they may have serious implications not only for the early intraoperative course but also for long-term outcome.

In patients with portal hypertension, the severity and natural history of some pulmonary abnormalities may be augmented such that it can be considered to be a contraindication to LT. Some abnormalities can, however, be resolved by LT, with these

Table 2	
Risk factors for the development of metabolic syndrome post-LT	
Pretransplant	
Candidate factors	Increased age at time of LT
	Male gender
	Increased BMI pre-LT
	Diabetes pre-LT
	Smoking history
	Etiology of the underlying liver disease (hepatitis C, cryptogenic cirrhosis, or alcohol have increased risk)
Donor Factors	Increased donor BMI
Posttransplant	Immunosuppressant regime
	>10% weight gain post-LT
	Incidence of rejection episodes (steroid boluses)
	Renal dysfunction post-LT

Abbreviation: BMI, body mass index.

abnormalities listed in special circumstances or Model for End-Stage Liver Disease (MELD) exception criteria for LT. Early identification and assessment of pulmonary abnormalities in patients with liver disease is therefore of the utmost importance. **Box 3** lists common pulmonary issues that can arise in LT candidates.

Hepatic Hydrothorax

Definition

- A collection of fluid in the pleural cavity in patients with liver cirrhosis and without primary cardiac, pulmonary, or pleural disease.

Box 3
Summary of pulmonary issues that may arise in patients with liver disease

Hepatic hydrothorax

- Unresponsive to diuretic therapy
- Transjugular intrahepatic portosystemic shunt contraindicated

Hepatopulmonary syndrome

Portopulmonary hypertension

Hemorrhagic hereditary telangiectasia

- Pulmonary AVMs
- High-output cardiac failure due to intrahepatic vascular malformations

Pulmonary nodules

- Inflammatory/infective
- Metastatic disease (care especially needed in patients with hepatocellular carcinoma)

Concomitant lung conditions that occur in general population

- Chronic obstructive pulmonary disease
- Interstitial lung disease (which may or may not be related to underlying liver disorder)
- Pulmonary fibrosis
- Recurrent pulmonary thromboembolism

Pathophysiology
- Ascitic fluid is drawn into pleural cavity because of the negative intrathoracic pressure that is generated during inspiration. Microscopic defects in diaphragm are also thought to play a role.[16]

Clinical features
- Occurs in 5% to 12% of patients with end-stage liver disease.
- Develops on the right side in approximately 85% of patients, whereas it is on the left side in approximately 13% and bilateral in 2%.
- Symptoms include breathlessness, cough, and/or chest discomfort.

Investigations
- Low O_2 pulse oximetry with confirmed hypoxia on arterial blood sample analysis (investigation results depend on the size of the effusion).
- CXR
- Diagnostic pleural fluid aspirate (with samples sent for biochemical, bacteriologic, and cytologic analysis). **Box 4** lists some characteristics of pleural fluid analysis in hepatic hydrothorax.

Management
- Treatment of hepatic hydrothorax is similar in principle to treatment of ascites.
- Dietary sodium is restricted to less than 2 g/d.
- Diuretic therapy is given (maximum dosage of 400 mg spironolactone and 160 mg furosemide daily).
- LT—just like the development of ascites, hepatic hydrothorax is a poor prognostic sign and should prompt early assessment for LT.
- TIPSS may be considered as a bridge to LT or in patients deemed unsuitable for LT. Pulmonary hypertension is, however, a contraindication to TIPPS insertion.
- About 20% of patients have a refractory hydrothorax, defined as patients with persistent hydrothorax despite diuretic therapy or those in whom diuretic dose is limited because of diuretic-related complications. Options for these patients include LT, repeated thoracentesis, and TIPSS placement.

Hepatopulmonary Syndrome

Definition
- HPS is defined as arterial deoxygenation induced by intrapulmonary vasodilatation associated with hepatic impairment.

Box 4
Characteristics of pleural fluid analysis in hepatic hydrothorax

Cell count less than 250 polymorphonuclear cells/mm^3

Protein less than 2.5 g/dL

Serum to pleural fluid albumin gradient greater than 1.1

Pleural fluid to serum total protein ratio less than 0.5

Pleural fluid to serum bilirubin ratio less than 0.6

Pleural fluid to serum lactate dehydrogenase ratio less than 0.6

Glucose level similar to that of serum

pH greater than 7.4

- It consists of a triad of
  1. Liver disease and/or portal hypertension
  2. Abnormal arterial oxygenation
  3. Intrapulmonary vasodilatation (defined as >3 cycles positive contrast-enhanced echocardiogram or abnormal extrapulmonary uptake of radioisotope after technetium Tc 99m macroaggregated albumin lung scan)

Pathophysiology
- Hypoxemia due to intrapulmonary vascular abnormalities that lead to arteriovenous (AV) shunting and V/Q mismatch.
- Increased production of nitrous oxide and endothelin 1 via endothelin b receptors, thought to be responsible for pulmonary vasodilatation.[17]

Clinical features
- There is a prevalence of 4% to 32% in patients assessed for LT.[18]
- Patients may be asymptomatic. They should be examined for hypoxemia and clubbing with or without cyanosis.
- A more specific symptom is platypnea (dyspnea that improves on lying flat), which is reflected in arterial blood sampling as orthodeoxia (hypoxia worsened by sitting or standing and improved by lying flat). Platypnea occurs because pulmonary arteriovenous malformations (AVMs) occur predominantly in the bases of the lung. Therefore, when standing, the gravitational effects result in blood pooling at the bases of the lung with resultant increased AV shunting.

Investigations
- Arterial blood gases (ABGs) at rest (may confirm hypoxia) with evidence of orthodeoxia (ie, ABGs performed at rest sitting and lying down)
- Echocardiography: positive bubble study confirms HPS

HPS staging

Mild: Pao_2 greater than or equal to 80 mm Hg

Moderate: Pao_2 greater than or equal to 60 mm Hg to less than 80 mm Hg

Severe: Pao_2 greater than or equal to 50 mm Hg to less than 60 mm Hg

Very severe: Pao_2 less than 50 mm Hg (Pao_2 arterial oxygen tension)

Management
- Response to 100% O_2 is variable.
- LT is the only established effective therapy.
  - But there is 30% mortality within 90 days if Pao_2 less than 50 mm Hg and high intrapulmonary shunt (>40%).[19] Although Pao_2 less than 50 mm Hg is regarded a relative contraindication to LT, studies[20] suggest LT remains a treatment option even in those with severe disease.

Portopulmonary Syndrome

Definition

Portopulmonary syndrome is defined as pulmonary arterial hypertension associated with portal hypertension with or without hepatic disease.

Diagnosis requires right heart catheterization and is defined hemodynamically as

- mPAP greater than 25 mm Hg at rest
- Pulmonary capillary wedge pressure less than 15 mm Hg
- Pulmonary vascular resistance (PVR) greater than 120 dyn s/cm^5

Pathophysiology
- Similar to primary pulmonary arterial hypertension with intense vasoconstriction of pulmonary capillaries with thickened, remodeled pulmonary vasculature.
- Mechanism not clearly understood. Vascular remodeling thought to be related to sheer stress to the pulmonary vasculature beds in addition to increased exposure of pulmonary vascular beds to vasomodulatory substances as a result of portosystemic shunting.

Clinical features
- Incidence of 4.5% to 8.5% has been reported in LT assessment patients.[21]
- Mean age of presentation is the fifth decade of life (cf primary pulmonary hypertension, which affects women more than men, in the fourth decade of life).
- Most patients are asymptomatic.
- Symptoms are often subtle or nonspecific, for example, dyspnea on exertion. Orthopnea, syncopy, and hemoptysis may be reported in advanced disease.
- O2 saturation at rest is often normal.
- Poor prognosis if left untreated; mean survival is 15 months.

Investigations
- Echocardiogram is the screening test (elevated pulmonary artery pressure [PAP], right ventricular impairment).
- Right heart catheterization is the gold standard in the diagnosis of portopulmonary syndrome. It provides assessment of disease severity, right heart function, and potential acute vasoreactivity.

PPH staging

Mild: mPAP 25 to 35 mm Hg

Moderate: mPAP 35 to 45 mm Hg

Severe: PAP greater than 45 mm Hg

Management
- Aim of treatment is to alleviate or ease symptoms to improve quality of life, improve survival, and facilitate safe LT.
- Treatment is the same as for primary pulmonary hypertension; therefore, close liaison with regional centers of expertise is required. **Box 5** lists differential diagnosis that should be considered.

Treatment options
- Anticoagulation is routinely used in patients with pulmonary hypertension because of increased risk of in situ pulmonary thrombi due to altered blood flow through the pulmonary vasculature.
- Vasodilatory medicines (eg, prostacyclin derivatives, endothelin receptor antagonists, phosphodiesterase type V inhibitors) with responsiveness prognostically useful when looking at reversibility posttransplant.

Box 5
Differential diagnosis of pulmonary hypertension

Primary

  Idiopathic pulmonary arterial hypertension

Secondary

  Pulmonary arterial hypertension associated with

- Primary lung conditions with or without chronic hypoxia

    Interstitial lung disease

    Chronic obstructive pulmonary disease

    Chronic recurrent pulmonary thromboembolism

    Obstructive sleep apnea

- Cardiac causes

    Valvular heart disease

    Left-sided heart disease

- Portal hypertension
- Connective tissue disorders, for example, systemic lupus erythematosis
- Human immunodeficiency virus infection

- LT is safe if mPAP can be improved to less than 35 mm Hg with PVR reduced to less than 400 dyn s/cm^5 (MELD listing exception criteria).
- mPAP greater than 50 mm Hg is an absolute contraindication to LT.[22]

Table 3 highlights some differences between HPS and PPH.

Hemorrhagic Hereditary Telangiectasia

Definition

- A rare autosomal dominant multisystemic condition. Characterized by the development of AVMs, which can occur in the skin, mucous membranes, gastrointestinal tract, liver, lungs, and brain.

This condition is diagnosed according to the presence of 4 criteria, known as the Curacao criteria (**Box 6**).[23] If 3 or 4 are met, patient has definite hemorrhagic hereditary telangiectasia (HHT).

Diagnosis is mainly clinical, but genetic testing also has a role.

- Index case mainly helpful in allowing genetic testing of relatives (especially minors).
- About 75% of cases: deletion/duplication analysis of the coding exons on the endoglin gene (ENG, HHT1) and the activin A receptor type II-like 1 gene (ACVRL1, HHT2).

Clinical features

- Hepatic vascular malformations (AVMs) occur in 32% to 78% of HHT,[24] with greater than 90% patients symptomatic.
- Patients may develop complications of hepatic AVMs:
  - High-output heart failure due to increased preload (exertional dyspnea, orthopnea, edema)

Table 3
HPS versus PPH

	HPS	PPH
Symptoms	Often asymptomatic Platypnea	Dyspnea on exertion orthopnea syncopy
Clinical findings	Low oxygen saturations Finger clubbing Cyanosis	Hypoxemia especially with exertion RV heave Loud P2 TR murmur
Diagnosis	Positive bubble echocardiographic study	ECG: R axis deviation RVH, R atrial enlargement Echo: elevated PAP Right heart catheterization
Treatment	Liver transplant	Management same as primary pulmonary hypertension **OLT contraindicated if PAP>40 mm Hg**

Abbreviations: ECG, electrocardiography; RV, right ventricle; RVH, right ventricular hypertrophy; TR, tricuspid regurgitation.

- ○ Portal hypertension (variceal hemorrhage, ascites)
- ○ Biliary ischemia (jaundice, fever, abdominal pain)
- ○ Hepatic encephalopathy
- ○ Steal syndrome (intestinal ischemia)
- Pulmonary AVMs occur in 15% to 50% of patients with HHT, with a small proportion of patients developing pulmonary hypertension.

Investigations
- Doppler ultrasonography or computed tomography (CT) of the abdomen is used to identify hepatic AVMs. It is also common to find incidental nodules on scans, as these patients have high incidence of focal nodule hyperplasia.
- Transthoracic echocardiography (? evidence of pulmonary hypertension, ? presence of high-output cardiac failure).
- Lung AVMs may be suspected because of the abnormal appearance of the lungs on a CXR or hypoxia on pulse oximetry or ABG determination.
- Bubble contrast echocardiography may be used as a screening tool, but it can miss smaller AVMs and does not identify the site of AVMs. High-resonance CT scanning of chest should be considered if the results of bubble echocardiography are positive.
- Right heart catheterization may also be required.
- CT of the brain should be performed to exclude any cerebral AVMs.

Box 6
Curacao Criteria for clinical diagnosis of HHT

Criteria

1. Spontaneous and recurrent epistaxis

2. Multiple telangiectasias at typical sites: lips, nose, oral cavity

3. Proven visceral AVMs (liver, lung, brain, spine)

4. First-degree family member has confirmed diagnosis of HHT

Management

- International consensus is that LT assessment should be considered for patients with HHT with
  - Ischemic biliary necrosis
  - Intractable heart failure
  - Intractable portal hypertension
- Embolization of intrahepatic vascular malformations is not advised because, although effective at improving symptoms related to high-output cardiac failure and mesenteric steal syndrome, there is a high incidence of ischemic biliary complications requiring urgent LT.[24]
- LT results in symptom resolution in the majority. Patients have, however, a longer hospital stay with high incidence of postoperative complications; 5-year survival is 83%.
- Pulmonary AVMs can be treated with coil embolotherapy with or without pulmonary vasoactive therapy if there is evidence of pulmonary hypertension.

Concomitant Lung Conditions

As the population ages, increasing numbers of transplant assessment candidates are of an advancing age and therefore have increased comorbidity at presentation for LT.

- Due to the high incidence of smoking, chronic obstructive pulmonary disease is commonly seen in greater than 50% of assessment patients. However, no definite guidelines exist to guide when patients are too high an operative risk to prohibit safe LT. Smoking cessation should be aggressively encouraged in all transplant candidates.
- Interstitial lung disease, which may or may not be related to underlying liver disorder, is also seen. Again, no specific guidance exists, but standard assessment of anesthetic risk should be sought.

REFERENCES

1. Dec GW, Kondo N, Farrell ML, et al. Cardiovascular complications following liver transplantation. Clin Transplant 1995;9:463–71.
2. Carey WD, Dumont JA, Pimentel RR, et al. The prevalence of coronary artery disease in liver transplant candidates over age of 50. Transplantation 1995;59:859–64.
3. Lee SS, Marty J, Mantz J, et al. Desensitization of myocardial β-adrenergic receptors in cirrhotic rats. Hepatology 1990;12:481–5.
4. Ward CA, Liu H, Lee SS. Altered cellular calcium regulatory systems in a rat model of cirrhotic cardiomyopathy. Gastroenterology 2001;121(5):1209–18.
5. Kazankov K, Holland-Fischer P, Andersen NH, et al. Resting myocardial dysfunction in cirrhosis quantified by tissue Doppler imaging. Liver Int 2011;31(4):534–40.
6. Desai MS, Zainuer S, Kennedy C, et al. Cardiac structural and functional alterations in infants and children with biliary atresia, listed for liver transplantation. Gastroenterology 2011;141(4):1264–72.
7. Zambruni A, Trevisani F, Caraceni P, et al. Cardiac electrophysiological abnormalities in patients with cirrhosis. J Hepatol 2006;44(5):994–1002.
8. Moller S, Henriksen JH. Cirrhotic cardiomyopathy. J Hepatol 2010;53(1):179–90.
9. Torregrosa M, Aguade S, Dos L, et al. Cardiac alterations in cirrhosis: reversibility after liver transplant. J Hepatol 2005;42:68–74.

10. Mohamed R, Forsey PR, Davis MK, et al. Effect of liver transplantation on QT interval prolongation and autonomic dysfunction in end stage liver disease. Hepatology 1996;23(5):1128–34.
11. Pagadala M, Dasarathy S, Eghtesad B, et al. Posttransplant metabolic syndrome: an epidemic waiting to happen. Liver Transpl 2009;15:1662–70.
12. Poordad F, Gish R, Wakil A, et al. De novo non-alcoholic fatty liver disease following orthotopic liver transplantation. Am J Transplant 2003;3:1413–7.
13. Anstee QM, Targher G, Day CP. Progression of NAFLD to diabetes mellitus, cardiovascular disease or cirrhosis. Nat Rev Gastroenterol Hepatol 2013;10(6): 330–44.
14. Johnston SD, Morris JK, Cramb R, et al. Cardiovascular morbidity and mortality after orthotopic liver transplantation. Transplantation 2002;73(6):901–6.
15. Plotkin JS, Johnson LB, Rustgi V, et al. Coronary artery disease and liver transplantation: the state of the art. Liver Transpl 2000;4(Suppl 1):S53–6.
16. Krok KL, Cardenas A. Hepatic hydrothorax. Semin Respir Crit Care Med 2012;33: 3–10.
17. Grace JA, Angus PW. Hepatopulmonary syndrome: update on recent advances in pathophysiology, investigation, and treatment. J Gastroenterol Hepatol 2013; 28(2):213–9.
18. Rodríguez-Roisin R, Krowka MJ. Hepatopulmonary syndrome–a liver-induced lung vascular disorder. N Engl J Med 2008;358(22):2378–87.
19. Swanson KL, Wiesner RH, Krowka MJ. Natural history of hepatopulmonary syndrome: impact of liver transplantation. Hepatology 2005;41:1122–9.
20. Gupta S, Castel H, Rao RV, et al. Improved survival after liver transplantation in patients with hepatopulmonary syndrome. Am J Transplant 2010;10(2).354–63.
21. Safadar Z, Bartolome S, Sussman N. Portopulmonary hypertension: an update. Liver Transpl 2012;18(8):881–91.
22. Krowka MJ, Plevak DJ, Findlay JY, et al. Pulmonary hemodynamics and perioperative cardiopulmonary-related mortality in patients with portopulmonary hypertension undergoing liver transplantation. Liver Transpl 2000;6(4):443–50.
23. Shovlin CL, Guttmacher AE, Buscarini E, et al. Diagnostic criteria for hereditary hemorrhagic telangeictasia (Rendu-Osler-Weber syndrome). Am J Med Genet 2000;91(1):66–7.
24. Faughnan ME, Palda VA, Garcia-Tsao G, et al. International guidelines for the diagnosis and management of hereditary hemorrhagic telangiectasia. J Med Genet 2011;48:73–87.

Renal Dysfunction in End-Stage Liver Disease and Post–Liver Transplant

Marcelo S. Sampaio, MD, PhD[a], Paul Martin, MD, FRCP, FRCPI[b],
Suphamai Bunnapradist, MD[a],*

KEYWORDS

- Renal failure • Liver-kidney transplant • Liver transplant

KEY POINTS

- Renal dysfunction is common in ESLD patients.
- A 24-hour urine collection or cystatin C are better alternatives to estimate GFR rather than serum creatinine.
- NGAL may be a better marker to differentiate intrinsic renal injury from HRS.

INTRODUCTION

Acute kidney injury (AKI) is associated with poor outcomes and increased mortality in the setting of liver disease.[1–3] The prevalence of renal dysfunction in orthotropic liver transplant (OLT) recipients has ranged between 17% and 95% depending on the study.[4,5] The etiologies of renal dysfunction in patients with end-stage liver disease (ESLD) differ from the posttransplant period. This article discusses renal injury in the patient with cirrhosis and in the ESLD patient, the evaluation of kidney function in pretransplant liver candidates, renal-replacement therapy (RRT) as a treatment of kidney injury or as a bridge to liver transplant, indications for OLT versus a combined liver-kidney transplant (CLKT), and kidney injury in the post–liver transplant period.

Fede and colleagues[6] reported a seven-fold increase in mortality, with 50% of death in the first month in patients with cirrhosis who developed renal failure. Prognosis also varies with the cause of renal dysfunction. Three-month probability of survival was 73% for parenchymal nephropathy, 46% for hypovolemia-associated renal failure, 30% for renal injury associated with infection, and 15% for hepatorenal syndrome

The authors have nothing to disclose.
[a] Division of Nephrology, Department of Medicine, Kidney and Pancreas Transplant Program, David Geffen School of Medicine at UCLA, 1015 Gayley Avenue, Suite 220, Los Angeles, CA 90024, USA; [b] Division of Hepatology, Miller School of Medicine, University of Miami, 1500 NW 12 Avenue, Jackson Medical Tower E-1101, Miami, FL 33136, USA
* Corresponding author. 1015 Gayley Avenue, Suite 220, Los Angeles, CA 90024.
E-mail address: bunnapradist@mednet.ucla.edu

(HRS) in a single-center study from Spain.[7] Management of AKI complicating advanced liver disease involves mitigation of risk factors, hemodynamic support, and RRT, whereas evaluating the need for liver transplant in a cirrhotic patient with prolonged renal insufficiency or in dialysis a CLKT may be indicated. Although successful liver transplantation reverses renal dysfunction from HRS, posttransplant kidney dysfunction may occur. Calcineurin inhibitor (CNI) nephrotoxicity is observed in most patients maintained on calcineurin and may lead to renal dysfunction with renal failure after a nonrenal solid organ transplant.[8] Eighteen percent of liver transplant recipients develop significant chronic kidney disease (CKD) at 5-years posttransplant.[4] Reducing risk factors for renal dysfunction, the early identification of AKI, and the appropriate management of AKI and CKD may improve the long-term outcomes of patients with liver disease.

PATIENTS WITH CIRRHOSIS AND ESLD
Revised Definition of Renal Dysfunction in Patients with Liver Disease

In 2010 the definition of renal dysfunction in cirrhosis was revisited. Concerns about the inadequacy of serum creatinine to diagnosis and identify patients with cirrhosis in an early stage of kidney disease led to a panel of specialists selected from the Acute Dialysis Quality Initiative Working Group and from the International Ascites Club to propose an update in the definition of kidney dysfunction in cirrhosis (**Box 1**). The term "hepatorenal disorder" was created to characterize any renal dysfunction in the setting of advanced liver disease. The expectation with the new definition is to improve diagnosis, earlier identification, and treatment of the renal condition to positively impact outcomes, and to create a uniform standard to develop research.[9]

Estimating Renal Function in Patients with Cirrhosis and ESLD

The assessment of renal function in ESLD patients is challenging because of reduced muscle mass, the substrate for creatinine, leading to a spuriously low serum creatinine despite a decreased glomerular filtration rate (GFR). Elevated bilirubin levels also falsely lower the serum creatinine by affecting the assay. A 24-hour urine collection for creatinine clearance has been shown to overestimate GFR by 30% to 40%, mainly in those with low GFR.[10] The gold standard for measurement of GFR is inulin or iohexol clearance, but these tests are cumbersome. Cystatin C has emerged as an alternative to estimate GFR. It is a low-molecular-weight protein produced by all nucleated cells. Cystatin C is freely filtered by the glomerulus but neither reabsorbed nor secreted. It is catabolized completely in the proximal tubule, and its serum concentration has been shown to estimate GFR at least as accurately as serum creatinine.[11] The serum

---

Box 1
Diagnostic criteria of kidney dysfunction in cirrhosis (hepatorenal disorders)

Acute kidney injury: Rise in serum creatinine of $\geq$50% from baseline or a rise of serum creatinine by $\geq$0.3 mg/dL in less than 48 hours. HRS type I is a specific form of acute kidney injury.

Chronic kidney disease: Glomerular filtration rate of less than 60 mL/min for greater than 3 months calculated using MDRD6 (Modification of Diet in Renal Disease) formula. HRS type II is a specific form of chronic kidney disease.

Acute-on-chronic kidney disease: Rise in serum creatinine of $\geq$50% from baseline or a rise of serum creatinine by $\geq$0.3 mg/dL in less than 48 hours in a patient with cirrhosis whose glomerular filtration rate is less than 60 mL/min for greater than 3 months calculated using MDRD6 formula.

concentration of cystatin C is independent of muscle mass and not affected by serum bilirubin levels.[12] In a recent study, Souza and colleagues[13] have shown that cystatin C–based equations are more accurate than the plasma creatinine-based equations to predict GFR in candidates for liver transplant with cirrhosis. Similar studies in ESLD patients to assess the accuracy of cystatin C in predicting estimated glomerular filtration rate (eGFR) are still needed. The inability to accurately estimate GFR also contributes to untoward effects from medications. Many medications are renally excreted and require dose adjustment based on eGFR, and they may be administered at inappropriately high doses in patients with cirrhosis because of the inaccuracy of serum creatinine.

TYPES OF RENAL DYSFUNCTION
Prerenal Azotemia

Prerenal azotemia results from renal hypoperfusion and is the most common cause of acute renal dysfunction in ESLD patients.[14] Patients with cirrhosis have multiple potential risk factors that can contribute to prerenal azotemia, including hypovolemia from diuretic use, diarrhea from lactulose, and gastrointestinal hemorrhage. Patients with cirrhosis have a progressive rightward shift of the renal vasculature autoregulation curve with progression of the disease, with renal blood flow more sensitive to a decrease in systemic blood pressure.[15] Medications that affect the hemodynamics of renal vasculature, such as nonsteroidal anti-inflammatory drugs and angiotensin-converting enzyme inhibitors, can induce or contribute to prerenal azotemia. Arterial blood pressure is an independent predictor of survival in patients with cirrhosis.[16] Caution should be taken when prescribing angiotensin-converting inhibitors and β-blockers to avoid hypotension. One-year survival was 70% and 40% with mean arterial blood pressure of greater than 82 mm Hg and lower, respectively.[17]

The HRS

The HRS is functional prerenal azotemia unique to patients with liver failure. HRS, typically seen only in the presence of ascites, can be precipitated by spontaneous bacterial peritonitis and other infections, overvigorous diuresis, and large-volume paracentesis (in general >4 L) without albumin infusion. The pathophysiology of HRS is complex including splanchnic vasodilation caused by portal hypertension. The shear stress on splanchnic vessels increases production of vasodilators, including nitric oxide.[9] Bacterial translocation from the gut to mesenteric lymph nodes may also play a role in the physiopathology of splanchnic vasodilatation by increasing local inflammation and cytokines production[18] and increased mesenteric angiogenesis. With the development of portosystemic shunts the "splanchnic vasodilators" may also lead to systemic vasodilatation. Vasodilatation leads to decreased effective circulatory volume, and overactivation of the renin-angiotensin-aldosterone system and sympathetic nervous system. The compensatory vasoconstrictive effects of the renin-angiotensin-aldosterone system and adrenergic hormones can cause renal ischemia and HRS.[19] In addition, decreased effective circulatory volume increases sodium and water retention by the kidneys worsening ascites and edema. The two types of HRS are differentiated based on their time course. Type I HRS is defined as a doubling of the initial serum creatinine to a level greater than 2.5 mg/dL in less than a 2-week period, whereas type II HRS is characterized by ascites that is resistant to diuretics with moderate renal dysfunction that is slowly progressive.[20] Development of HRS suggests a poor prognosis with median survival time of 2 weeks in type I HRS and 6 months in type II HRS not responsive to treatment.[21] The diagnosis of HRS is one of exclusion, and true intravascular volume depletion must be ruled out before the diagnosis can be made (**Box 2**). New urine biomarkers are being investigated to assist in the differential diagnosis of AKI in patients with cirrhosis.[22] So far, NGAL among many seems to be the most promising marker.[19,23–25]

Treatment of HRS is challenging. Reversal of precipitating factors, namely infection and hypovolemia, in conjunction with vasoconstrictors are part of the strategy. HRS treatment is based on the theory that administration of vasoconstrictors ameliorates arterial vasodilatation and increases effective circulatory volume and renal blood flow (**Box 3**). Terlipressin, a synthetic analogue of lysine-vasopressin, in conjunction with albumin infusion is the treatment of choice outside the United States for HRS. A randomized, double-blind, placebo-controlled prospective trial examining the effects of terlipressin on HRS resulted in a significant reversal of renal dysfunction in 34% of the treated group versus 13% in the placebo group.[26] A recent meta-analysis associated the use of terlipressin with a 24% reduction in mortality.[27,28] According to the European Association for the Study of Liver Guidelines, terlipressin is generally started at a dose of 1 mg every 4 to 6 hours with increase to 2 mg if no response by the third treatment day, and is frequently combined with albumin infusion (1 g/kg on Day 1 followed by 40 g/day).[10] However, terlipressin is not yet licensed in the United States. The American Association for the Study of Liver Disease recommends treatment of HRS with albumin infusion, octreotide, and midodrine, or albumin infusion and norepinephrine/vasopressin depending on the severity or setting of the liver disease.[16,18,29,30] A small uncontrolled study in seven patients with HRS showed that transjugular intrahepatic portosystemic shunt improved renal function and renal plasma flow with decreased plasma renin activity, aldosterone, and norepinephrine in six patients. Use of transjugular intrahepatic portosystemic shunt, however, needs to be carefully considered in a decompensated patient with cirrhosis because of the risk of precipitating hepatic encephalopathy. The American Association for the Study of Liver Disease Guidelines does not currently endorse transjugular intrahepatic portosystemic shunt for treatment of HRS based on current evidence.[31]

Intrinsic Renal Disease

Patients with ESLD are also at risk for intrinsic renal disease (**Box 4**, **Table 1**). Acute tubular necrosis (ATN) is the most common intrinsic renal disease in patients with cirrhosis and can be precipitated by systemic hypotension (eg, gastrointestinal hemorrhage, overuse of diuretics, and large-volume paracentesis); antibiotics or intravenous contrast nephrotoxicity; or prolonged ischemia, such as with HRS or shock. Patients at highest risk for developing contrast-induced nephropathy (CIN) include

---

Box 2
Diagnostic criteria for hepatorenal syndrome

- Presence of cirrhosis with ascites
- Serum creatinine greater than 1.5 mg/dL
- No improvement of creatinine after 2 days of fluid or albumin challenge (1 g/kg body weight/day up to a maximum of 100 g/day) and withdrawal of diuretics
- Absence of shock
- No recent administration of nephrotoxic medications
- Lack of intrinsic kidney disease as evidenced by bland urinalysis and normal renal ultrasound

Data from Barri YM, Sanchez EQ, Jennings LW, et al. Acute kidney injury following liver transplantation: definition and outcome. Liver Transpl 2009;15(5):475–83.

Box 3
Management of hepatorenal syndrome

1. Rule out intravascular depletion with a fluid (1.5 L of normal saline infusion) or albumin (1 g/kg/day for 2 days with doses divided into 3 to 4 doses/day, maximum 100 g/day) challenge.

2. If there is no improvement in renal function, start treatment with vasoconstrictors, such as midodrine and octreotide or terlipressin, plus albumin. Start midodrine, 7.5 mg, orally three times daily and octreotide, 100 μg, subcutaneously three times daily, or start terlipressin, 0.5 mg, intravenously every 6 hours if available. Give 25 to 50 g of albumin daily.

3. Titrate midodrine and octreotide to raise mean arterial pressure by at least 15 mm Hg. Midodrine can be increased up to 15 mg three times daily and octreotide to 200 μg three times daily.

4. Titrate terlipressin to decrease the creatinine by at least 25% by doubling the dose every 2 days for maximum dose of 12 mg/day.

5. Continue treatment until reversal of HRS (creatinine <1.5 mg/dL). Treatment needs to be restarted if HRS recurs.

6. Can stop treatment if there is no response in the first 3 days or if creatinine does not decrease by at least 50% in the first 7 days at maximum doses. Albumin can be discontinued if serum albumin greater than 4.5 g/dL or there are signs of volume overload.

---

those with pre-existing renal dysfunction, diabetes, or volume depletion. A retrospective analysis showed that the incidence of CIN in hospitalized patients with cirrhosis was 25% with ascites noted as a significant risk factor.[32] Use of nonionic, whether low or iso-osmolal agents, may diminish risk of CIN in high-risk patients. Patients who are at risk for development of CIN should be given isotonic saline or bicarbonate intravenous fluids before and after the study unless contraindicated. Evidence for use of N-acetylcysteine in protecting against CIN is conflicting[33–35] but given its low toxicity and cost it may be used starting the day before the study.

Acute interstitial nephritis (AIN) is another potential cause of AKI in the patient with cirrhosis. Causes of AIN include drug hypersensitivity reaction, infection, immune-mediated diseases, and glomerular disease, although many cases remain idiopathic. ESLD patients often receive antibiotics, many of which have been implicated in AIN.

Box 4
Evaluation of intrinsic renal disease

1. Rule out prerenal azotemia by checking fractional excretion of sodium and/or fractional excretion of urea (both low in prerenal azotemia).

2. Consider exposure to nephrotoxic agents, such as antibiotics and intravenous contrast, or hypotensive episodes that can cause acute tubular necrosis.

3. Urinalysis for pyuria, eosinophils, microscopic hematuria, dysmorphic red blood cells, red blood cell casts, and proteinuria to rule out acute interstitial nephritis and vasculitides.

4. Send serologic work-up (C3, C4, cryocrit) to rule out glomerulonephritis if urinalysis is concerning for glomerular disease.

5. Consider renal biopsy if cause unclear.

6. Administer N-acetylcysteine, 1200 mg, orally twice a day for 48 hours with intravenous fluids if patient requires a computed tomography study with intravenous contrast. Ideally, two doses should be given before administration of contrast.

7. Evaluate need for dialysis and supportive therapies.

Table 1
Diagnostic criteria and management of intrinsic renal disease

Renal Disease	Diagnostic Criteria	Risk Factors	Treatment
Acute tubular necrosis	Bland urinalysis, fractional excretion of sodium >1%	Hypotension, nephrotoxic medications, intravenous contrast, prolonged ischemia caused by hepatorenal syndrome or shock	Supportive care to treat underlying cause
Acute interstitial nephritis	Classic triad of rash, fever, and eosinophilia; sterile pyuria, eosinophiliuria	β-Lactam antibiotics, cephalosporins, sulfonamides, nonsteroidal anti-inflammatory drugs, infection	Discontinue offending agent
IgA nephropathy	Microscopic hematuria, proteinuria occasionally	Cirrhosis, particularly alcoholic	Supportive care
Membranous nephropathy	Proteinuria, hypocomplementemia, supepithelial deposits on kidney biopsy	Hepatitis B and C infections	Antiviral medications (lamivudine, interferon-α)
Membranoproliferative glomerulonephritis/cryoglobulinemia	Proteinuria, dysmorphic red cells on urinalysis, hypocomplementemia, positive cryocrit, subendothelial deposits on kidney deposit with immune complex deposition	Hepatitis B and C infections	Antiviral medications (interferon-α, ribavirin)

The most common drugs implicated in causing AIN include penicillins, cephalosporins, sulfonamides, and nonsteroidal anti-inflammatory drugs.[36] Proton pump inhibitors may also be associated with AIN.[37–41] The classic triad of rash, fever, and eosinophilia is seen in less than 30% of patients and the most common presentation is of sterile pyuria in the setting of renal injury. The main treatment consists of discontinuation of the suspected drug. Also, some authors advocate the early use of glucocorticoids, although there are no randomized controlled studies to prove their benefit.[42–44]

IgA nephropathy has been associated with cirrhosis, particularly alcoholic, but its role in contributing to renal dysfunction is unclear.[45] An observational study of renal biopsies obtained at time of liver transplantation in 30 patients with hepatitis C–related cirrhosis suggested the incidence of IgA nephropathy was 23%.[46] Impaired transport of IgA immune complexes from blood to bile by the Kupffer cells in the liver is thought to be the cause of increased IgA deposition in the kidneys.[47] Treatment options remain limited, even in primary IgA nephropathy.

Glomerulonephritis can complicate chronic hepatitis B and C infection. Patients with hepatitis C virus (HCV) may develop mixed cryoglobulinemia with associated membranoproliferative glomerulonephritis (MPGN).[48] The incidence of MPGN was found to be 40% in HCV patients who underwent intraoperative renal biopsy at time of liver transplantation.[46] Cryoglobulinemic vasculitis is seen in less than 10% of HCV patients, and one-third of those with cryoglobulinemia have MPGN. Most HCV patients with cryoglobulinemia do not exhibit clinical manifestations, but approximately one-third have arthralgias, purpura, and asthenia.[49] Serologic markers include low C3 and C4 levels with elevated rheumatoid factor and cryoglobulins.[50] Treatment of hepatitis C with antiviral therapy, including pegylated interferon α and ribavirin, and achievement of virologic response has been shown to improve cryoglobulinemia and lessen renal dysfunction.[51,52] Excellent results with combined and interferon-free regimens based on the use of sofusbuvir, simeprevir, and other oral agents for the treatment of hepatitis C were recently published expanding options to treat hepatitis C.[53–59] Rituximab has also been reported to decrease cryoglobulins, rheumatoid factor, and proteinuria in six patients with hepatitis C–associated cryoglobulinemia.[60]

Hepatitis B virus (HBV) can be associated with membranous nephropathy, MPGN, and polyarteritis nodosa. Previous studies have shown that hepatitis B envelope antigen is present in the subepithelial deposits seen in HBV-associated membranous nephropathy (HBVMN).[61] Spontaneous remission of nephrotic syndrome has been reported in 30% to 60% of patients, and seroconversion to anti–hepatitis B envelope antigen is associated with remission of proteinuria. Treatment with interferon-α yielded reduction in proteinuria and HBV DNA levels in 8 of 15 patients treated. All of the treatment responders were noted to have HBVMN, whereas the nonresponders mostly had MPGN.[62] Lamivudine has also been used to treat HBVMN. A case control trial of 10 patients treated with lamivudine compared with 12 control patients found that the treatment group had reduction in proteinuria and resolution of HBV DNA.[63] In the control group, 42% subsequently developed severe renal dysfunction requiring dialysis, whereas none in the treatment group required renal replacement after 3 years of follow-up. Newer analogs of nucleoside, entecavir, and tenofovir, more potent antiviral agents than lamivudine and adefovir, are now licensed to treat HBV infection.[64,65] Although there are no randomized clinical studies examining treatment of hepatitis B–associated glomerulonephritis, antiviral therapy is clearly indicated in patients with replicating HBV and glomerulonephritis.

ROLE OF RRT

RRT, such as hemodialysis (HD), is often required in sicker OLT candidates as they become more overtly decompensated. For patients who required RRT preoperatively, 35% survived to liver transplant or discharge, whereas 65% died while waiting for transplant in the hospital, but the 1-year mortality after transplant in those that started RRT was 30% compared with 9.7% for patients who did not need RRT before transplant.[3] Indications for RRT in ESLD patients are essentially similar to other patients (eg, acidemia, electrolyte derangements, volume overload, and uremia refractory to medical management). However, there are some key differences in ESLD patients. Respiratory alkalosis typically develops in patients with cirrhosis and can cause a compensatory metabolic acidosis, which may be mistaken for acidemia unless a blood gas analysis is performed. Uremic encephalopathy may be difficult to differentiate from hepatic encephalopathy. The hemodynamic stability of ESLD patients also impacts RRT because patients frequently become hypotensive during treatment. Continuous RRT, or continuous venovenous HD, may be required if patients have severe hypotension, hyponatremia, or cerebral edema. The amount of fluid removed and electrolyte corrections that are achieved with continuous RRT occur over a 24-hour period versus a 3-hour period with single-pass HD, so hemodynamically unstable patients tolerate continuous RRT better. However, if rapid adjustments in fluid status or electrolytes are needed, such as in severe acidemia or hyperkalemia, single-pass HD is the preferred modality. The role of alternative methods of RRT, such as molecular readsorbent recirculation system (MARS [Gambro, Sweden] system) or fractioned plasma separation and adsorption (PROMETHEUS [Fresenius, Germany] system) is still unclear. They may be important as a bridge for the liver transplant, but studies are needed to create evidence-based arguments for routine recommendation.[18,27]

EVALUATION FOR CLKT

Since the introduction of the model of ESLD system in 2002, the rate of CLKT has tripled from 134 patients in 2001 to 399 patients in 2006, reflecting the importance of creatinine in this model of organ allocation.[66] Compared with isolated liver transplant recipients, CLKT recipients with end-stage renal disease (ESRD) had higher posttransplant survival at 1 year, but CLKT recipients without ESRD fared no better than liver transplant alone recipients.[67] There is concern that CLKT may be recommended for liver transplant candidates with potentially reversible renal failure (eg, HRS and ATN). A renal biopsy to assess chronicity of renal dysfunction is the gold standard but is daunting in a patient with cirrhosis and coagulopathy. Intraoperative renal biopsy has been proposed as a tool to evaluate necessity of CLKT, but there is currently no consensus or criteria to determine which patients to biopsy.[68] Renal ultrasound to assess kidney size and echogenicity of the cortex can help determine the potential reversibility of renal dysfunction. Generally, if dialysis has been required for more than a few weeks before liver transplant, renal recovery is much less likely after OLT, and CLKT needs to be considered. A consensus panel of experts was convened in 2007 to discuss indications for CLKT, establish a registry, and recommend standard listing criteria. Recommendations for CLKT were revised in a new summit and were published in 2012 (**Box 5**).[10,69] An algorithm has been recommended for evaluation and selection of CLKT patients (**Box 6**).[70]

KIDNEY INJURY IN THE POST–LIVER TRANSPLANT PERIOD

Postoperatively, multiple risk factors can cause renal dysfunction in liver transplant recipients. Management of postoperative renal dysfunction is summarized in **Box 7**.

Box 5
Recommendations for combined liver-kidney transplant

1. End-stage renal disease patients with cirrhosis and symptomatic portal hypertension or hepatic vein wedge pressure with gradient greater than 10 mm Hg.

2. Patients with ESLD and CKD with GFR $\leq$30 mL/min.

3. Patients with AKI, including HRS, with creatinine $\geq$2.0 mg/dL and dialysis dependence for $\geq$8 weeks.

4. Patients with ESLD and evidence of CKD with renal biopsy showing greater than 30% glomerulosclerosis or fibrosis.

Other indications for granting exceptions include comorbidities, such as diabetes, hypertension, or other pre-existing renal disease, along with proteinuria, kidney size, and duration of creatinine $\geq$2.0 mg/dL.

1. Candidates with persistent AKI for greater than 4 weeks with one of the following:

   a. Stage 3 AKI as defined by modified RIFLE, ie, a three-fold increase in Serum creatinine (Scr) from baseline, Scr greater than 4.0 mg/dL with an acute increase of greater than 0.5 mg/dL or RRT

   b. eGFR $\leq$35 mL/min (MDRD-6 [Modification of Diet in Renal Disease] equation) or GFR $\leq$25 mL/min (iothalamate clearance)

2. Candidates with CKD, as defined by the National Kidney Foundation, for 3 months with one of the following:

   a. eGFR $\leq$40 mL/min (MDRD-6 equation) or GFR $\leq$30 mL/min (iothalamate clearance)

   b. Proteinuria >2 g/day

   c. Kidney biopsy showing greater than 30% global glomerulosclerosis or greater than 30% interstitial fibrosis

   d. Metabolic disease

Data from Eason JD, Gonwa TA, Davis CL, et al. Proceedings of Consensus Conference on Simultaneous Liver Kidney Transplantation (SLK). Am J Transplant 2008;8(11):2243–51; and Nadim MK, Sung RS, Davis CL, et al. Simultaneous liver-kidney transplantation summit: current state and future directions. Am J Transplant 2012;12(11):2901–8.

ATN can result from induction of anesthesia, surgical technique, hemodynamic instability requiring use of vasopressors, intraoperative bleeding, and large volume of transfused blood products. A single-center study involving 250 liver transplants found that a higher transfusion requirement of packed red blood cells (3.8 L vs 2.29 L) was associated with early onset renal dysfunction.[71] More patients with early renal dysfunction did have hypotension (20.9% vs 7.7%) compared with patients who developed late renal dysfunction. A Spanish study of 184 OLT recipients found that prolonged treatment with dopamine, pretransplant AKI, low serum albumin, and severity of graft dysfunction all contributed to early postoperative renal dysfunction.[72] Efforts to minimize risk factors for renal dysfunction perioperative and immediately postoperative by stabilizing hemodynamics, minimizing bleeding and blood transfusion products, and using different surgical techniques are essential.

CNI is the backbone of immunosuppressive treatment in liver transplant. On 2012, according to Organ Procurement and Transplantation Network/Scientific Registry of Transplant Recipients (OPTN/SRTR), 80% of liver transplant recipients were using tacrolimus alone or in combination with mycophenolate at 1 year after the transplant.[73] Although CNIs have lowered rates of acute rejection and improved patient and graft outcomes, they are also associated with nephrotoxicity, hyperglycemia, hyperlipidemia, and hypertension. CNIs can cause AKI by afferent arteriole vasoconstriction producing prerenal ischemia, and prolonged ischemia can lead to ATN. Chronic nephrotoxicity caused by CNIs is reflected in tubular atrophy, interstitial fibrosis, and glomerulosclerosis on kidney biopsy.[74] The use of a CNI-free regimen is challenging, and so far few studies have shown successful switch to another class of drug with complete CNI withdrawal, but yet with short follow-up. The trend in liver transplant is to use regimens that minimize the use of CNIs by addition of or substitution with Mycophenolate Mofetil (MMF) or mammalian target of rapamycin inhibitors. Many studies have shown the potential renal benefit for OLT recipients justifying a combined

---

Box 6
Evaluation and selection of potential CLKT patients

1. Clinical assessment:

   a. Past medical history: history of diabetes, hypertension, or CKD, baseline serum creatinine levels, urinalysis

   b. History of present illness: current medications (diuretics, nonsteroidal anti-inflammatory drugs, lactulose), gastrointestinal issues (nausea, vomiting, diarrhea), paracentesis, infections (peritonitis, urinary tract infection), recent use of intravenous contrast

   c. Physical examination: assessment of volume status, edema, ascites, 24-hour urine output

2. Laboratory evaluation:

   a. Serum creatinine and electrolytes, cystatin C

   b. Spot urine creatinine, sodium, and protein to calculate fractional excretion of sodium and estimate the amount of proteinuria per day

   c. Urinalysis and sediment for hematuria, proteinuria, white blood cells, red blood cells, and casts

   d. Serology for antibodies, complement, cryoglobulinemia, and rheumatoid factor in patients with proteinuria, active sediment, hepatitis B or hepatitis C infections

3. Glomerular filtration measurement:

   a. Creatinine clearance by 24-hour urine collection

   b. Cockgroft-Gault and Modification of Diet in Renal Disease formulas

   c. Inulin, iohexol, or I-125–iothalamate clearance

4. Renal ultrasound to assess kidney size, echogenicity of the cortex, and to exclude hydroenphrosis

5. Renal biopsy:

   a. Suspect glomerular disease, tubular injury, or inflammation based on history and laboratory evaluation

   b. Assess degree of tubular atrophy, interstitial fibrosis, glomerulosclerosis, and arteriosclerosis

6. Management of renal failure:

   a. Correction of prerenal factors, hypovolemia, and other offending agents: discontinue diuretics and nephrotoxic drugs, give intravenous hydration and albumin; evaluate for gastrointestinal bleeding

   b. Treatment of hepatorenal syndrome

   c. Treatment of infection

   d. Renal-replacement therapy if necessary

7. List for CLKT if:

  a. Candidates with persistent AKI for ≥4 weeks with one of the following:

   i. Stage 3 AKI as defined by modified RIFLE, ie, a three-fold increase in Serum creatinine (Scr) from baseline, Scr greater than 4.0 mg/dL with an acute increase of ≥0.5 mg/dL or RRT

   ii. eGFR ≤35 mL/min (MDRD-6 [Modification of Diet in Renal Disease] equation) or GFR ≤25 mL/min (iothalamate clearance)

  b. Candidates with CKD, as defined by the National Kidney Foundation, for 3 months with one of the following:

   i. eGFR ≤40 mL/min (MDRD-6 equation) or GFR ≤30 mL/min (iothalamate clearance)

   ii. Proteinuria >2 g/day

   iii. Kidney biopsy showing greater than 30% global glomerulosclerosis or greater than 30% interstitial fibrosis

   iv. Metabolic disease

Data from Papafragkakis H, Martin P, Akalin E. Combined liver and kidney transplantation. Curr Opin Organ Transplant 2010;15(3):263–8.

therapy approach. In 2012, more than 70% of the liver recipients received CNI with MMF as a primary therapy. By the end of the first transplant year, 40% of the liver recipients were treated with a combination of CNI and MMF, and 35% with tacrolimus alone with or without concomitant use of steroid.[73] A comprehensive review of the multiple clinical trials involving CNI minimization has been published by Trotter and colleagues.[75] One important observation, however, from a recent publication is that a regimen with sirolimus combined with reduced dose of tacrolimus was associated with higher rates of graft loss, death, and sepsis when compared with the conventional dose of tacrolimus alone.[76] However, the use of everolimus with reduced tacrolimus exposure helped to preserve renal function after a 3-year follow-up.[77,78] For OLT recipients with renal dysfunction, consideration can be given to minimize the dose of CNI or switch to MMF or everolimus early. Although, a study using belatacept early on after transplant was recently published and suggested that belatacept in addition

---

Box 7
Management of postoperative liver transplant renal dysfunction

1. Consider delayed use, minimization, or withdrawal of calcineurin inhibitor if patient has baseline renal dysfunction.

2. If patient has AKI associated with hemolytic anemia and thrombocytopenia, the differential diagnosis includes thrombotic microangiopathy, which may require initiation of plasmapheresis.

3. Monitor blood glucose and blood pressure on a regular basis, and treat aggressively based on goals for nontransplant patients.

4. If patient has unexplained kidney disease, consider checking BK virus in blood and urine. If positive, consider kidney biopsy to evaluate for viral inclusion bodies. Treatment strategies include decreasing immunosuppression and giving intravenous immunoglobulin, leflunomide, or cidofovir if patient with definite BK nephropathy.

5. Patients who develop ESRD may be a candidate for a kidney transplant and should be referred for evaluation.

to MMF may be safely used as a bridge to CNI therapy in liver recipients with postoperative renal dysfunction, the use of belatacept in liver transplant is contraindicated due to an increase risk of graft loss and death.[79]

Thrombotic microangiopathy (TMA) of the kidneys has also been associated with CNI use and renal dysfunction in transplant recipients. TMA is a syndrome characterized by hemolytic anemia, thrombocytopenia, renal dysfunction, fevers, and occasionally neurologic deficits. On biopsy, arteriolar thrombi with intimal edema and fibrinoid necrosis of the vessel wall can be seen.[80] Mortality is high, 50% at 3 years in renal transplant patients with TMA.[81] The association between CNI and TMA may be related to direct endothelial injury.[82] Kidney biopsies performed in nonrenal transplant recipients who had prolonged AKI after transplant or sudden unexplained AKI found a prevalence of 13% in liver transplant patients.[8] Patients with TMA in this cohort also had the lowest long-term kidney survival compared with other etiologies of renal dysfunction. Empiric treatment for posttransplant TMA includes therapeutic plasma exchange and discontinuation or exchange of CNI. A case series of renal transplant patients showed that after switching from cyclosporine to tacrolimus, 81% of recipients had good graft function 1 year after an episode of TMA.[83] In bone marrow transplant recipients, however, response rates to plasma exchange have been reported to be less than 50%.[80]

New-onset diabetes mellitus after transplant (NODAT) and hypertension also contribute to renal dysfunction in liver transplant recipients. Review of the Organ Procurement and Transplant Network/United Network for Organ Sharing database revealed that the incidence of NODAT in liver transplant recipients was 26.4%.[84] Risk factors for development of NODAT included older age, African American race, hepatitis C infection, tacrolimus use, steroids on discharge, and high body mass index. Hypertension has also been shown to be associated with CNI use.[85] Renal insufficiency, NODAT, and posttransplant hypertension have all been identified as risk factors for mortality after liver transplant.[86] Although there are no formal transplant studies recommending blood pressure goals, results from large studies summarized in the Joint National Committee on Prevention, Detection, Evaluation, and Treatment of High Blood Pressure have been extrapolated for liver transplant recipients.[87] Goal blood pressure for patients with renal dysfunction is less than 125/75 and for all other patients is less than 130/80. First-line therapy includes lifestyle modification, such as weight loss and low-sodium diet. Pharmacologic therapies include initiation of calcium channel blockers initially in patients without proteinuria. Use of nondihydropyridine calcium channel blockers, such as verapamil or diltiazem, can increase CNI levels. Recipients with proteinuria should be started on angiotensin-converting enzyme inhibitors or angiotensin-receptor blockers with close monitoring of potassium and renal function. Diabetic nephropathy presents initially with microalbuminuria, and efforts to minimize proteinuria with angiotensin-converting enzyme inhibitors or angiotensin-receptor blockers have been shown to retard progression of renal disease in nontransplant patients.

Polyomavirus infection, notably BK virus, can occur with immunosuppression because it remains latent in B lymphocytes and the kidney after primary infection. Its role in nephropathy of renal transplant patients is well established. However, it is unclear if BK virus also causes nephropathy in liver transplant recipients. A study in 41 post-OLT patients showed a prevalence of BK viruria in 24.2% of patients, but presence or absence of viruria was not associated with a decline in eGFR.[88] An analysis of nonrenal solid organ transplant patients with unexplained chronic renal dysfunction showed that 15% had BK viruria.[89] Although the significance of BK virus and kidney dysfunction in liver transplant recipients is not known at this time, it is a possibility that should be considered if renal disease remains unexplained.

Hepatitis C may recur after transplant and my affect both liver and kidney graft survival.[90] Hepatitis C treatment is recommended before the transplant because use of interferon is associated with an increased risk of rejection and profound anemia. The development of the antiviral sofosbuvir and the promising combination sofosbuvir-ledipasvir[91] or daclatasvir-sofosbuvir[92] may allow treatment of hepatitis C recipients in the posttransplant period with interferon-free regimens and possibly improve their outcomes.

OLT recipients who subsequent develop ESRD are potentially candidates for kidney-after-liver transplantation. There was a 330% increase in the number of renal transplant listings from 1995 to 2008 in ex-OLT recipients.[93] In 2008, 124 kidney-after-liver transplants were performed in the United States, which comprised 0.9% of all kidney transplants.[94] Kidney transplant does provide a survival benefit compared with remaining on dialysis after OLT.[93] Overall graft survival in kidney-after-liver recipients was less than kidney-alone recipients at 1, 3, and 5 years, but death-censored graft survival was similar between the two groups.[93]

SUMMARY

Renal dysfunction is common in ESLD patients. A 24-hour urine collection or cystatin C are better alternatives to estimate GFR rather than serum creatinine. NGAL may be a better marker to differentiate intrinsic renal injury from HRS. Preoperatively, the most common causes of renal dysfunction are prerenal azotemia and ATN. Efforts to keep patients hemodynamically stable and refrain from using nephrotoxic agents are important. Hepatitis B and C are known to cause glomerulonephritis, which may be treatable if recognized early. A CLKT should be considered in patients whose renal function will likely not recover. After a liver transplant, consideration should be given to reduce exposure to CNI. Future studies are needed to explore potential strategies to reduce or eliminate CNI renal toxicity, such as regimens with everolimus. Aggressive control of NODAT and blood pressure management may aid in slowing down progression of CKD. TMA and BK virus are also potential contributors to nephropathy, which is often seen in renal and bone marrow transplant recipients. With the introduction of sofosbuvir and its combination with ledispavir or daclatasvir the treatment of hepatitis C in the posttransplant period looks promising. A kidney-after-liver transplant can be beneficial in OLT recipients who develop ESRD.

REFERENCES

1. Gonwa TA, McBride MA, Anderson K, et al. Continued influence of preoperative renal function on outcome of orthotopic liver transplant (OLTX) in the US: where will MELD lead us? Am J Transplant 2006;6(11):2651–9.
2. Fraley DS, Burr R, Bernardini J, et al. Impact of acute renal failure on mortality in end-stage liver disease with or without transplantation. Kidney Int 1998;54(2): 518–24.
3. Wong LP, Blackley MP, Andreoni KA, et al. Survival of liver transplant candidates with acute renal failure receiving renal replacement therapy. Kidney Int 2005; 68(1):362–70.
4. Ojo AO, Held PJ, Port FK, et al. Chronic renal failure after transplantation of a nonrenal organ. N Engl J Med 2003;349(10):931–40.
5. Barri YM, Sanchez EQ, Jennings LW, et al. Acute kidney injury following liver transplantation: definition and outcome. Liver Transpl 2009;15(5):475–83.
6. Fede G, D'Amico G, Arvaniti V, et al. Renal failure and cirrhosis: a systematic review of mortality and prognosis. J Hepatol 2012;56(4):810–8.

7. Martin-Llahi M, Guevara M, Torre A, et al. Prognostic importance of the cause of renal failure in patients with cirrhosis. Gastroenterology 2011;140(2):488–96.e4.

8. Schwarz A, Haller H, Schmitt R, et al. Biopsy-diagnosed renal disease in patients after transplantation of other organs and tissues. Am J Transplant 2010; 10(9):2017–25.

9. Wong F, Nadim MK, Kellum JA, et al. Working party proposal for a revised classification system of renal dysfunction in patients with cirrhosis. Gut 2011;60(5): 702–9.

10. Nadim MK, Sung RS, Davis CL, et al. Simultaneous liver-kidney transplantation summit: current state and future directions. Am J Transplant 2012;12(11):2901–8.

11. Hojs R, Bevc S, Ekart R, et al. Serum cystatin C-based equation compared to serum creatinine-based equations for estimation of glomerular filtration rate in patients with chronic kidney disease. Clin Nephrol 2008;70(1):10–7.

12. Orlando R, Mussap M, Plebani M, et al. Diagnostic value of plasma cystatin C as a glomerular filtration marker in decompensated liver cirrhosis. Clin Chem 2002; 48(6 Pt 1):850–8.

13. Souza VD, Hadj-Aissa A, Dolomanova O, et al. Creatinine- versus cystatine C-based equations in assessing the renal function of candidates for liver transplantation with cirrhosis. Hepatology 2014;59(4):1522–31.

14. Garcia-Tsao G, Parikh CR, Viola A. Acute kidney injury in cirrhosis. Hepatology 2008;48(6):2064–77.

15. Stadlbauer V, Wright GA, Banaji M, et al. Relationship between activation of the sympathetic nervous system and renal blood flow autoregulation in cirrhosis. Gastroenterology 2008;134(1):111–9.

16. Runyon BA. Introduction to the revised American Association for the Study of Liver Diseases Practice Guideline management of adult patients with ascites due to cirrhosis 2012. Hepatology 2013;57(4):1651–3.

17. Llach J, Gines P, Arroyo V, et al. Prognostic value of arterial pressure, endogenous vasoactive systems, and renal function in cirrhotic patients admitted to the hospital for the treatment of ascites. Gastroenterology 1988;94(2):482–7.

18. Fagundes C, Gines P. Hepatorenal syndrome: a severe, but treatable, cause of kidney failure in cirrhosis. Am J Kidney Dis 2012;59(6):874–85.

19. Verna EC, Wagener G. Renal interactions in liver dysfunction and failure. Curr Opin Crit Care 2013;19(2):133–41.

20. Salerno F, Gerbes A, Gines P, et al. Diagnosis, prevention and treatment of hepatorenal syndrome in cirrhosis. Gut 2007;56(9):1310–8.

21. Guevara M, Gines P. Hepatorenal syndrome. Dig Dis 2005;23(1):47–55.

22. Belcher JM, Parikh CR, Garcia-Tsao G. Acute kidney injury in patients with cirrhosis: perils and promise. Clin Gastroenterol Hepatol 2013;11(12):1550–8.

23. Belcher JM, Sanyal AJ, Peixoto AJ, et al. Kidney biomarkers and differential diagnosis of patients with cirrhosis and acute kidney injury. Hepatology 2013. [Epub ahead of print]. http://dx.doi.org/10.1002/hep.26980.

24. Fagundes C, Pepin MN, Guevara M, et al. Urinary neutrophil gelatinase-associated lipocalin as biomarker in the differential diagnosis of impairment of kidney function in cirrhosis. J Hepatol 2012;57(2):267–73.

25. Verna EC, Brown RS, Farrand E, et al. Urinary neutrophil gelatinase-associated lipocalin predicts mortality and identifies acute kidney injury in cirrhosis. Dig Dis Sci 2012;57(9):2362–70.

26. Sanyal AJ, Boyer T, Garcia-Tsao G, et al. A randomized, prospective, double-blind, placebo-controlled trial of terlipressin for type 1 hepatorenal syndrome. Gastroenterology 2008;134(5):1360–8.

27. Fabrizi F, Aghemo A, Messa P. Hepatorenal syndrome and novel advances in its management. Kidney Blood Press Res 2013;37(6):588–601.

28. Fabrizi F, Dixit V, Messa P, et al. Terlipressin for hepatorenal syndrome: a meta-analysis of randomized trials. Int J Artif Organs 2009;32(3):133–40.

29. Angeli P, Volpin R, Gerunda G, et al. Reversal of type 1 hepatorenal syndrome with the administration of midodrine and octreotide. Hepatology 1999;29(6):1690–7.

30. Skagen C, Einstein M, Lucey MR, et al. Combination treatment with octreotide, midodrine, and albumin improves survival in patients with type 1 and type 2 hepatorenal syndrome. J Clin Gastroenterol 2009;43(7):680–5.

31. Boyer TD, Haskal ZJ. The role of transjugular intrahepatic portosystemic shunt in the management of portal hypertension. Hepatology 2005;41(2):386–400.

32. Lodhia N, Kader M, Mayes T, et al. Risk of contrast-induced nephropathy in hospitalized patients with cirrhosis. World J Gastroenterol 2009;15(12):1459–64.

33. Alonso A, Lau J, Jaber BL, et al. Prevention of radiocontrast nephropathy with N-acetylcysteine in patients with chronic kidney disease: a meta-analysis of randomized, controlled trials. Am J Kidney Dis 2004;43(1):1–9.

34. Isenbarger DW, Kent SM, O'Malley PG. Meta-analysis of randomized clinical trials on the usefulness of acetylcysteine for prevention of contrast nephropathy. Am J Cardiol 2003;92(12):1454–8.

35. Marenzi G, Assanelli E, Marana I, et al. N-acetylcysteine and contrast-induced nephropathy in primary angioplasty. N Engl J Med 2006;354(26):2773–82.

36. Michel DM, Kelly CJ. Acute interstitial nephritis. J Am Soc Nephrol 1998;9(3): 506–15.

37. Blank ML, Parkin L, Paul C, et al. A nationwide nested case-control study indicates an increased risk of acute interstitial nephritis with proton pump inhibitor use. Kidney Int 2014. http://dx.doi.org/10.1038/ki.2014.74. Advance online publication March 19, 2014 [Epub ahead of print].

38. Berney-Meyer L, Hung N, Slatter T, et al. Omeprazole-induced acute interstitial nephritis: a possible Th1-Th17 mediated injury? Nephrology (Carlton) 2014; 19(6):359–65.

39. Harmark L, van der Wiel HE, de Groot MC, et al. Proton pump inhibitor-induced acute interstitial nephritis. Br J Clin Pharmacol 2007;64(6):819–23.

40. Simpson IJ, Marshall MR, Pilmore H, et al. Proton pump inhibitors and acute interstitial nephritis: report and analysis of 15 cases. Nephrology (Carlton) 2006;11(5):381–5.

41. Geevasinga N, Coleman PL, Webster AC, et al. Proton pump inhibitors and acute interstitial nephritis. Clin Gastroenterol Hepatol 2006;4(5):597–604.

42. Praga M, Gonzalez E. Acute interstitial nephritis. Kidney Int 2010;77(11):956–61.

43. Gonzalez E, Gutierrez E, Galeano C, et al. Early steroid treatment improves the recovery of renal function in patients with drug-induced acute interstitial nephritis. Kidney Int 2008;73(8):940–6.

44. Appel GB. The treatment of acute interstitial nephritis: more data at last. Kidney Int 2008;73(8):905–7.

45. Pouria S, Feehally J. Glomerular IgA deposition in liver disease. Nephrol Dial Transplant 1999;14(10):2279–82.

46. McGuire BM, Julian BA, Bynon JS Jr, et al. Brief communication: glomerulonephritis in patients with hepatitis C cirrhosis undergoing liver transplantation. Ann Intern Med 2006;144(10):735–41.

47. Amore A, Coppo R, Roccatello D, et al. Experimental IgA nephropathy secondary to hepatocellular injury induced by dietary deficiencies and heavy alcohol intake. Lab Invest 1994;70(1):68–77.

48. Roccatello D, Fornasieri A, Giachino O, et al. Multicenter study on hepatitis C virus-related cryoglobulinemic glomerulonephritis. Am J Kidney Dis 2007; 49(1):69–82.
49. Perico N, Cattaneo D, Bikbov B, et al. Hepatitis C infection and chronic renal diseases. Clin J Am Soc Nephrol 2009;4(1):207–20.
50. Mackelaite L, Alsauskas ZC, Ranganna K. Renal failure in patients with cirrhosis. Med Clin North Am 2009;93(4):855–69, viii.
51. Alric L, Plaisier E, Thebault S, et al. Influence of antiviral therapy in hepatitis C virus-associated cryoglobulinemic MPGN. Am J Kidney Dis 2004;43(4):617–23.
52. Misiani R, Bellavita P, Fenili D, et al. Interferon alfa-2a therapy in cryoglobulinemia associated with hepatitis C virus. N Engl J Med 1994;330(11):751–6.
53. Asselah T. Sofosbuvir-based interferon-free therapy for patients with HCV infection. J Hepatol 2013;59(6):1342–5.
54. Gane EJ, Stedman CA, Hyland RH, et al. Nucleotide polymerase inhibitor sofosbuvir plus ribavirin for hepatitis C. N Engl J Med 2013;368(1):34–44.
55. Lawitz E, Mangia A, Wyles D, et al. Sofosbuvir for previously untreated chronic hepatitis C infection. N Engl J Med 2013;368(20):1878–87.
56. Jacobson IM, Gordon SC, Kowdley KV, et al. Sofosbuvir for hepatitis C genotype 2 or 3 in patients without treatment options. N Engl J Med 2013;368(20):1867–77.
57. Hagan LM, Sulkowski MS, Schinazi RF. Cost analysis of sofosbuvir/ribavirin versus sofosbuvir/simeprevir for genotype 1 HCV in interferon ineligible/intolerant individuals. Hepatology 2014. [Epub ahead of print]. http://dx.doi.org/10.1002/hep.27151.
58. Hussar DA, Jin ZJ. New drugs: simeprevir, sofosbuvir, and dolutegravir sodium. J Am Pharm Assoc (2003) 2014;54(2):202–7.
59. Izumi N, Hayashi N, Kumada H, et al. Once-daily simeprevir with peginterferon and ribavirin for treatment-experienced HCV genotype 1-infected patients in Japan: the CONCERTO-2 and CONCERTO-3 studies. J Gastroenterol 2014; 49(5):941–53.
60. Roccatello D, Baldovino S, Rossi D, et al. Long-term effects of anti-CD20 monoclonal antibody treatment of cryoglobulinaemic glomerulonephritis. Nephrol Dial Transplant 2004;19(12):3054–61.
61. Bhimma R, Coovadia HM. Hepatitis B virus-associated nephropathy. Am J Nephrol 2004;24(2):198–211.
62. Conjeevaram HS, Hoofnagle JH, Austin HA, et al. Long-term outcome of hepatitis B virus-related glomerulonephritis after therapy with interferon alfa. Gastroenterology 1995;109(2):540–6.
63. Tang S, Lai FM, Lui YH, et al. Lamivudine in hepatitis B-associated membranous nephropathy. Kidney Int 2005;68(4):1750–8.
64. Carey I, Harrison PM. Monotherapy versus combination therapy for the treatment of chronic hepatitis B. Expert Opin Investig Drugs 2009;18(11): 1655–66.
65. Pipili CL, Papatheodoridis GV, Cholongitas EC. Treatment of hepatitis B in patients with chronic kidney disease. Kidney Int 2013;84(5):880–5.
66. Tanriover B, Mejia A, Weinstein J, et al. Analysis of kidney function and biopsy results in liver failure patients with renal dysfunction: a new look to combined liver kidney allocation in the post-MELD era. Transplantation 2008;86(11): 1548–53.
67. Locke JE, Warren DS, Singer AL, et al. Declining outcomes in simultaneous liver-kidney transplantation in the MELD era: ineffective usage of renal allografts. Transplantation 2008;85(7):935–42.

68. Chopra A, Cantarovich M, Bain VG. Simultaneous liver and kidney transplants: optimizing use of this double resource. Transplantation 2011;91(12):1305–9.
69. Eason JD, Gonwa TA, Davis CL, et al. Proceedings of consensus conference on simultaneous liver kidney transplantation (SLK). Am J Transplant 2008;8(11): 2243–51.
70. Papafragkakis H, Martin P, Akalin E. Combined liver and kidney transplantation. Curr Opin Organ Transplant 2010;15(3):263–8.
71. Lebron Gallardo M, Herrera Gutierrez ME, Seller Perez G, et al. Risk factors for renal dysfunction in the postoperative course of liver transplant. Liver Transpl 2004;10(11):1379–85.
72. Cabezuelo JB, Ramirez P, Rios A, et al. Risk factors of acute renal failure after liver transplantation. Kidney Int 2006;69(6):1073–80.
73. Kim WR, Smith JM, Skeans MA, et al. OPTN/SRTR 2012 annual data report: liver. Am J Transplant 2014;14(Suppl 1):69–96.
74. Flechner SM, Kobashigawa J, Klintmalm G. Calcineurin inhibitor-sparing regimens in solid organ transplantation: focus on improving renal function and nephrotoxicity. Clin Transplant 2008;22(1):1–15.
75. Trotter JF, Grafals M, Alsina AE. Early use of renal-sparing agents in liver transplantation: a closer look. Liver Transpl 2013;19(8):826–42.
76. Asrani SK, Wiesner RH, Trotter JF, et al. De novo sirolimus and reduced-dose tacrolimus versus standard-dose tacrolimus after liver transplantation: the 2000-2003 phase II prospective randomized trial. Am J Transplant 2014;14(2): 356–66.
77. Sterneck M, Kaiser GM, Heyne N, et al. Everolimus and early calcineurin inhibitor withdrawal: 3-year results from a randomized trial in liver transplantation. Am J Transplant 2014;14(3):701–10.
78. Saliba F, De Simone P, Nevens F, et al. Renal function at two years in liver transplant patients receiving everolimus: results of a randomized, multicenter study. Am J Transplant 2013;13(7):1734–45.
79. LaMattina JC, Jason MP, Hanish SI, et al. Safety of belatacept bridging immunosuppression in hepatitis C-positive liver transplant recipients with renal dysfunction. Transplantation 2014;97(2):133–7.
80. Batts ED, Lazarus HM. Diagnosis and treatment of transplantation-associated thrombotic microangiopathy: real progress or are we still waiting? Bone Marrow Transplant 2007;40(8):709–19.
81. Reynolds JC, Agodoa LY, Yuan CM, et al. Thrombotic microangiopathy after renal transplantation in the United States. Am J Kidney Dis 2003;42(5): 1058–68.
82. Ruggenenti P. Post-transplant hemolytic-uremic syndrome. Kidney Int 2002; 62(3):1093–104.
83. Zarifian A, Meleg-Smith S, O'Donovan R, et al. Cyclosporine-associated thrombotic microangiopathy in renal allografts. Kidney Int 1999;55(6):2457–66.
84. Kuo HT, Sampaio MS, Ye X, et al. Risk factors for new-onset diabetes mellitus in adult liver transplant recipients, an analysis of the Organ Procurement and Transplant Network/United Network for Organ Sharing database. Transplantation 2010;89(9):1134–40.
85. Perez MJ, Garcia DM, Taybi BJ, et al. Cardiovascular risk factors after liver transplantation: analysis of related factors. Transplant Proc 2011;43(3):739–41.
86. Watt KD, Pedersen RA, Kremers WK, et al. Evolution of causes and risk factors for mortality post-liver transplant: results of the NIDDK long-term follow-up study. Am J Transplant 2010;10(6):1420–7.

87. Guckelberger O. Long-term medical comorbidities and their management: hypertension/cardiovascular disease. Liver Transpl 2009;15(Suppl 2):S75–8.
88. Salama M, Boudville N, Speers D, et al. Decline in native kidney function in liver transplant recipients is not associated with BK virus infection. Liver Transpl 2008;14(12):1787–92.
89. Barton TD, Blumberg EA, Doyle A, et al. A prospective cross-sectional study of BK virus infection in non-renal solid organ transplant recipients with chronic renal dysfunction. Transpl Infect Dis 2006;8(2):102–7.
90. Carbone M, Mutimer D, Neuberger J. Hepatitis C virus and nonliver solid organ transplantation. Transplantation 2013;95(6):779–86.
91. Lawitz E, Poordad FF, Pang PS, et al. Sofosbuvir and ledipasvir fixed-dose combination with and without ribavirin in treatment-naive and previously treated patients with genotype 1 hepatitis C virus infection (LONESTAR): an open-label, randomised, phase 2 trial. Lancet 2014;383(9916):515–23.
92. Sulkowski MS, Gardiner DF, Rodriguez-Torres M, et al. Daclatasvir plus sofosbuvir for previously treated or untreated chronic HCV infection. N Engl J Med 2014; 370(3):211–21.
93. Srinivas TR, Stephany BR, Budev M, et al. An emerging population: kidney transplant candidates who are placed on the waiting list after liver, heart, and lung transplantation. Clin J Am Soc Nephrol 2010;5(10):1881–6.
94. Gonwa TA, McBride MA, Mai ML, et al. Kidney transplantation after previous liver transplantation: analysis of the organ procurement transplant network database. Transplantation 2011;92(1):31–5.

Acute-On-Chronic Liver Failure

Sumeet K. Asrani, MD, MSc[a], Jacqueline G. O'Leary, MD, MPH[b],*

KEYWORDS

- Acute-on-chronic liver failure • Acute liver failure • Organ failure
- Liver transplantation • Cirrhosis

KEY POINTS

- Acute-on-chronic liver failure (ACLF) is characterized by a precipitating event in patients with underlying chronic liver disease, leading to acute deterioration of liver function and often ending in multiorgan system failure.
- The physiology of ACLF can be divided into a 4-part model: (1) predisposition, (2) injury caused by the precipitating event, (3) response to the injury, and (4) organ failure.
- The definition of ACLF, like the definition of acute liver failure, requires liver dysfunction, and the prognosis depends on the number of extrahepatic organs involved (ie, renal, cerebral, circulatory, and pulmonary). Increasing numbers of organ failures with underlying cirrhosis usually portends progressively worse outcomes.
- Acute renal failure in patients with cirrhosis is associated with an almost 8-fold increased risk of death; smaller increases ($\geq$0.3 mg/dL) in creatinine level, some of which occur lower than the 1.0 mg/dL creatinine cutoff for MELD (Model for End-Stage Liver Disease) point allocation, have significant prognostic implications.
- ACLF carries a high mortality in wait-listed patients, and those who survive require prompt transplantation.

INTRODUCTION

According to the US Centers for Disease Control, chronic liver disease and cirrhosis is the 12th leading cause of death in the United States, and liver disease–related mortality has remained unchanged over the last 3 decades, despite dramatic improvements in general medical care, hepatology care, and post–liver transplant outcomes achieved during that time.[1] Chronic liver disease is not only a significant cause of morbidity and mortality but it accounts for a substantial portion of health care

Financial Disclosures: None relevant to the article.

[a] Division of Hepatology, Baylor University Medical Center, 3410 Worth Street, Suite 860, Dallas, TX 75246, USA; [b] Division of Hepatology, Hepatology Research, Annette C. & Harold C. Simmons Transplant Institute, Baylor University Medical Center, 3410 Worth Street, Suite 860, Dallas, TX 75246, USA
* Corresponding author.
E-mail address: Jacquelo@BaylorHealth.edu

Clin Liver Dis 18 (2014) 561–574
http://dx.doi.org/10.1016/j.cld.2014.05.004
1089-3261/14/$ – see front matter © 2014 Elsevier Inc. All rights reserved.

liver.theclinics.com

expenditure in the United States and worldwide.[2] Therefore, to improve prognostication and outcomes in patients with chronic liver disease, the current terminology that defines liver dysfunction must first be evaluated. Although liver dysfunction was often discussed as compensated versus decompensated cirrhosis, quantitation of liver dysfunction was first reasonably and accurately accomplished by the Child-Turcott-Pugh (CTP) score and is now accomplished in a more granular manner by the Model for End-Stage Liver Disease (MELD) score.[3,4] However, when a cirrhotic patient experiences an acute event, such as an infection, their pre-event MELD score does not accurately predict their mortality risk. The concept of acute-on-chronic liver disease emerged, because cirrhotics often experience a nonlinear progression in their liver disease (**Fig. 1**).[5–7] However, this notion has struggled to achieve universal acceptance as a uniform entity. In an effort to understand the concept and describe its implication peritransplant, it is important to distinguish acute-on-chronic liver failure (ACLF) from decompensation.

ACLF IS NOT DECOMPENSATED CIRRHOSIS

ACLF is a distinct entity from compensated and decompensated liver disease (presence of ascites, hepatorenal syndrome, variceal hemorrhage, hepatic encephalopathy, or synthetic dysfunction). In a population-based study, persons with compensated cirrhosis had a 5-fold, and persons with decompensated cirrhosis had a 10-fold, increased risk of death compared with the general population.[8] Most of the deaths among patients with compensated cirrhosis occurred because of a transition to decompensation and resultant complications. However, unlike the simple features of ascites, encephalopathy, hepatorenal syndrome, variceal hemorrhage, and hepatic synthetic dysfunction that characterize hepatic decompensation, ACLF focuses on the acute events (**Box 1**) that move patients from low-risk to high-risk of organ failure and death.

PHYSIOLOGY OF ACLF

Borrowing from the sepsis literature, Jalan and colleagues[6] parsed the pathophysiologic basis of ACLF into a 4-part model: (1) predisposition, (2) injury caused by

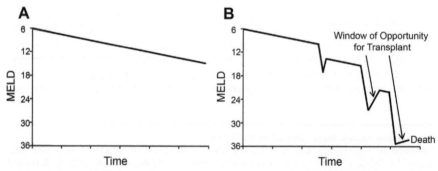

Fig. 1. (*A*) Few patients with cirrhosis experience a smooth and steady increase in MELD score over time. (*B*) Most patients have a background slope of slowly increasing MELD score, which is punctuated by ACLF events, which early on result in recovery, but later on result in longer periods of illness, less recovery potential, and a higher risk of multiorgan system failure. After the acute event has resolved, there is a window of opportunity to transplant patients while their MELD is high enough to receive priority, but they are no longer too sick for transplant.

Box 1
Events known to precipitate ACLF

- Acute alcoholic hepatitis
- Acute hepatotrophic viral infection
  - Acute hepatitis A
  - Reactivation hepatitis B
  - Acute hepatitis D in the presence of hepatitis B
  - Acute hepatitis E
- Drug-induced liver injury
- Gastrointestinal bleeding
- Infection
- Ischemia
  - Hypotension
  - Surgery
  - Trauma
- Portal vein thrombosis

---

precipitating event, (3) response to injury, and (4) organ failure.[5,7,9,10] In their model, predisposition refers to underlying cirrhosis and concomitant illnesses. Patients with advanced liver dysfunction measured by either MELD or CTP are at greater risk to experience a precipitating event. In patients with a high MELD score, this finding is coupled with an impaired hepatic reserve.

Injury may be caused by one of many insults (see **Box 1**). All causes can cause ACLF; however, there are geographic differences in prevalence: reactivation of hepatitis B and development of acute hepatitis A, D, and E are important causes of ACLF in Asian centers, whereas acute alcoholic hepatitis and infections are more common precipitants of ACLF in Western centers. Despite continent-wide differences, an identifiable precipitating injury remains unknown in many cases.

Because most events that precipitate ACLF, regardless of the continent, are ischemic or infectious in nature, the inflammatory response plays a critical role in the outcome of ACLF. Given that about half of admitted cirrhotics have evidence of infection, and a further 25% develop nosocomial infections with high inpatient mortality, infection plays an overwhelming factor in the natural history of ACLF.[11–13] Overt bacterial infection and possibly covert bacterial translocation with subsequent systemic inflammatory response may be responsible for transition from a compensated to decompensated state.[6] The inflammatory response is important: a robust response is measured by an increased C-reactive protein (CRP) level or an increased leukocyte count and is associated with worse outcomes.[14] It is unclear whether the inflammation is a response to the inciting event or a part of the inciting event. On the other hand, failure of the immune response is also important, given the higher mortality associated with nosocomial or second infections.[12,15]

Organ failure is the last component of ACLF; increasing numbers of organ failures (ie, renal, cerebral, circulatory, and pulmonary) portend progressively worse outcomes in patients with underlying cirrhosis.[14,15] The definition of ACLF, like the definition of acute liver failure (ALF), requires liver disease and dysfunction but is prognostically based on extrahepatic organ failures, which are discussed separately.

Renal

Acute renal failure in patients with cirrhosis is associated with an almost 8-fold increased risk of death,[16] which is reflected by the prominence of serum creatinine in the MELD score.[17] The cause of renal dysfunction, in addition to the serum creatinine level, determines prognosis; hepatorenal syndrome and infection-related renal dysfunction portend a worse prognosis than chronic renal failure.[18] However, the MELD score does not differentiate between causes of renal failure or incorporate differences in baseline creatinine.[19] Recent data have shown that smaller increases (≥0.3 mg/dL) in creatinine level, some of which occur lower than the 1.0 mg/dL creatinine cutoff for MELD point allocation, have significant prognostic implications.[20,21] The chance for recovery is partially related to the absolute change in creatinine, and the risk for death does not completely abate, even if patients experience resolution of their acute renal failure (**Fig. 2**).[20] This situation has resulted in novel categorizations

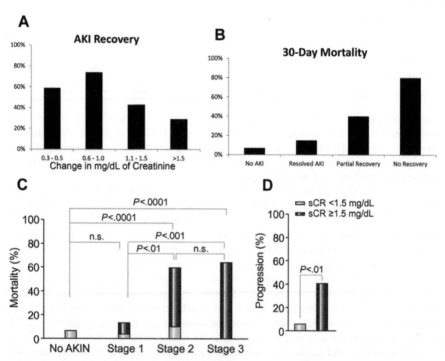

Fig. 2. (A, B) Acute kidney injury (AKI) was defined as an absolute increase in serum creatinine (sCR) level 0.3 mg/dL or greater in less than 48 hours or a 50% increase in serum creatinine from baseline. (A) The chance for renal recovery was proportional to the absolute change in creatinine, and (B) the 30-day mortality was lowest in patients without AKI, and greatest in those without renal recover. (C, D) Similar findings were seen with the Acute Kidney Injury Network (AKIN) staging system (see **Table 1**). Progression was less likely in patients whose peak creatinine level was less than 1.5 mg/dL. n.s., not significant. ([A, B] *Adapted from* Wong F, O'Leary JG, Reddy KR, et al. North American Consortium for Study of End-Stage Liver Diseases. New consensus definition of acute kidney injury accurately predicts 30-day mortality in patients with cirrhosis and infection. Gastroenterology 2014;145:1280–8, with permission; and [C, D] *Reproduced from* Piano S, Rosi S, Maresio G, et al. Evaluation of the Acute Kidney Injury Network criteria in hospitalized patients with cirrhosis and ascites. J Hepatol 2013;59:486, with permission.)

of renal dysfunction in patients with cirrhosis being proposed and validated beyond just hepatorenal syndrome.[20–22] These scores (**Table 1**) acknowledge the importance of earlier diagnosis for acute kidney injury and do not require the absence of chronic renal disease. Unlike hepatorenal syndrome, the adoption of these new scoring systems in clinical trials of novel therapeutics will facilitate earlier implementation of therapy and, it is hoped, improve clinical outcomes.

Brain

Akin to ALF, but in contrast to chronic decompensation, patients with ACLF can develop cerebral edema. The resultant increase in intracranial pressure can be reversed with liver transplantation (LT). Brain edema may be caused by the synergy between increased ammonia and the inflammatory response that is often super-imposed on an additional hepatic injury.[6] The role of rifaximin as a potential reducer of bacterial translocation, with subsequent diminution of inflammation, is hypothe-sized to be of benefit but remains untested in persons with ACLF.[6]

Circulatory

ACLF is characterized by a paralysis of immune response similar to changes seen in severe sepsis.[23] Patients with ACLF usually first experience the systemic inflammatory response system (SIRS) and second, the compensatory antiinflammatory response system (CARS). Unlike SIRS, CARS downregulates antigen presentation, causes

Table 1
Definitions of renal dysfunction in patients with cirrhosis

	Hepatorenal Syndrome	Acute Kidney Injury Network	International Ascites Club and Adult Dialysis Quality Initiative
Cirrhosis required	Yes	Yes	Yes
Absence of underlying renal disease	Required	Not required	Not required, Acute-on-chronic kidney disease defined
Minimum serum creatinine level	≥1.5	Stage 2 and 3 yes, serum creatinine ≥1.5	No
Stages/Types	Yes	Yes	No
Criteria	(1) Ascites, (2) no improvement after 2 d of diuretic withdrawal and volume expansion, (3) no shock, (4) no nephrotoxic drugs; type 1: doubling in serum creatinine level to ≥2.5 in <14 d	Stage 1 = ≥0.3 mg/dL in <48 h or increase 1.5–2 × baseline Stage 2 = increase 2–3 × baseline Stage 3 = increase >3 × baseline or >4.0 mg/dL with an acute ≥0.5 mg/dL increase	Acute kidney injury: ≥0.3 mg/dL in <48 h or >50% over baseline. Chronic renal disease: estimated glomerular filtration rate <60 mL/min for >3 mo by Modification of Diet in Renal Disease 6 formula

macrophage deactivation, results in antiinflammatory cytokine production, and can result in anergy.[24–26] Therefore, once ACLF occurs, patients are at risk for additional infections.[12] There is a strong correlation between ACLF, previous history of acute decompensation, leukocyte count, and risk of death (**Fig. 3**).[14]

The increased infectious risk is often coupled to cardiac dysfunction; there may be failure to appropriately increase the cardiac output in response to the insult. This finding is in contrast to chronic decompensated cirrhosis, in which cardiac output is appropriately increased. Inotrope support is often needed, similar to persons with ALF. The appropriate inotrope is unknown; however, norepinephrine has been shown in small studies to improve renal function in patients with hepatorenal syndrome and therefore may be beneficial.[27,28]

Pulmonary

The impact of pulmonary compromise on mortality in ACLF is highlighted by its incorporation into the Chronic Liver Failure (CLIF)–Sequential Organ Failure Assessment (SOFA) and the sepsis-related ACLF (S-ACLF) scores.[14,15] Although some patients are intubated for airway protection for severe encephalopathy, several other pulmonary complications can occur. Hepatic hydrothorax can result in pulmonary compromise and, like ascites, can become infected. Transfusion-related acute lung injury likely occurs more often than it is diagnosed[29] and may increase the systemic inflammation present during ACLF. Therefore, minimizing transfusions, when appropriate, is essential.

However, most pulmonary complications that result in ACLF are infectious. Numerous factors increase this risk of aspiration, including diminished airway protection from encephalopathy, increased intra-abdominal pressure from ascites, and endoscopy for gastrointestinal bleeding. In addition, bacterial colonization more commonly occurs with microaspiration or translocation because of overutilization of proton pump inhibitors.[30,31] As a result, respiratory tract infections represent 14% to 48% of infections in cirrhotic patients[32]; however, they disproportionately increase a cirrhotic patient's risk of death.[12,32]

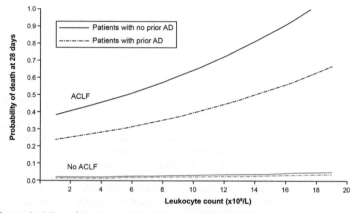

Fig. 3. The probability of death at 28 days is shown based on the presence of ACLF, a previous history of acute decompensation (AD), and leukocyte count. (*Reproduced from* Moreau R, Jalan R, Gines P, et al. Acute-on-chronic liver failure is a distinct syndrome that develops in patients with acute decompensation of cirrhosis. Gastroenterology 2013;144:1433; with permission.)

DEFINITIONS OF ACLF

The most widely accepted definition of ACLF suggested by an American Association for the study of Liver Diseases (AASLD)/European Association for the Study of the Liver (EASL) consortium is the presence of a precipitating event (identified or surreptitious) in patients with underlying chronic liver disease, leading to acute deterioration of liver function and often ending in multiorgan dysfunction characterized by a high short-term mortality (**Table 2**).[5–7] However, 3 separate definitions are described derived from multicenter efforts from the Asia Pacific Region (Asia Pacific Association for the Study of the Liver [APASL]),[33] Europe (EASL-CLIF)[14] as well as North America (North American Consortium for the Study of End-Stage Liver Disease [NACSELD])[15] groups.[34]

APASL

APASL, which comprises experts within the Asia Pacific Region, defined ACLF as an "acute hepatic insult manifesting as jaundice (bilirubin level >5 mg/dL) and coagulopathy (international normalized ratio >1.5) complicated within 4 weeks by ascites and/or encephalopathy in a patient with previously diagnosed or undiagnosed chronic liver disease."[33] Reactivation of hepatitis B as well as super infection with hepatitis E virus were the predominant causes, and the presence of cirrhosis was not required. The investigators questioned whether sepsis acted as an initial precipitating event or played a role in the progression of ACLF, and debate occurred over whether surgery and variceal bleeding should be included as potential precipitants.

EASL-CLIF

Moreau and colleagues,[14] on behalf of EASL-CLIF, recently reported a novel scoring system for ACLF (**Fig. 4**). In their study population, 31% of patients had ACLF, most of whom had ACLF in the setting of alcoholic liver disease. Bacterial infections were the number 1 precipitating event, although no precipitant was found in 44% of cases.

The most common cause of death was multiorgan system failure. Cirrhotics with ACLF had a mortality of 34% versus 1.9% for patients with decompensation without ACLF. The type of organ failure (renal failure carried the highest risk) was a risk factor for mortality, and mortality increased as the number of organs with dysfunction increased. ACLF was defined by occurrence of acute decompensation, organ failure, and mortality within 28 days of greater than 15% and characterized into 3 grades (see **Fig. 4**).[14] The 28-day mortality was 5%, 22%, 32%, and 77% for grades 0, 1, 2, and 3, respectively. Patients with increased leukocyte counts and plasma CRP levels did worse; infection or inflammatory response was one of the most important risk factors for poor outcomes after ACLF.[14,35]

Table 2
Differences in definitions of ACLF

	APASL Definition	AASLD/EASL Consensus
Duration	<4 wk	Not defined
Chronic liver disease	Any fibrosis stage	Cirrhosis only
Most common precipitant	Hepatotrophic viruses	Infections
Other agreed precipitants	Alcohol, drug-induced liver injury, ischemia	
Variceal bleeding	No consensus	Yes
Infection	No	Yes

Adapted from Bajaj JS. Defining acute-on-chronic liver failure: will east and west ever meet? Gastroenterology 2013;144(7):1337; with permission.

A

Organ/system	0	1	2	3	4
Liver (bilirubin, mg/dL)	<1.2	≥1.2 to <2.0	≥2.0 to <6.0	≥6.0 to <12.0	**≥12.0**
Kidney (creatinine, mg/dL)	<1.2	≥1.2 to <2.0	**≥2.0 to <3.5**	**≥3.5 to <5.0**	**≥5.0**
				or use of renal replacement therapy	
Cerebral (HE grade)	No HE	I	II	III	IV
Coagulation (international normalized ratio)	<1.1	≥1.1 to <1.25	≥1.25 to <1.5	≥1.5 to <2.5	**≥2.5 or platelet count ≤20—10⁹/L**
Circulation (mean arterial pressure, mm Hg)	≥70	<70	**Dopamine ≤5 or dobutamine or terlipressin**	**Dopamine >5 or E ≤0.1 or NE ≤0.1**	**Dopamine >15 or E >0.1 or NE >0.1**
Lungs					
PaO/Fio₂ or	>400	>300 to ≤400	>200 to ≤300	>100 to ≤200	**≤100**
Spo₂/Fio₂	>512	>357 to ≤512	>214 to ≤357	>89 to ≤214	**≤89**

B

ACLF Grade	Criteria	Additional Criteria
ACLF grade 1	Single renal failure	None
	Single liver, coagulation, circulation or respirtory failure	Creatinine 1.5-1.9 mg/dL and/or mild-moderate encephaloapthy
	Single cerebral failure	Creatinine 1.5-1.9 mg/dL
ACLF grade 2	2 organ failures	None
ACLF grade 3	≥3 organ failures	None

C

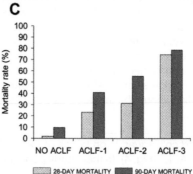

Fig. 4. (*A*) CLIF-SOFA score is used to categorize patients into (*B*) grades of ACLF. (*C*) Patient's risk of mortality is based on their ACLF grade. Bold type in panel (*A*) indicates organ failure. E, epinephrine; HE, hepatic encephalopathy; NE, norepinephrine. (*From* Moreau R, Jalan R, Gines P, et al, CANONIC Study Investigators of the EASL–CLIF Consortium. Acute-on-chronic liver failure is a distinct syndrome that develops in patients with acute decompensation of cirrhosis. Gastroenterology 2013;144(7):1428.e6; with permission.)

NACSELD

NACSELD recently examined survival in S-ACLF.[15] Overall organ failures were purposefully simply defined: circulatory failure was shock, cerebral failure was West Haven grade 3 or 4 hepatic encephalopathy, renal failure was need for dialysis, and pulmonary failure was need for mechanical ventilation. S-ACLF was defined as 2 or more organ failures, and 30-day mortality increased with the number of extrahepatic organ failures present: 8%, 27%, 49%, 64%, and 77% for 0, 1, 2, 3, and 4, respectively (**Fig. 5**). Independent predictors of ACLF were nosocomial infections, nonspontaneous bacterial peritonitis as the first infection, low mean arterial pressure, and admission MELD score. In addition to the S-ACLF score, second infections, MELD, and admission white blood cell count were independent predictors of 30-day mortality, whereas a higher admission serum albumin level was protective.

Regional Differences in Defining ACLF

Several differences exist in the definition of ACLF, partly contingent on regional variation in causes of ACLF. First, most patients had reactivation of hepatitis B in the APASL group, alcohol-related cirrhosis in the EASL-CLIF group and hepatitis C in

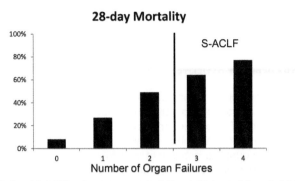

Fig. 5. NACSELD defined S-ACLF as 2 or more organ failures. (*Adapted from* Bajaj JS, O'Leary JG, Reddy KR, et al, on behalf of NACSELD. Survival in infection-related acute-on-chronic liver failure is defined by extra-hepatic organ failures. Hepatology 2014 Feb 20. http://dx.doi.org/10.1002/hep.27077. [Epub ahead of print]; with permission.)

the NACSELD group. Second, definitions proposed by APASL suggest a duration of the inciting event to be less than 4 weeks, with manifestations of ACLF being characterized by ascites and encephalopathy. However, Western centers place less emphasis on deterioration of liver function and more emphasis on development of extrahepatic organ failure. Third, whereas APASL and NACSELD definitions rely on presenting factors (eg, multiorgan system failure), the EASL-CLIF definition includes the outcome (mortality >15%) in the definition. Fourth, the definition of underlying liver disease also varies across the groups. Chronic liver disease is enough to qualify for the APASL definition, whereas EASL-CLIF and NACSELD require the presence of cirrhosis. Fifth, renal failure and infection play a more prominent role in EASL-CLIF and NACSELD compared with viral hepatitis in APASL definitions.

PREDICTIVE MODELS

Several models may help predict outcomes in patients with ACLF. Certain models were developed to be cause specific. Patients with acute alcoholic hepatitis are at a higher risk for ACLF compared with other hospitalized cirrhotic patients.[14] For this disorder, MELD predicts early mortality but has not been validated in patients with ACLF.[36,37] The Lille model assesses short-term prognosis in patients with alcoholic hepatitis treated with steroids.[38] For cirrhotics undergoing surgery, who are at risk for an ischemic or infectious insult that can result in ACLF, a combination of the MELD score, age, and American Society of Anesthesiologists classification are predictive of short-term mortality.[39]

Other models are not disease specific and capture risk of mortality based on liver function, such as the CTP or MELD score. Given that multiorgan failure is common, models that address end-organ dysfunction such as the SOFA as well as the Acute Physiology Age and Chronic Health Evaluation have been used. Moreau and colleagues[14] examined the sequential SOFA score modified to include factors associated with liver disease (SOFA-CLIF), as discussed earlier (see **Fig. 4**). In contrast to elaborate models, Bajaj and colleagues,[15] using data from the NACSELD data set, showed that extent of multiorgan failure was sufficient to predict short-term mortality in patients with S-ACLF (see **Fig. 5**).

Although laboratory and clinical models may predict outcome, stool analysis may as well. Analysis of the gut microbiome, using the cirrhosis/dysbiosis ratio (CDR), shows a progressive decrease in the CDR with worsening liver dysfunction, which is predictive of short-term organ failure and death.[40] This finding requires validation in additional studies.

ACLF IN PRETRANSPLANT PATIENTS

Data on ACLF and outcomes among cirrhotics awaiting LT are sparse. Given the high short-term mortality, persons who may be candidates for transplant with ACLF need to be evaluated rapidly. Finkenstedt and colleagues[41] examined ACLF on the waiting list in a single-center European cohort between 2002 and 2010 using the APASL definition (n = 144). Although no precipitant was found in 40%, infection and bleeding were the most common precipitants identified. The mean MELD score was 28, hepatorenal syndrome developed in 53%, wait-list mortality was 54% (median survival was 54 days), and only 10 persons survived without LT over a median follow-up of 1.5 years. Patients with better renal function and lower CRP levels were more likely to receive an LT compared with those with sepsis or those needing mechanical ventilation. Most patients who underwent LT had it occur during their ACLF event. Although it was not explicitly stated, there seemed to be increased short-term mortality; however, there was no difference in long-term (1-year, 3-year, and 5-year) posttransplant mortality between those transplanted with and without ACLF.

Bahirwani and colleagues[42] examined patients at a large American transplant center with ACLF (defined as an increase in MELD score of >5 points within 4 weeks of LT) between 2002 and 2006. There was no significant difference in 3-year renal function, risk of recurrent cirrhosis, graft loss, and death between those transplanted with and without ACLF. However, both studies lacked a comparison with a MELD-matched cohort without ACLF.

MEDICAL THERAPY

There is no ACLF-specific treatment. Appropriate intensive care management of patients with ACLF is the mainstay of treatment, as recently reviewed.[5] Management of ACLF is contingent on first addressing the precipitating event. For example, in the setting of acute alcoholic hepatitis, administration of prednisolone early in the course may play a critical role if warranted by the disease severity and absence of contraindications. Administration of tenofovir for ACLF caused by reactivation of hepatitis B may lead to improved survival.[43] However, a major impact in ACLF risk reduction will be achieved only through novel infection prevention strategies. Although antibiotic-based gastrointestinal bleeding prophylaxis and spontaneous bacterial peritonitis prophylaxis remain essential, ideally the future of ACLF prevention would be with non-antibiotic-related preventative interventions.

Liver Assist Devices

The role of liver assist devices in ACLF management remains unclear.[44] MARS (Gambro, Rostock, Germany), a nonbiological molecular adsorbent recirculating system, was examined in a multicenter study of 180 patients with ACLF complicated with either hepatorenal syndrome, hepatic encephalopathy, or worsening hyperbilirubinemia who were randomized to receive standard medical therapy with or without MARS. Patients assigned to MARS showed significant improvement in bilirubin, creatinine, and hepatic encephalopathy, but at 28 days, a survival benefit was not observed.[45] Similarly, in a study of the nonbiological device Prometheus (Fresenius Medical Care, Bad Homburg, Germany) (which uses fractional plasma separation absorption and dialysis), an overall survival benefit was not observed in patients with

ACLF, but it was seen in subgroup analysis of persons with type I hepatorenal syndrome and MELD scores greater than 30.[44]

ACLF AND OUTCOMES AFTER LT

The decision to proceed with LT in an individual recipient is based on organ availability, recipient disease severity, and the absence of contraindications. It is unclear whether criteria that are applicable to ALF are appropriate for ACLF. There is no specific priority assigned to persons with ACLF above and beyond the inevitable increase in MELD that occurs with ACLF. Recent data suggest that candidates with the highest MELD scores (>36) should be assigned either similar or higher priority than status 1 patients given their significant wait-list mortality.[46] However, the presence of cerebral edema, active infection, and hemodynamic instability, often present in persons with ACLF, remains an obvious contraindication to transplantation. Therefore, timing of transplant is critical. There is a lack of accurate laboratory parameters or biomarkers that signal the earliest safe window of transplant opportunity.

Living donor LT has been used in patients with ACLF caused by hepatitis B reactivation.[47,48] In a single-center analysis in Hong Kong of 32 patients with ACLF between 1996 and 2002,[49] living donor LT was used for patients with ACLF in the intensive care unit with a mean MELD score of 36. Overall operative morbidity was significant (59%), resulting in a 38-day mean length of stay. Patient and graft survival were both 88% at a median follow-up of almost 2 years, and was similar to a reference group who underwent elective living donor with lower MELD scores.

The role of simultaneous liver-kidney transplantation (SLKT) in patients with ACLF and renal dysfunction was recently examined in 133 patients with a mean MELD of 32 undergoing deceased donor transplantation at a single Chinese center between 2001 and 2009.[50] Patients were divided into 3 groups: (1) those with ACLF without renal dysfunction who underwent LT (5-year survival = 72%), (2) those with ACLF with renal dysfunction who underwent LT (5-year survival = 56%), and (3) those with ACLF with renal dysfunction who underwent SLKT (5-year survival = 82%). Many key factors about these patients remain unclear, such as how many patients had acute versus chronic kidney disease and how long the renal dysfunction was present before transplant.[51] Therefore validation is essential.

UNRESOLVED QUESTIONS

Despite the progress in defining ACLF, several questions remain. First, an element of reversibility is proposed among persons with ACLF who are successfully navigated through the acute decompensation. Theoretically, once the acute insult is managed, the long-term prognosis should be similar between MELD-matched patients with and without ACLF. However, this theory has not been well studied, and there is likely a point of no return, which is yet to be defined. Second, definitions from the various groups need to be aligned with the establishment of a common understanding of the underlying substrate (chronic liver disease vs compensated cirrhosis vs decompensated cirrhosis). Third, it is unclear whether all renal dysfunction in patients with ACLF is reversible.[6] Recent investigations have highlighted the importance of the cause, severity, and duration of renal dysfunction as critical determinants of outcome; even persons with normal renal function before ACLF can develop irreversible renal dysfunction after LT.[52–54] Whether this finding is more pronounced in persons with ACLF is unknown. Last, the best way to improve ACLF outcomes is likely through prevention.[55] Because the most common precipitant of ACLF is infection, development of accurate risk stratification schemes followed by implementation of novel (preferably nonantibiotic) prevention strategies is desperately needed.

REFERENCES

1. Asrani SK, Larson JJ, Yawn B, et al. Underestimation of liver-related mortality in the United States. Gastroenterology 2013;145:375–82.e1–2.
2. Kim WR, Brown RS Jr, Terrault NA, et al. Burden of liver disease in the United States: summary of a workshop. Hepatology 2002;36:227–42.
3. Pugh RN, Murray-Lyon IM, Dawson JL, et al. Transection of the oesophagus for bleeding oesophageal varices. Br J Surg 1973;60:646–9.
4. Malinchoc M, Kamath PS, Gordon FD, et al. A model to predict poor survival in patients undergoing transjugular intrahepatic portosystemic shunts. Hepatology 2000;31:864–71.
5. Olson JC, Wendon JA, Kramer DJ, et al. Intensive care of the patient with cirrhosis. Hepatology 2011;54:1864–72.
6. Jalan R, Gines P, Olson JC, et al. Acute-on chronic liver failure. J Hepatol 2012;57(6):1336–48.
7. Rosselli M, MacNaughtan J, Jalan R, et al. Beyond scoring: a modern interpretation of disease progression in chronic liver disease. Gut 2013;62:1234–41.
8. Fleming KM, Aithal GP, Card TR, et al. All-cause mortality in people with cirrhosis compared with the general population: a population-based cohort study. Liver Int 2012;32:79–84.
9. Olson JC, Kamath PS. Acute-on-chronic liver failure: what are the implications? Curr Gastroenterol Rep 2012;14:63–6.
10. Olson JC, Kamath PS. Acute-on-chronic liver failure: concept, natural history, and prognosis. Curr Opin Crit Care 2011;17:165–9.
11. Jalan R, Fernandez J, Wiest R, et al. Bacterial infections in cirrhosis. A Position Statement based on the EASL Special Conference 2013. J Hepatol 2014;60:1310–24.
12. Bajaj JS, O'Leary JG, Reddy KR, et al, NACSELD. Second infections independently increase mortality in hospitalized patients with cirrhosis: the North American Consortium for the Study of End-Stage Liver Disease (NACSELD) experience. Hepatology 2012;56:2328–35.
13. Fernandez J, Acevedo J, Castro M, et al. Prevalence and risk factors of infections by multiresistant bacteria in cirrhosis: a prospective study. Hepatology 2012;55:1551–61.
14. Moreau R, Jalan R, Gines P, et al. Acute-on-chronic liver failure is a distinct syndrome that develops in patients with acute decompensation of cirrhosis. Gastroenterology 2013;144:1426–37, 1437.e1–9.
15. Bajaj JS, O'Leary JG, Reddy KR, et al, on behalf of NACSELD. Survival in infection-related acute-on-chronic liver failure is defined by extra-hepatic organ failures. Hepatology 2014. [Epub ahead of print].
16. Fede G, D'Amico G, Arvaniti V, et al. Renal failure and cirrhosis: a systematic review of mortality and prognosis. J Hepatol 2011;56(4):810–8.
17. Kamath PS, Wiesner RH, Malinchoc M, et al. A model to predict survival in patients with end-stage liver disease. Hepatology 2001;33:464–70.
18. Martin-Llahi M, Guevara M, Torre A, et al. Prognostic importance of the cause of renal failure in patients with cirrhosis. Gastroenterology 2011;140:488–96.e4.
19. Francoz C, Prie D, Abdelrazek W, et al. Inaccuracies of creatinine and creatinine-based equations in candidates for liver transplantation with low

creatinine: impact on the model for end-stage liver disease score. Liver Transpl 2010;16:1169–77.

20. Wong F, O'Leary JG, Reddy KR, et al, North American Consortium for Study of End-Stage Liver Disease. New consensus definition of acute kidney injury accurately predicts 30-day mortality in patients with cirrhosis and infection. Gastroenterology 2013;145:1280–8.e1.

21. Wong F, Nadim MK, Kellum JA, et al. Working Party proposal for a revised classification system of renal dysfunction in patients with cirrhosis. Gut 2011; 60:702–9.

22. Piano S, Rosi S, Maresio G, et al. Evaluation of the Acute Kidney Injury Network criteria in hospitalized patients with cirrhosis and ascites. J Hepatol 2013;59: 482–9.

23. Wasmuth HE, Kunz D, Yagmur E, et al. Patients with acute on chronic liver failure display 'sepsis-like' immune paralysis. J Hepatol 2005;42:195–201.

24. Oberholzer A, Oberholzer C, Moldawer LL. Sepsis syndromes: understanding the role of innate and acquired immunity. Shock 2001;16:83–96.

25. Bone RC. Toward a theory regarding the pathogenesis of the systemic inflammatory response syndrome: what we do and do not know about cytokine regulation. Crit Care Med 1996;24:163–72.

26. Ward NS, Casserly B, Ayala A. The compensatory anti-inflammatory response syndrome (CARS) in critically ill patients. Clin Chest Med 2008;29:617–25, viii.

27. Singh V, Ghosh S, Singh B, et al. Noradrenaline vs. terlipressin in the treatment of hepatorenal syndrome: a randomized study. J Hepatol 2012;56: 1293–8.

28. Duvoux C, Zanditenas D, Hezode C, et al. Effects of noradrenalin and albumin in patients with type I hepatorenal syndrome: a pilot study. Hepatology 2002;36: 374–80.

29. Vlaar AP, Juffermans NP. Transfusion-related acute lung injury: a clinical review. Lancet 2013;382:984–94.

30. Bajaj JS, Ratliff SM, Heuman DM, et al. Proton pump inhibitors are associated with a high rate of serious infections in veterans with decompensated cirrhosis. Aliment Pharmacol Ther 2012;36:866–74.

31. Bernard B, Cadranel JF, Valla D, et al. Prognostic significance of bacterial infection in bleeding cirrhotic patients: a prospective study. Gastroenterology 1995; 108:1828–34.

32. Christou L, Pappas G, Falagas ME. Bacterial infection-related morbidity and mortality in cirrhosis. Am J Gastroenterol 2007;102:1510–7.

33. Sarin SK, Kumar A, Almeida JA, et al. Acute-on-chronic liver failure: consensus recommendations of the Asian Pacific Association for the Study of the Liver (APASL). Hepatol Int 2009;3:269–82.

34. Bajaj JS. Defining acute-on-chronic liver failure: will East and West ever meet? Gastroenterology 2013;144:1337–9.

35. Wang FS, Zhang Z. Liver: how can acute-on-chronic liver failure be accurately identified? Nat Rev Gastroenterol Hepatol 2013;10:390–1.

36. Dunn W, Jamil LH, Brown LS, et al. MELD accurately predicts mortality in patients with alcoholic hepatitis. Hepatology 2005;41:353–8.

37. Dunn W, Angulo P, Sanderson S, et al. Utility of a new model to diagnose an alcohol basis for steatohepatitis. Gastroenterology 2006;131:1057–63.

38. Louvet A, Naveau S, Abdelnour M, et al. The Lille model: a new tool for therapeutic strategy in patients with severe alcoholic hepatitis treated with steroids. Hepatology 2007;45:1348–54.

39. Teh SH, Nagorney DM, Stevens SR, et al. Risk factors for mortality after surgery in patients with cirrhosis. Gastroenterology 2007;132(4):1261–9.
40. Bajaj JS, Heuman DM, Hylemon PB, et al. Altered profile of human gut microbiome is associated with cirrhosis and its complications. J Hepatol 2013; 60(5):940–7.
41. Finkenstedt A, Nachbaur K, Zoller H, et al. Acute-on-chronic liver failure: excellent outcomes after liver transplantation but high mortality on the wait list. Liver Transpl 2013;19:879–86.
42. Bahirwani R, Shaked O, Bewtra M, et al. Acute-on-chronic liver failure before liver transplantation: impact on posttransplant outcomes. Transplantation 2011;92:952–7.
43. Garg H, Sarin SK, Kumar M, et al. Tenofovir improves the outcome in patients with spontaneous reactivation of hepatitis B presenting as acute-on-chronic liver failure. Hepatology 2011;53:774–80.
44. Hassanein TI, Schade RR, Hepburn IS. Acute-on-chronic liver failure: extracorporeal liver assist devices. Curr Opin Crit Care 2011;17:195–203.
45. Banares R, Nevens F, Larsen FS, et al, RELIEF study group. Extracorporeal albumin dialysis with the molecular adsorbent recirculating system in acute-on-chronic liver failure: the RELIEF trial. Hepatology 2013;57:1153–62.
46. Sharma P, Schaubel DE, Gong Q, et al. End-stage liver disease candidates at the highest model for end-stage liver disease scores have higher wait-list mortality than status-1A candidates. Hepatology 2012;55:192–8.
47. Chok KS, Fung JY, Chan SC, et al. Outcomes of living donor liver transplantation for patients with preoperative type 1 hepatorenal syndrome and acute hepatic decompensation. Liver Transpl 2012;18:779–85.
48. Chan AC, Fan ST, Lo CM, et al. Liver transplantation for acute-on-chronic liver failure. Hepatol Int 2009;3:571–81.
49. Liu CL, Fan ST, Lo CM, et al. Live-donor liver transplantation for acute-on-chronic hepatitis B liver failure. Transplantation 2003;76:1174–9.
50. Xing T, Zhong L, Chen D, et al. Experience of combined liver-kidney transplantation for acute-on-chronic liver failure patients with renal dysfunction. Transplant Proc 2013;45:2307–13.
51. Nadim MK, Sung RS, Davis CL, et al. Simultaneous liver-kidney transplantation summit: current state and future directions. Am J Transplant 2012;12:2901–8.
52. Nadim MK, Genyk YS, Tokin C, et al. Impact of the etiology of acute kidney injury on outcomes following liver transplantation: acute tubular necrosis versus hepatorenal syndrome. Liver Transpl 2012;18:539–48.
53. Moreau R, Lebrec D. Acute renal failure in patients with cirrhosis: perspectives in the age of MELD. Hepatology 2003;37:233–43.
54. Asrani SK, Kim WR, Heimbach JH, et al. Acute tubular necrosis in present in the majority of patients undergoing liver transplantation. Hepatology 2011;54:159A.
55. Bajaj JS, O'Leary JG, Wong F, et al. Bacterial infections in end-stage liver disease: current challenges and future directions. Gut 2012;61:1219–25.

Hepatitis Viruses and Liver Transplantation

Evolving Trends in Antiviral Management

Elizabeth C. Verna, MD, MS

KEYWORDS

- Liver transplant • HCV • HEV • HBV • Antiviral therapy

KEY POINTS

- Viral hepatitis-related end-stage liver disease and hepatocellular carcinoma (HCC) remain the most common indications for liver transplant (LT) throughout the world.
- The profound improvement in post-LT outcomes in patients with hepatitis B virus (HBV) due to the development of effective antiviral strategies is one of the most dramatic success stories in liver transplantation.
- The management of LT recipients with hepatitis C virus (HCV) is evolving rapidly.
- The ideal strategy to prevent recurrence of HCV after LT would be antiviral treatment with cure while on an LT waitlist, thus potentially eliminating the risk of recurrent HCV.

Viral hepatitis-related end-stage liver disease and HCC remain the most common indications for LT throughout the world. This review focuses on recent updates in antiviral management of 3 viral hepatidities: hepatitis C, B, and E. Each of these potentially chronic viral infections is in a different phase of understanding of their impact on the LT population and the ability to prevent recurrent or progressive disease. The profound improvement in post-LT outcomes in patients with HBV due to the development of effective antiviral strategies is one of the most dramatic success stories in liver transplantation. By comparison, peri-LT treatment of HCV is in its infancy, although rapidly accumulating data on novel and interferon (IFN)-free direct-acting antiviral (DAA) regimens will soon permanently alter the natural history of HCV in LT recipients. Finally, data have emerged that hepatitis E virus (HEV) is more common in LT recipients throughout the world than previously understood, and although HEV can cause chronic hepatitis and progressive graft failure in this setting, the incidence, natural history, and optimal treatment strategy for HEV in this setting remain uncertain.

Disclosure: None.
Division of Digestive and Liver Diseases, Center for Liver Disease and Transplantation, Columbia University College of Physicians and Surgeons, 622 West 168th Street, New York, NY 10032, USA
E-mail address: ev77@columbia.edu

Clin Liver Dis 18 (2014) 575–601
http://dx.doi.org/10.1016/j.cld.2014.05.002
1089-3261/14/$ – see front matter © 2014 Elsevier Inc. All rights reserved.

ANTIVIRAL MANAGEMENT OF HEPATITIS C VIRUS IN LIVER TRANSPLANT RECIPIENTS

The management of LT recipients with HCV is evolving rapidly. Despite marked improvements in the ability to cure patients of HCV infection, HCV-related end-stage liver disease remains the leading indication for LT, and, due to recurrence of HCV in the liver allograft, death and graft failure are more common in this population compared with HCV-negative recipients (**Fig. 1**).[1] Successful antiviral treatment with sustained virologic response (SVR) improves post-LT survival (**Fig. 2**),[2–4] but, until now, HCV treatment in patients on a waitlist to prevent recurrence or on immunosuppression after LT was hindered by significant toxicities and disappointing response rates. There is a variety of new DAAs recently approved or in clinical trials that will soon lead to a marked improvement in SVR rates with shorter duration of therapy. Although these agents are not yet well tested or approved for use in waitlisted or post-LT patients, strategies to eradicate the virus in the pre- and post-LT setting will play a key role in improving outcomes and are now included in the recently published joint American Association for the Study of Liver Disease (AASLD) and Infectious Diseases Society of America (IDSA) recommendations for the treatment of HCV.[5]

The Diagnosis of HCV Recurrence

The natural history of HCV-related liver disease is accelerated in the post-LT setting, including rapid progression to cirrhosis (10%–25% of patients within 5–10 years), rapid decompensation once cirrhosis occurs (40% with clinical decompensation within 1 year), and thus poor survival.[6] The overall 1-, 3-, and 5-year survival rates United States national data between 1997 and 2010 were recently reported to be 87%, 78%, and 70%, respectively.[7]

Risk factors for severe or rapid recurrence of advanced fibrosis include most prominently donor age, with an increase in risk of graft loss with donors as young as in their fourth decade.[1] Additional risk factors include graft characteristics, such as the donor risk index[8] and HCV serostatus[9]; recipient characteristics, such as female gender[10] and race/ethnicity[11,12]; and post-LT factors, including biliary complications,[13] treated

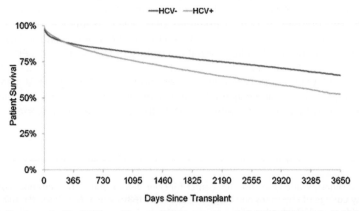

Fig. 1. Patient survival in HCV-positive and HCV-negative recipients from a report on the Scientific Registry of Transplant Recipients (SRTR) database for liver transplantation between 1999 and 2008. (*From* Thuluvath PJ, Guidinger MK, Fung JJ, et al. Liver transplantation in the United States, 1999–2008. Am J Transplant 2010;10:1003–19; with permission.)

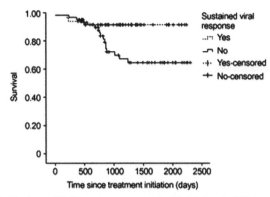

Fig. 2. After the initiation of HCV treatment, survival is higher in HCV-positive LT recipients who achieve SVR, with 1-, 3-, and 5-year survival rates of 96%, 94%, and 94%, respectively, compared to 97%, 73% and 68%, respectively in nonresponders (*P* = .012). (*From* Berenguer M, Aguilera V, Rubin A, et al. Comparison of two non-contemporaneous HCV-liver transplant cohorts: strategies to improve the efficacy of antiviral therapy. J Hepatol 2012;56:1310–6; with permission.)

rejection,[14,15] and choice of baseline immunosuppressive regimen.[16–19] Interesting work on the impact of donor and recipient genetic polymorphisms for genes, including interleukin 28B,[20] Toll-like receptor 4,[21] and the 7-gene signature, termed, *cirrhosis risk score*,[22] has also been reported.

Assessment of fibrosis progression is essential in the management of LT recipients with HCV. Fibrosis progresses at an accelerated rate compared with the non-LT setting (with median annual rates of progression from 0.2 to 0.8 Metavir stages per year compared with 0.1–0.2 stages per year pre-LT[23]), however, it remains unpredictable and nonlinear. Liver histology is the gold standard for fibrosis assessment because there is poor correlation between liver test elevations and histology. Given the significant toxicities and limited efficacy of the historically available pegylated-IFN (P-IFN)–based regimens, treatment has generally been reserved for those patients with histologically significant recurrence (ie, F≥2). For these reasons, many centers perform post-LT protocolized liver biopsies. The ideal biopsy frequency is unknown, but most centers advocate for annual assessment.

Given the limitations of surveillance with serial liver biopsy, including procedural complications, sampling error, and the complexities of biopsy interpretation in the post-LT setting, there is great interest in the development and validation of noninvasive fibrosis markers. Although not yet routinely used in the clinic, several more specific combinations of serologic fibrosis markers have been tested with variable accuracy in determining the current stage of disease or predicting disease progression.[23] Data may be more promising in the use of imaging to assess fibrosis stage. Ultrasound and magnetic resonance elastography may correlate well with liver histology and portal pressure measurements both before and after LT. In a recent systematic review pooling 5 studies of patients with recurrent HCV, ultrasound elastography had a sensitivity and specificity of 83% each for the diagnosis of significant fibrosis and 98% and 84% for the diagnosis of cirrhosis, respectively.[24] Transient elastography performed at 1 year post-LT also predicts patient and graft outcomes post-LT and could be considered when risk stratifying patients for treatment.[25]

Whether noninvasive testing, including serum markers, will replace biopsy for HCV surveillance, or whether all patients will soon be treated with a safe and effective antiviral regimen immediately before or after LT and no longer require surveillance, remains to be seen. Although experience with DAA regimens in these high-risk settings remains limited and the cost of some regimens remains prohibitive for many patients, monitoring for progression remains an important indicator of which patients must be prioritized for treatment. In addition, reliable noninvasive tests to differentiate the causes of liver test elevation, including HCV recurrence, rejection, and fatty liver disease, are lacking, rendering liver biopsy an essential tool in the management of these patients.

Antiviral Treatment to Prevent HCV Recurrence

Treatment on the liver transplant waitlist

The ideal strategy to prevent recurrence of HCV after LT would be antiviral treatment with cure while on an LT waitlist, thus potentially eliminating the risk of recurrent HCV. Treatment with IFN-based regimens in this setting, however, especially in patients with decompensated liver disease, is often ineffective and poses significant risk. Most patients cannot tolerate the full dose and duration of treatment in this setting, and serious adverse events (SAEs) are common, including exacerbation of encephalopathy, serious infection, and death, with an up to 10% treatment-related mortality. Thus, alternative strategies, such as the low accelerating dose regimen (LADR), have been developed, whereby patients are started at low doses of P-IFN and ribavirin, titrated up to their maximally tolerated dose, with the goal of either completing the regimen or truncating therapy through transplant with viral suppression (**Table 1**).[26,27] With this approach, treatment response rates may be higher with fewer adverse events, although early discontinuation of therapy remains common. In patients transplanted with an undetectable viral load while on treatment, the post-LT SVR (pTVR) rates may be as high as 80%. This approach is of particular use when the timing of LT can be reasonably predicted, such as in the setting of living donation or Model for End-Stage Liver Disease exception points. When implemented in a randomized controlled trial within the National Institutes of Health–sponsored Adult-to-Adult Living Donor Liver Transplantation Cohort Study (A2ALL),[27] the overall pTVR rate was 28% (18% for genotypes 1/4/6 and 39% for genotypes 2/3) in treated patients, and pTVR was significantly associated with pre-LT treatment duration.

The immediate pre-LT setting may be ideal to investigate the use of potent combinations of DAAs as LT during even brief periods of viral clearance may lead to cure. Data are limited on pre-LT treatment with the first two first-generation NS3/4A protease inhibitors, boceprevir and telaprevir. When used in combination with P-IFN and ribavirin, response rates in patients with compensated cirrhosis are superior to those seen with P-IFN and ribavirin alone, with on-treatment response and SVR rates approaching 70%.[28–30] Patients with decompensated liver disease awaiting transplantation were, however, generally not included in these larger studies, and SAEs (seen in 40%), including severe infection, clinical decompensation, or death (6.4%), have been observed in patients with compensated cirrhosis treated with triple therapy.[28] These severe complications were most common in patients with thrombocytopenia (platelets <100,000/mm^3) and hypoalbuminemia (<35 g/dL).

There is 1 multicenter observational report of 29 patients on an LT waitlist with genotype 1 HCV treated with protease inhibitor–based triple therapy. The overall 12 week SVR (SVR12) was 52% (see **Table 1**).[31] Among the 12 patients who were transplanted, however, the pTVR rate was 67% and as high as 89% in patients who were undetectable at the time of LT. Although these response rates represent a marked improvement over treatment with P-IFN and ribavirin dual therapy, there were significant toxicities observed, including 31% with SAEs and 1 on-treatment death.

Table 1
Studies of HCV treatment on the liver transplantation waitlist

Study	Patients	Design	Treatment	Response	Safety
Thomas et al,[141] 2003	N = 20 GT1-4	Prospective cohort	IFN-α2b 5 MU/d	pTVR 4/20 (20%)	No infections, hospitalizations, or deaths
Forns et al,[142] 2003	N = 30 Expected time to LT <4 mo, GT1-3	Prospective cohort	IFN-α2b 3 MU/d + Riba 800 mg/d	pTVR 6/30 (20%)	No deaths, 4 hepatic decompensation, 2 sepsis, 6 early treatment discontinuation
Everson et al,[26] 2005	N = 124 GT1-6	Observational cohort	P-IFN + Riba in LADR protocol for up to 48 wk	SVR 13% GT1 and 50% other GT; pTVR in 12/15 with LT while undetectable	12% SAE, 4 (3%) died
Carrion et al,[143] 2009	N = 102 (51 treated, 51 untreated matched controls) GT1-4	Retrospective case-control	P-IFN-α2a + Riba	29% Undetectable at LT, 20% SVR overall	Bacterial infections more common in treated patients compared with untreated controls, 4 deaths on waitlist in treated group
Everson et al,[27] 2013	N = 47 (31 treated, 16 controls) LDLT or HCC, GT1-4	Randomized controlled trial	P-IFN + Riba in LADR protocol for up to 48 wk	SVR12 19% in treated arm, pTVR 28% (18% GT1/4/6, 39% GT2/3)	SAEs similar in treated (68%) and untreated controls (55%, P = .30)
Verna et al,[31] 2013	N = 28 GT1	Multicenter observational cohort	Tel or Boc + P-IFN + Riba for up to 48 wk	Overall SVR12 51%, pTVR 67% (89% if undetectable at LT)	31% SAE, 1 on-treatment death
Curry et al,[32] 2013[a]	N = 36 GT1-3, HCC	Single-arm trial	SOF 400 mg/d + Riba (1000–1200 mg/d) for up to 48 wk	Of those with undetectable RNA at LT, pTVR12 rate of 69% (27% recurred, 4% early post-LT death)	1 SAE (anemia)

Abbreviations: Boc, boceprevir; GT, genotype; LDLT, living donor liver transplant; P-IFN, peculated-interferon; Riba, ribavirin; SAE, serious adverse event; SOF, sofosbuvir; Tel, telaprevir.

[a] Preliminary results reported in abstract form only; final results not yet available.

With the recent approval of the next generation of DAAs, IFN-free pre-LT treatment options with improved safety profiles are available. Special attention must be paid to the potential impact of moderate or severe hepatic impairment on the pharmacokinetics of these agents as they become available. Simeprevir, for example, is not recommended for use in patients with moderate or severe hepatic impairment. Interim analysis of the ongoing phase 2 open-label study of the nucleotide analogue, NS5B polymerase inhibitor sofosbuvir (400 mg daily), with ribavirin (1000–1200 mg daily) for up to 48 weeks, in waitlisted patients was recently reported. Of the 37 patients with undetectable viral loads at transplant, the pTVR rate was 62% (10 patients experienced post-LT recurrence).[32] All of the patients in this trial had HCC with generally well-compensated cirrhosis, and 25% had HCV genotype 2 or 3. It is possible that longer duration of treatment or a combination of DAAs (currently being studied) will reduce the rate of relapse. The pangenotypic activity and favorable safety profile, however, render this regimen a significant step forward. Although there is no untreated or standard of care control arm in this study, there was only 1 SAE reported in their interim analysis (anemia), perhaps rendering this regimen or other IFN-free combinations most attractive when available. As a result of these preliminary results, treatment of listed patients with HCC with sofosbuvir and ribavirin for up to 48 weeks is included in the Food and Drug Administration (FDA) label and has been recommended by the joint AASLD/IDSA guidelines.[5] It has yet to be established whether successful treatment of patients with decompensated cirrhosis may lead to improvement in liver function (and possibly elimination of the need for LT), as in cases of HBV-related cirrhosis.

Prophylactic and preemptive HCV treatment

Prophylactic and preemptive strategies are not currently recommended. Unlike in patients with HBV, there is no clear role for HCV immunoglobulin. The results of an ongoing randomized phase 2 trial of HCV immunoglobulin from pooled HCV-infected donors are awaited, as an adjunct to pre-LT treatment with the goal of minimizing post-LT relapse and recurrence.

The use of P-IFN and ribavirin in the early post-LT period prior to histologically significant recurrent disease is historically poorly tolerated and not recommended. A minority of patients have the clinical and blood count stability to start IFN and ribavirin in the first several months post-LT, and in the most comprehensive randomized controlled trial of this treatment strategy compared with treatment of histologically recurrent disease, there was no improvement in outcomes in preemptively treated patients (significant recurrence by 120 weeks was 62% vs 65%, respectively, and there were no differences in patient and graft survival).[33] When safe and potent combinations of DAAs are available to LT recipients, for those patients who are not cured prior to LT, early post-LT preemptive therapy prior to significant recurrent liver disease may become the new standard.

Antiviral Therapy for the Treatment of Significant Recurrent HCV

HCV treatment with SVR is a key goal in the management of post-LT patients because it is clearly associated with improved survival.[34,35] Disease stabilization and/or regression of fibrosis over time may occur in up to 75% of patients with SVR compared with 50% in controls in 1 large single-center study.[35] Although this field is rapidly evolving, due to the limitations and toxicities of preemptive treatments available, antiviral treatment is currently recommended in patients with established recurrent disease.

Until now, studies of post-LT treatment have generally led to disappointing SVR rates, likely due to the high proportion of patients with genotype 1 or previous nonresponse, the poor tolerability of P-IFN and ribavirin, and concomitant immuno-suppression, which have an impact on viral kinetics and render interpretation of traditional stopping rules complex. When more than 40 treatment trials of P-IFN or IFN with ribavirin were pooled, the composite SVRs were 27% and 24%, respectively.[36] Pooled discontinuation rates were 24% and 26%, respectively. With only approximately one-quarter of patients achieving SVR with this regimen and the rapid fibrosis and graft loss that can occur in these patients, there is an urgent need to bring safe and effective DAA regimens to the post-LT population.

Telaprevir and boceprevir are not FDA approved for post-LT patients. Because these 2 protease inhibitors are cytochrome P450 3A4 substrates and inhibitors, significant interactions exist with essential immunosuppressive agents, including calcineurin inhibitors (**Table 2**),[37,38] mTOR inhibitors,[39] and, to a lesser extent, prednisone. Many centers, however, cautiously used these agents once available in post-LT patients with few other options, and response rates have been reported on several hundred patients in observational cohorts throughout the world (**Table 3**).[40–42] In the latest American experience to date, a multicenter observational cohort described 81 patients with high early on-treatment response rates (73% undetectable HCV RNA at 12 weeks) and SVR12 rate of 63% overall.[41] Calcineurin inhibitor dosing was dramatically altered by the addition of telaprevir (mean dose 1/0.06 mg for tacrolimus and 200/50 mg for cyclosporine), and on-treatment adverse events included 7 deaths, 3% treated for acute rejection, and a one third with worsening of kidney function. Similar results were reported in a multicenter European cohort of 37 patients, where the overall SVR12 rate was 50% among the 12 patients with sufficient follow-up.[40] Treatment toxicities are a significant issue in all of these cohorts, including several deaths, up to 27% with infections, 35% to 50% requiring blood transfusion, a significant incidence of renal dysfunction, and up to one-third of patients requiring hospitalization.[40–42] The patients treated in these observational studies were at significant risk of adverse events, however, because many had advanced recurrent fibrosis (including several with cholestatic hepatitis) and were nonresponders to IFN-based post-LT treatment. The final results of the formal clinical trial of telaprevir-based triple therapy with pharmacokinetic analysis (the REFRESH study) have yet to be reported.[43] Although these studies demonstrate improved efficacy, the need for IFN, significant medication interactions, lack of efficacy in non–genotype 1 patients, and persistently inadequate overall response rates render these regimens an only marginal improvement in the treatment armamentarium.

Table 2
Drug-drug interactions between available direct-acting antivirals and the calcineurin inhibitors cyclosporine and tacrolimus

DAA	Cyclosporine		Tacrolimus	
	Impact on AUC[a]	Dose Adjustment	Impact on AUC	Dose Adjustment
Telaprevir[37]	↑ 4.6-Fold	↓ 2-Fold	↑ 70-Fold	↓ 35-Fold
Boceprevir[38]	↑ 2.7-Fold	↓ 4-Fold	↑ 17-Fold	↓ 5-Fold
Sofosbuvir[144]	No change	None	No change	None
Simeprevir[145]	↑ 19%	None	↓ 17%	None

Abbreviation: AUC, area under the curve.
[a] Impact on AUC in healthy volunteers.
Adapted from Lens S, Gambato M, Londono M, et al. Interferon-free regimens in the liver-transplant setting. Sem Liv Dis 2014;34:58–71.

Table 3
Direct-acting antivirals for the treatment of recurrent HCV after liver transplantation

Study	Patients	Design	Treatment	Response	Safety
Burton et al,[41] 2014	N = 81 GT1	Multicenter observational cohort	Tel or Boc + P-IFN + Riba for up to 48 wk total	SVR12 in 28/50 (63%) with sufficient follow-up	7 Deaths, 15% early discontinuation due to AE
Brown et al,[43] 2013[a]	N = 46 GT1	Open-label trial	Tel + P-IFN + Riba for 48 wk total	Undetectable HCV RNA 53% at 4 wk, 60% at 12 wk. No SVR data reported	No deaths or rejection. 48% Anemia, 22% worsened renal function, 22% infection
Faisal et al,[42] 2013[a]	N = 76 GT1	Multicenter observational cohort	Tel or Boc + P-IFN + Riba	28/37 (76%) EOTR	10 Early discontinuations for AE, 1 death
Fontana et al,[46] 2013	N = 1 GT1b CH	Case report	Dac 20 mg/d + P-IFN + Riba 800 mg/d for 24 wk	SVR	
Fontana et al,[47] 2013	N = 1 GT1b CH	Case report	SOF 50 mg/d + Dac 60 mg/d for 24 wk	SVR	

Study	N/GT	Type	Treatment	Results	Adverse events
Coilly et al,[40] 2014	N = 37 GT1	Multicenter observational cohort	Tel or Boc + P-IFN + Riba for up to 48 wk	SVR12 in 50% among the 12 patients with f/u (Tel 20%, Boc 71%)	14% Treatment d/c due to AE, 27% infection, 8% died
Pellicelli et al,[48] 2014[a]	N = 12 GT1,4 Severe recurrent HCV	Compassionate use cohort	SOF + Dac ± Riba	HCV RNA undetectable in 9/11 (82%) at week 4 and in 7/7 (100%) at week 12.	3 Died, 4 with SAEs
Samuel et al,[44] 2014[a]	N = 40 GT1-4	Open-label trial	SOF + Riba for 24 wk	Interim SVR4 rate is 77% (27/35)	6 (15%) SAEs, no death, no rejection
Forns et al,[45] 2014[a]	N = 87	Compassionate use cohort	SOF + Riba ± P-IFN for up to 48 wk	Preliminary SVR12 rate 54% for SOF + Riba and 44% for SOF + Riba + P-IFN; 70% with clinical improvement on treatment	13 (17%) Died, all due to liver disease; 29 (33%) with SAEs, none attributable to study drug
Kwo et al,[146] 2014[a]	N = 34 GT1	Open-label trial	ABT-450/R/ABT-267 + ABT-333 + Riba for 24 wk	RVR 100% (34/34), EOTR 100% (13/13), SVR4 92% (12/13), 1 relapse	One with early discontinuation due to AE, no acute rejection

Abbreviations: AE, adverse event; Boc, boceprevir; CH, cholestatic hepatitis; Dac, daclatasvir; d/c, discontinuation; GT, genotype; P-IFN, peculated-interferon; Riba, ribavirin; SAE, serious adverse event; SOF, sofosbuvir; Tel, telaprevir.
[a] Preliminary results reported in abstract form, final results not yet available.

With the recent approval of sofosbuvir and simeprevir, it is now a reality that IFN-free potent DAA combinations with minimal medication interactions (see **Table 3**) are available for these difficult to treat patients. These medicines have not been extensively studied in LT recipients, however, and may have limited applicability in patients with significant renal (sofosbuvir) or hepatic (simeprevir) impairment. In a preliminary report of a phase 2 open-label study of LT recipients who received sofosbuvir and ribavirin for 24 weeks, 100% of the 40 patients evaluated achieved rapid virologic response (RVR) and end-of-treatment response (EOTR). Only 77% remained undetectable for 4 week SVR (SVR4), however, and SVR12 rates were not reported.[44] This study included patients with genotypes 1–4 and some patients with early recurrent disease (only 66% with Metavir stage 3–4), rendering this population somewhat easier to treat than many post-LT patients who need therapy the most. Preliminary analysis of a sofosbuvir compassionate use program for patients with severe HCV recurrence who were treated with sofosbuvir and ribavirin with or without P-IFN for up to 48 weeks are also available.[45] Of the 87 patients whose outcomes were recently reported, preliminary SVR12 rates were 54% for patients treated with sofosbuvir and ribavinin and 44% for those treated with sofosbuvir, ribavirin, and P-IFN; 53 (70%) had clinical improved on treatment, 10 (13%) had disease stabilized, and 13 (17%) died due to complications of liver disease. Although safety seems better with the sofosbuvir and ribavirin regimen (33% with SAEs in the preliminary analysis, none due to study drug), the efficacy of IFN-free regimens in patients with recurrent advanced disease must be improved. There are also several reports of successful viral eradication with experimental daclatasvir-based regimens (with P-IFN and ribavirin[46] or with sofosbuvir[47,48]), and trials of several other IFN-free combinations are ongoing in LT recipients. Finally, due to the promising reports of sofosbuvir in combination with simeprevir for genotype 1 patients in the non-LT setting (the COSMOS trial),[49] this IFN-free regimen has also been advocated for in LE recipients.[5]

As a result of these limited data, the approach to post-LT patients may soon be similar to the non-LT setting. Given the risks of IFN in LT recipients, the AASLD/IDSA statement currently recommends IFN-free regimens as first-line therapy in all post-LT patients.[5] For genotype 1, despite the lack of any clinical trials in LT recipients, they recommend sofosbuvir with simeprevir, with or without ribavirin for those with compensated liver disease. For genotypes 2 and 3, sofosbuvir with ribavirin is the preferred regimen. They state that there are no data on which to base treatment recommendations for genotypes 4–6, although many currently treat genotype 4 patients with sofosbuvir-based therapy, which includes IFN, if possible. Despite these recommendations, it must be stressed that DAA-based treatment in this setting is off-label and based on little or no safety or efficacy data in LT recipients. Treatment data from the non-LT setting must be applied to the LT population with caution. It remains unknown what the impact of immunosuppression; aggressive forms of recurrence, such as cholestatic hepatitis; and the high viral loads and thus possibly increased risk of selection of resistant strains will have on treatment success.

RECENT ADVANCES IN THE ANTIVIRAL MANAGEMENT OF LIVER TRANSPLANT RECIPIENTS WITH HEPATITIS B

Despite significant progress in the treatment of HBV, HBV-related end-stage liver disease and HCC remain important indications for LT throughout the world. Since the introduction of effect prophylactic and preventative regimens (ie, hepatitis B immune globulin [HBIG] and subsequently nucleos(t)ide analogues [NAs]), outcomes in patients transplanted for complications of HBV-related liver disease have dramatically improved. In the early years of transplantation, 5-year survival was only approximately 50% for HBV-infected patients, prompting many centers to view HBV as a contraindication to LT. Remarkably, 1- and 3-year post-LT survival rates are among the highest for any transplant indication, at approximately 90% and 85%, respectively.[50] This section on the management of HBV in LT recipients focuses on new advances in management, including antiviral strategies to prevent recurrent disease and the diagnosis and treatment of de novo or reactivated HBV, particularly in the case of allografts from hepatitis B core antibody (HBcAb)-positive donors.

Antiviral Strategies to Prevent HBV Recurrence

Prevention of HBV reinfection of the graft includes antiviral therapy starting in the pre-LT setting and continuing post-LT, with or without the addition of HBIG. The goal of pre-LT treatment is the optimization of liver function prior to LT, in some cases obviating a transplant, and/or to prevent HBV reinfection in the allograft. Once a transplant occurs, NAs with or without HBIG are used to provide ongoing prevention of recurrence. Unlike in the case of HCV, antiviral therapy for HBV is currently viewed as potentially indefinite.

HBV treatment on the transplant waitlist

All patients with indications for LT and detectable HBV DNA should be started on antiviral therapy. The choice of antiviral agents in the pre-LT setting includes several potent agents with high barriers to resistance and acceptable side-effect profiles, including most prominently tenofovir and entecavir. Lamivudine and adefovir are not ideal first-line agents in this setting, given the need for long-term therapy in these patients and the high rates of resistance and, in the case of adefovir, considerable risk of nephrotoxicity (up to 20% in pre- and post-LT patients).[51–53] Entecavir and tenofovir have both been studied in patients with advanced liver disease and may have similar efficacy in terms of viral suppression as well as stabilization or improvement in liver function.[51,54] Some experts also advocate for the use of de novo combination therapy, such as tenofovir-emtricitabine, to further minimize the risk of resistance; however, data to support this approach are lacking, except perhaps in patients with very high HBV DNA levels. In the only study to compare these agents directly, 112 patients with HBV and decompensated liver disease were randomized to entecavir, tenofovir, or tenofovir-emtricitabine.[54] The rates of viral suppression to less than 400 copies/mL by 48 weeks (73%, 71%, and 88%, respectively) and decrease in Child-Turcotte-Pugh score of at least 2 units (42%, 26%, and 48%, respectively) were statistically similar between all 3 treatment groups. HBeAg seroconversion was more common in the tenofovir (21%) and tenofovir-emtricitabine (13%) groups, however, than in those on entecavir (0%).

HBV reinfection prevention strategies after liver transplantation and the evolving role of HBIG

Antiviral therapy with NAs should be continued indefinitely in the post-LT setting, with or without the addition of HBIG. With the use of these agents, the reinfection rate is consistently below 10%. Prevention of reinfection remains an important goal because it not only lowers the risk of HBV-related liver dysfunction but also decreases the risk of HCC recurrence.[55]

HBIG immunoprophylaxis has been central to post-LT regimens since Samuel and colleagues[56] initially demonstrated a dramatic reduction in the risk of reinfection (from 75% to 36%) and improvement in patient survival, a finding that has since been confirmed.[57–61] HBIG is a polyclonal preparation of pooled human anti-HBs antibody, generally given as an intravenous bolus in the anhepatic phase followed by daily doses for the first week, then either monthly or based on an anti-HBs titer threshold (100–500 IU/L) thereafter. When lamivudine was approved, lamivudine monotherapy was then attempted but with unacceptable recurrence rates. Combination NA and HBIG is associated with lower recurrence rates, however, than either agent alone.[62–64] Thus, combination HBIG and NA has been the standard of care for prophylaxis for some time.

Despite the widespread use of these preventative protocols, however, the optimal dose, frequency, duration, and route of administration of HBIG are unknown, and practices vary widely by center. The high cost, inconvenience of parenteral administration, and limited availability in parts of the world have led investigators to attempt alternative protocols, including lower-dose or truncated HBIG combination regimens.[63,65–73] For example, Gane and colleagues[70] reported 147 patients who received lamivudine with low-dose (400–800 IU daily) HBIG intramuscularly daily in the first week and then monthly and found similar rates of HBV recurrence. Although this may have been a fairly low risk cohort (a majority of patients had undetectable HBV DNA at LT), the overall recurrence risk was only 1% at 1 year and 4% at 5 years, with a considerably cheaper HBIG regimen. Other investigators have compared multiple HBIG regimens in a retrospective series, including high- and low-dose, intravenous and intramuscular, and finite duration therapy, and were unable to demonstrate differences in recurrence between these groups.[72] Furthermore, small prospective studies have suggested that perhaps termination of HBIG several years after transplant while continuing NAs may not have a negative impact on outcomes. Teperman and colleagues[73] recently reported a trial where 40 post-LT patients who had been receiving combination treatment for a mean of 3.4 years were randomized to emtricitabine and tenofovir with continuation of HBIG or emtricitabine and tenofovir alone, and no patient experienced HBV recurrence by 72 weeks of follow-up. This suggests that in patients who are stable and without recurrence for several years post-LT, HBIG may no longer be necessary in this era of potent antivirals with a high barrier to resistance. HBV vaccination in the setting of HBIG withdrawal has led to variable response rates despite aggressive dosing of vaccines.[74–76] Finally, self-administered subcutaneous formations of HBIG are available and may offer similar protection against recurrence with considerable improvement in the convenience of the regimen.[77]

The optimal NA to use with HBIG in LT recipients also remains uncertain. There is emerging evidence that newer agents with high genetic barriers to resistance (tenofovir and entecavir) may offer greater protection against reinfection than lamivudine. In a recent systematic review, only 1% of patients treated with entecavir or tenofovir with HBIG (n = 303) experienced recurrence, compared with 6.1% of patients treated with lamivudine plus HBIG (n = 1889).[62] Thus, when resources are available, many centers now use entecavir- or tenofovir-containing regimens.

Treatment success with these newer NAs has also led some investigators to test whether HBIG may be eliminated from the regimen completely. In 1 single-center, open-label series of living donor liver transplant recipients, patients with HBV DNA levels less than 2000 IU/mL (75/89 patients included) were not given HBIG.[78] The rate of HBV recurrence, defined as HBV DNA positivity 6 months post-LT, was 8%, and recurrence was only seen in patients with noncompliance with antivirals or entecavir resistance in 1 case. All patients were salvaged by changing the antiviral regimen. Most recently, Fung and colleagues[79] treated a total of 362 patients with NA prophylaxis (49% lamivudine, 39% entecavir, and 12% lamivudine plus adefovir) without HBIG. The virologic relapse (defined as >1 log IU/mL increase in HBV DNA) rates at 3 years were significantly lower in the entecavir group (0%) compared with lamivudine (17%). The overall 8-year survival was 83% and was similar between groups. There were no HBV-related deaths in the cohort.

As a result of these observations, some centers have adopted a risk-based strategy, reserving high-dose and/or prolonged HBIG for patients at high risk of recurrence.[80] High-risk patients are generally those with high HBV DNA levels at LT, with HBeAg positivity, HBeAg negative but high viral load, hepatitis D (HDV) co-infection, or with known antiviral resistance. These patients are likely to benefit from combination therapy with a potent NA plus low-dose HBIG. Conversely, those at low risk of recurrence are patients with fulminant HBV or cirrhotic patients with low HBV DNA levels and HBeAg negativity. These patients can likely safely be treated with potent NA monotherapy or NA with fixed duration HBIG. What constitutes a high HBV DNA is debated and levels of approximately 5 log copies/mL have been shown to predict recurrence.[81] In this era of expanded antiviral options and a desire to reduce the risk of recurrence to approaching zero, however, much lower cutoffs, such as approximately 100 copies/mL, have been advocated.[80]

De Novo Infection and the Use of Hepatitis B Core Antibody-Positive Donors

Although the risk of acquiring HBV from HBcAb-positive grafts is low, rates vary greatly and, in the absence of prophylaxis, may be up to approximately 80%.[82–84] This risk may be lower in recipients who are anti-Hbs antibody and/or HBcAb positive prior to LT,[82,83,85–89] and vaccination of antibody-negative patients awaiting LT has been advocated despite suboptimal response rates.[89] In this era of potent NAs, whether this risk of de novo infection has a negative impact on patient outcomes remains debated, but elimination of these livers, especially in endemic areas, might have a significant impact on the donor pool. Thus, cautious use of these organs with the addition of antiviral prophylaxis continues to be an accepted approach. Several prophylactic regimens have been reported in small studies, including HBIG monotherapy, NA monotherapy, and combination HBIG and NA protocols. HBIG alone has been shown in small series to reduce the risk of de novo infection, especially in recipients with HBsAb. There are also several small studies of lamivudine monotherapy,[90] and in a systematic review of the use of lamivudine in hepatitis B surface antigen (HBsAg)-negative recipients of HBcAb-positive donors, de novo infection occurred in only 3.6% of patients.[90] This was statistically similar to rates seen in the patients who received combination HBIG and lamivudine (2.7%), suggesting that the addition of HBIG does not provide additional benefit.[90] Given the cost associated with HBIG administration, NA monotherapy is the preferred approach. Many centers are using entecavir or tenofovir to minimize the risk of resistance, although data on these regimens are limited.[91]

Reactivation of HBV in recipients with isolated HBcAb positivity, indicating previous exposure, who received HBV seronegative grafts has also been reported though the risk is low. In 1 small series of 22 patients who were HBcAb positive prior to LT, HBV DNA was found in the explanted liver in 5, and in 2 of these, 5 on post-LT biopsy.[92] None of these patients became HBsAg positive, however, and there is currently no evidence that antiviral prophylaxis is needed in this setting.

Treatment of Recurrent and De Novo HBV Infection After LT

The choice of antiviral therapy for post-LT patient with chronic HBV infection is dependent on each patient's treatment and prophylaxis history, resistance testing when available, and renal function. Long-term data on the safety and efficacy of NAs used in the post-LT setting are lacking and there are no randomized trials comparing different agents. Many centers are using entecavir or tenofovir, however, given the need or indefinite treatment and the high genetic barrier to resistance of these agents. For treatment-naïve patients and/or patients with no prior lamivudine or entecavir exposure, entecavir may be the most attractive choice, given the potential for nephrotoxicity with tenofovir in post-LT patients already at high risk of renal dysfunction.

HEPATITIS E VIRUS IN LIVER TRANSPLANT RECIPIENTS: AN EMERGING CAUSE OF GRAFT DYSFUNCTION?
The Evolving Epidemiology of HEV

HEV is a single-stranded RNA virus with 4 major genotypes (1–4) and a common cause of enterically transmitted viral hepatitis worldwide. Although HEV is endemic in developing regions, including Asia, Africa, the Middle East, and Central America, it is more common in developed countries than previously considered. The epidemiologic features of human disease are different in areas of high and low endemicity. In highly endemic areas, transmission is mostly between humans with frequent sporadic infection as well as outbreaks due to contamination of the water supply and/or natural or humanitarian disasters. Transmission with human illness in developed nations is rare and occurs in the setting of travel or migration of individuals from endemic regions (usually HEV genotypes 1 and 2) as well as rare autochthonous infections possibly representing transmission from animal reservoirs (genotypes 3 and 4). The seroprevalence in the Unites States may as high as approximately 20%, although rates vary depending on the assays used.[93,94]

Like hepatitis A virus (HAV), the presentation of acute HEV infection can range from subclinical to, rarely, acute liver failure. For HEV, the associated morbidity and morality seem particularly high in pregnant women. Unlike HAV, it is well established that HEV can persist as chronic infection, defined as ongoing detection of HEV RNA and/or anti-HEV IgM in serum or stool for at least 6 months (some investigators have proposed 3 months as adequate to establish chronicity[95]). Chronic HEV almost always occurs in the setting of immunosuppression, including solid organ transplantation,[96–104] human immunodeficiency virus,[105–109] and hematologic malignancies.[110–112] Unfortunately, chronic HEV in these settings may lead to significant liver dysfunction, rapid development of cirrhosis, and death, and experience with antiviral therapy is limited. Clearance with IFN and/or ribavirin-based antiviral therapies[113–120] as well as with lowering of immunosuppression in solid organ transplant recipients[121] have been successful in some reported cases.

One major limitation to the identification and treatment of acute and chronic HEV infection is the lack of widely available and reproducible diagnostic assays, likely leading to delayed or missed diagnoses, especially in low prevalence areas. Currently available diagnostic tests include indirect tests for the host immune response, such as enzyme immune assays for HEV IgG and IgM, and direct detection of the viral components, such as HEV RNA quantification and genotype sequencing. In immunocompetent patients, HEV IgM testing is generally recommended as the first-line test and is positive after a 2- to 6-week incubation period. Prior to this, HEV RNA may be detectable in the blood and/or stool at approximately 3 weeks after the onset of symptoms. There are currently no FDA-approved commercial tests for HEV, however, available in the United States. The commercially available IgG and IgM assays continue to be inadequate, with sensitivities of IgM ranging from 17% to 100% in patients with active infection, and significant discordance between assays.[122–126] The sensitivity of these tests are even lower in immunocompromised patients, in whom direct methods, such as RNA quantification, are more reliable,[123,126] although significant variation in the sensitivity of nucleic acid amplification assays has also been reported and there are currently no commercially available RNA assays.[127] Due to the poor sensitivity of the available serologic assays, the true prevalence of HEV is not known. New international standards for the HEV diagnostic assays have recently been proposed[128] but improvement in assay performance and reproducibility are needed.

HEV in Liver Transplant Recipients

Chronic HEV after liver transplantation was first reported by Kamar and colleagues[102] in 2008, when 57% of a group of 14 solid organ transplant recipients with acute HEV went on to develop chronic infection, including all 3 LT recipients (**Table 4**). Series of LT recipients with evidence of chronic HEV have been reported throughout the world, including patients identified in real time as well as retrospectively by testing stored samples.[113] The true prevalence and incidence of HEV in LT recipients remain uncertain given the diagnostic assay limitations described previously. The reported seroprevalence of HEV infection in LT recipients tested with HEV IgM, IgG, and/or RNA assays ranges from 1% to 16.3%, depending on the assay and region sampled.[100,129–132] This prevalence may be higher in patients with elevations in liver tests at 5% to 10%,[100,102,133] and approximately 50% to 60% of these patients may go on to chronic infection.[99,102,131] The prevalence of HEV IgG seems similar to the general population; thus, the overall risk remains low.[133] LT recipients may be at the highest risk of developing chronic infection,[99] however, and, therefore, the development of sequelae, including fibrosis and graft failure. Other risk factors for chronic infection in solid organ transplant recipients may include T-cell composition, tacrolimus use (compared with cyclosporine), and low platelet count.[99,102]

The natural history of chronic HEV in LT recipients is not well established, although several centers have reported progression to advanced fibrosis, cirrhosis, and either death or re-transplantation. In the largest cohort of transplant patients with HEV, 85 patients from 16 centers in Europe and the United States, 28 with liver transplants, were recently described.[99] All cases were HEV genotype 3, and HEV IgM seroconversion was detected in only 41% of patients tested. Chronic infection developed in 56 (66%) of the whole cohort and 23 (82%) of the LT recipients. Among those with chronic HEV, 32% cleared infection with reduction of immunosuppression alone and 20 (36%) underwent antiviral therapy with P-IFN (5), ribavirin (14), or combination therapy (1). At last follow-up, 14 had achieved SVR whereas 6 were viremic or on treatment. Overall, 8 (14%) of those with chronic infection developed cirrhosis and 2 underwent retransplantation.

A more detailed description of fibrosis progression is available for 27 solid organ transplant recipients (including 8 LT recipients) with acute HEV, 16 (56%) of whom went on to chronic HEV and had at least 6 months of follow-up.[121] With 1 to 5 liver biopsies performed per patient over a median of 22 months, the median (range) fibrosis score increased from 1 (0–2) to 2 (1–4) Metavir units, with 3 patients developing cirrhosis, 2 of whom subsequently decompensated and died.

In addition to progressive liver disease, extrahepatic manifestations of acute and chronic HEV are also reported in solid organ transplant recipients. In a cohort from the United Kingdom and France, neurologic complications were noted in 5.5% of patients with acute and chronic infection, including in 3 transplant recipients who were diagnosed with inflammatory polyradiculopathy, encephalitis, and ataxia/proximal myopathy.[134] All patients had genotype 3 HEV infection, with virus detectable in the cerebrospinal fluid analysis. Other investigators have reported Guillain-Barré syndrome in LT patients with HEV.[135] Kidney dysfunction has also been reported in solid organ transplant recipients with HEV, including decline in glomerular filtration rate, membranoproliferative glomerulonephritis, and nephrotic syndrome.[97,136]

Table 4
Reports of chronic HEV in liver transplant recipients: prevalence, treatment, and outcomes

Study	Country	Number of LT Recipients Studied	Prevalence of Any Positive HEV Test (n [%])[a]	Chronic HEV Infection (n)	Antiviral Treatment Regimen Reported	Outcomes
Kamar et al,[102] 2008	France	86	9 (10.4)	3	—	—
Haagsma et al,[129,147] 2009 & 2008	Netherlands	285	10 (3.9)	2	—	One developed HEV-related cirrhosis and underwent re-LT.
Pischke et al,[100] 2010	Germany	226	10 (4.0)	2	—	One progressed to advanced recurrent fibrosis.
Buti et al,[133] 2010	Spain	82[b]	3 (2.7)	0	—	—
Legrand-Abravanel et al,[131] 2011	France	171	22 (12.9)	16	—	Incidence of new infection in LT recipients 4.8 (2.2–7.4)/100 person years
Kamar et al,[118] 2010	France	3	—	3	Reduction in immunosuppression dose and P-IFN–α2a for 12 wk	SVR in 2/3 patients
Haagsma et al,[113] 2010	Netherlands	2	—	2	Reduction in immunosuppression dose and P-IFN–α2a	SVR in 1/2 patients; early discontinuation at 16 wk due to nonresponse in the second patient

Study	Country				Treatment	Outcome
Kamar et al,[99] 2011	Multinational	26	—	23	Reduction in immunosuppression, P-IFN–α2a, riba or combination therapy	32% with SVR with decreased IS alone, 38 patients with antiviral therapy, SVR in 4 of these[c]
Halac et al,[148] 2012[d]	Canada	80	22 (27.5)	—	—	One patient developed recurrent cirrhosis.
Lhomme et al,[98] 2012	France	3	—	2	—	Chemokine levels and HEV quasispecies diversification were associated with chronic infection and fibrosis progression, respectively.
Pas et al,[132] 2012	Netherlands	300	3 (1)	3	—	—
Pischke et al,[119] 2013	Germany	2	—	2	Reduction in immunosuppression	SVR in 2/2
Junge et al,[149] 2013[d]	Germany	22[b]	1 (4.5)	1	Reduction in immunosuppression and ribavirin for 6 mo	SVR in 1/1
Kamar et al,[120] 2014	France	10	—	10	Ribavirin monotherapy for a median of 3 mo	SVR in 46/59 (78%) with initial treatment, additional 2 with SVR with retreatment for relapse[c]

Abbreviations: P-IFN, peculated-interferon; riba, ribavirin.
[a] HEV testing includes HEV IgG, HEV IgM, and/or HEV RNA in fresh and/or stored serum samples.
[b] All patients included had elevated liver tests.
[c] Treatment response rates for all solid organ transplant recipients (including liver, heart, lung, and kidney) in these studies.
[d] Pediatric patients.

Successful treatment of chronic HEV post-LT has occurred in several centers (see **Table 4**). Post-LT treatment algorithms recently proposed include monitoring for the development of chronic infection, lowering of immunosuppression (perhaps with an emphasis on minimization of calcineurin exposure[137]), and, if still viremic, treatment with either ribavirin[120,138] or P-IFN[139] monotherapy for 12 weeks as the initial approach. Ribavirin monotherapy is more widely reported in the setting of solid organ transplant, perhaps due to concerns about IFN-related rejection in these groups, with response rates as high as 78%.[120] Successful retreatment with 3 to 6 months of ribavirin in the setting of relapse was also observed in this cohort.

Donor-Derived HEV Infection

Transmission of occult HEV infection was reported in which donor and recipient blood tested negative for evidence of HEV prior to LT, but HEV infection was identified in the work-up for post-LT hepatitis, progressive fibrosis, and graft failure.[140] Testing done in retrospect included the identification of high levels of HEV RNA in the donor liver tissue as well as positive HEV IgM and RNA in the recipient serum starting 150 days post-LT. Phylogenetic analysis then confirmed the donor and recipient were infected with the

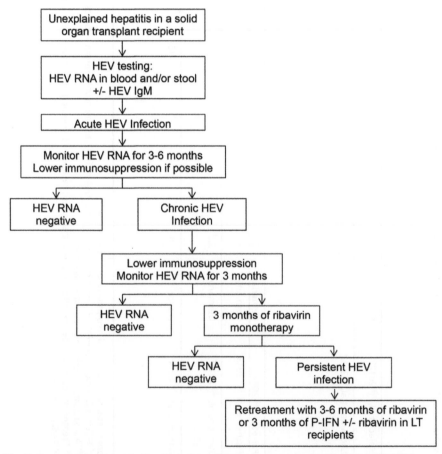

Fig. 3. Proposed treatment algorithm for solid organ transplant recipients with HEV.

same strain. Routine screening of blood and organ donors in the United States has not been recommended.

SUMMARY AND RECOMMENDATIONS

In summary, HEV testing in LT recipients with unexplained acute or chronic hepatitis should be considered (**Fig. 3**). If HEV testing is performed, it should include direct assays, such as blood or stool HEV RNA, and if positive, patients should be assessed for the development of chronic infection. If chronic infection is established, immunosuppression should be decreased, if possible, and patients should be monitored closely for the development of recurrent fibrosis. If chronic infection persists, antiviral treatment should be considered, although with limited data regarding the optimal regimen. Given the side effects and risk of rejection associated with IFN, ribavirin monotherapy for 3 months may be the preferred initial treatment.

REFERENCES

1. Thuluvath PJ, Guidinger MK, Fung JJ, et al. Liver transplantation in the United States, 1999-2008. Am J Transplant 2010;10:1003–19.
2. Picciotto FP, Tritto G, Lanza AG, et al. Sustained virological response to antiviral therapy reduces mortality in HCV reinfection after liver transplantation. J Hepatol 2007;46:459–65.
3. Berenguer M, Palau A, Aguilera V, et al. Clinical benefits of antiviral therapy in patients with recurrent hepatitis C following liver transplantation. Am J Transplant 2008;8:679–87.
4. Bizollon T, Pradat P, Mabrut JY, et al. Benefit of sustained virological response to combination therapy on graft survival of liver transplanted patients with recurrent chronic hepatitis C. Am J Transplant 2005;5:1909–13.
5. Recommendations for testing, managing, and treating hepatitis C. Available at: http://wwwhcvguidelinesorg. Accessed March 3, 2014.
6. Berenguer M, Prieto M, Rayon JM, et al. Natural history of clinically compensated hepatitis C virus-related graft cirrhosis after liver transplantation. Hepatology 2000;32:852–8.
7. Afzali A, Berry K, Ioannou GN. Excellent posttransplant survival for patients with nonalcoholic steatohepatitis in the United States. Liver Transpl 2012;18:29–37.
8. Maluf DG, Edwards EB, Stravitz RT, et al. Impact of the donor risk index on the outcome of hepatitis C virus-positive liver transplant recipients. Liver Transpl 2009;15:592–9.
9. Lai JC, O'Leary JG, Trotter JF, et al. Risk of advanced fibrosis with grafts from hepatitis C antibody-positive donors: a multicenter cohort study. Liver Transpl 2012;18:532–8.
10. Lai JC, Verna EC, Brown RS Jr, et al. Hepatitis C virus-infected women have a higher risk of advanced fibrosis and graft loss after liver transplantation than men. Hepatology 2011;54(2):418–24.
11. Verna EC, Valadao R, Farrand E, et al. Effects of ethnicity and socioeconomic status on survival and severity of fibrosis in liver transplant recipients with hepatitis C virus. Liver Transpl 2012;18:461–7.
12. Saxena V, Lai JC, O'Leary JG, et al. Donor-recipient race mismatch in African-American liver transplant patients with chronic hepatitis C. Liver Transpl 2012;18(5):524–31.

13. Verna EC, De Martin E, Burra P, et al. The impact of hepatitis C and biliary complications on patient and graft survival following liver transplantation. Am J Transplant 2009;9:1398–405.

14. Berenguer M, Prieto M, Cordoba J, et al. Early development of chronic active hepatitis in recurrent hepatitis C virus infection after liver transplantation: association with treatment of rejection. J Hepatol 1998;28:756–63.

15. Sheiner PA, Schwartz ME, Mor E, et al. Severe or multiple rejection episodes are associated with early recurrence of hepatitis C after orthotopic liver transplantation. Hepatology 1995;21:30–4.

16. Berenguer M, Aguilera V, Prieto M, et al. Significant improvement in the outcome of HCV-infected transplant recipients by avoiding rapid steroid tapering and potent induction immunosuppression. J Hepatol 2006;44:717–22.

17. Irish WD, Arcona S, Bowers D, et al. Cyclosporine versus tacrolimus treated liver transplant recipients with chronic hepatitis C: outcomes analysis of the UNOS/OPTN database. Am J Transplant 2011;11:1676–85.

18. Watt KD, Dierkhising R, Heimbach JK, et al. Impact of sirolimus and tacrolimus on mortality and graft loss in liver transplant recipients with or without hepatitis C virus: an analysis of the Scientific Registry of Transplant Recipients Database. Liver Transpl 2012;18:1029–36.

19. Bahra M, Neumann UI, Jacob D, et al. MMF and calcineurin taper in recurrent hepatitis C after liver transplantation: impact on histological course. Am J Transplant 2005;5:406–11.

20. Charlton MR, Thompson A, Veldt BJ, et al. Interleukin-28B polymorphisms are associated with histological recurrence and treatment response following liver transplantation in patients with hepatitis C virus infection. Hepatology 2011;53:317–24.

21. Dhillon N, Walsh L, Kruger B, et al. A single nucleotide polymorphism of Toll-like receptor 4 identifies the risk of developing graft failure after liver transplantation. J Hepatol 2010;53:67–72.

22. do ON, Eurich D, Schmitz P, et al. A 7-gene signature of the recipient predicts the progression of fibrosis after liver transplantation for hepatitis C virus infection. Liver Transpl 2012;18:298–304.

23. Berenguer M, Schuppan D. Progression of liver fibrosis in post-transplant hepatitis C: mechanisms, assessment and treatment. J Hepatol 2013;58(5):1028–41.

24. Adebajo CO, Talwalkar JA, Poterucha JJ, et al. Ultrasound-based transient elastography for the detection of hepatic fibrosis in patients with recurrent hepatitis C virus after liver transplantation: a systematic review and meta-analysis. Liver Transpl 2012;18:323–31.

25. Crespo G, Lens S, Gambato M, et al. Liver stiffness 1 year after transplantation predicts clinical outcomes in patients with recurrent hepatitis C. Am J Transplant 2014;14:375–83.

26. Everson GT, Trotter J, Forman L, et al. Treatment of advanced hepatitis C with a low accelerating dosage regimen of antiviral therapy. Hepatology 2005;42:255–62.

27. Everson GT, Terrault NA, Lok AS, et al. A randomized controlled trial of pretransplant antiviral therapy to prevent recurrence of hepatitis C after liver transplantation. Hepatology 2013;57:1752–62.

28. Hezode C, Fontaine H, Dorival C, et al. Triple therapy in treatment-experienced patients with HCV-cirrhosis in a multicentre cohort of the French Early Access Programme (ANRS CO20-CUPIC) - NCT01514890. J Hepatol 2013;59(3):434–41.

29. Colombo M, Fernandez I, Abdurakhmanov D, et al. Safety and on-treatment efficacy of telaprevir: the early access programme for patients with advanced hepatitis C. Gut 2013. [Epub ahead of print]. http://dx.doi.org/10.1136/gutjnl-2013-305667.

30. Ogawa E, Furusyo N, Nakamuta M, et al. Telaprevir-based triple therapy for chronic hepatitis C patients with advanced fibrosis: a prospective clinical study. Aliment Pharmacol Ther 2013;38:1076–85.

31. Verna EC, Shetty K, Lukose T, et al. High post-transplant virologic response in hepatitis C virus infected patients treated with pre-transplant protease inhibitor-based triple therapy. Liver Int 2014 Jun 6. http://dx.doi.org/10.1111/liv.12616.

32. Curry MP, Forns X, Chung RT, et al. Pretransplant sofosbuvir and ribavirin to prevent recurrence of HCV infection after liver transplantation. Hepatology 2013;58:314S–5S.

33. Bzowej N, Nelson DR, Terrault NA, et al. PHOENIX: a randomized controlled trial of peginterferon alfa-2a plus ribavirin as a prophylactic treatment after liver transplantation for hepatitis C virus. Liver Transpl 2011;17:528–38.

34. Crespo G, Carrion JA, Coto-Llerena M, et al. Combinations of simple baseline variables accurately predict sustained virological response in patients with recurrent hepatitis C after liver transplantation. J Gastroenterol 2013;48(6):762–9.

35. Berenguer M, Aguilera V, Rubin A, et al. Comparison of two non-contemporaneous HCV-liver transplant cohorts: strategies to improve the efficacy of antiviral therapy. J Hepatol 2012;56:1310–6.

36. Wang CS, Ko HH, Yoshida EM, et al. Interferon-based combination anti-viral therapy for hepatitis C virus after liver transplantation: a review and quantitative analysis. Am J Transplant 2006;6:1586–99.

37. Garg V, van Heeswijk R, Lee JE, et al. Effect of telaprevir on the pharmacokinetics of cyclosporine and tacrolimus. Hepatology 2011;54:20–7.

38. Hulskotte E, Gupta S, Xuan F, et al. Pharmacokinetic interaction between the hepatitis C virus protease inhibitor boceprevir and cyclosporine and tacrolimus in healthy volunteers. Hepatology 2012;56:1622–30.

39. O'Leary JG, McKenna GJ, Klintmalm GB, et al. Effect of telaprevir on the pharmacokinetics of sirolimus in liver transplant recipients. Liver Transpl 2013;19:463–5.

40. Coilly A, Roche B, Dumortier J, et al. Safety and efficacy of protease inhibitors to treat hepatitis C after liver transplantation: a multicenter experience. J Hepatol 2014;60:78–86.

41. Burton JR Jr, O'Leary JG, Verna EC, et al. A US multicenter study of hepatitis C treatment of liver transplant recipients with protease-inhibitor triple therapy. J Hepatol 2014 May 3. [Epub ahead of print]. http://dx.doi.org/10.1016/j.jhep.2014.04.037.

42. Faisal N, Renner EL, Bilodeau M, et al. Protease inhibitor-based triple therapy is highly effective in liver transplant recipients with genotype 1 hepatitis C recurrence: a Canadian multicenter experience. Hepatology 2013;58:238A.

43. Brown KA, Fontana RJ, Russo MW, et al. Twice-daily Telaprevir in combination with Pefinterferon Alpha-2a/Ribavirin in genotype 1 HCV Liver transplant recipients: interim week 16 safety and efficacy results of the prospective, multicenter REFRESH study. Hepatology 2013;58:209A.

44. Samuel D, Charlton M, Gane E, et al. Sofosbuvir and Ribavirin for the treatment of recurrent hepatitis C infection after liver transplantation: results of a prospective, multicenter study. J Hepatol 2014;60:S499.

45. Forns X, Prieto M, Charlton M, et al. Sofosbuvir compassionate use progran for patients wtih severe recurrent hepatitis C including fibrosing cholestatic hepatitis following liver transplantation. J Hepatol 2014;60:S26.

46. Fontana RJ, Hughes EA, Appelman H, et al. Case report of successful peginterferon, ribavirin, and daclatasvir therapy for recurrent cholestatic hepatitis C after liver retransplantation. Liver Transpl 2012;18:1053–9.

47. Fontana RJ, Hughes EA, Bifano M, et al. Sofosbuvir and daclatasvir combination therapy in a liver transplant recipient with severe recurrent cholestatic hepatitis C. Am J Transplant 2013;13:1601–5.

48. Pellicelli AM, Lionetti R, Montalbano M, et al. Sofosbuvir and Daclatasvir for recurrent hepatitis C after liver transplantation: potent antiviral activity but lack of clinical benefit if treatment is given too late. J Hepatol 2014;60:S532.

49. Jacobson IM, Ghalib RM, Rodriguez-Torres M. SVR results of a once-daily regimen of simeprevir (TMC435) plus sofosbuvir (GS-7977) with or without ribavirin in cirrhotic and non-cirrhotic HCV genotype 1 treatment-naive and prior null responder patients: the COSMOS study. Hepatology 2013;58.

50. Singal AK, Guturu P, Hmoud B, et al. Evolving frequency and outcomes of liver transplantation based on etiology of liver disease. Transplantation 2013;95:755–60.

51. Liaw YF, Raptopoulou-Gigi M, Cheinquer H, et al. Efficacy and safety of entecavir versus adefovir in chronic hepatitis B patients with hepatic decompensation: a randomized, open-label study. Hepatology 2011;54:91–100.

52. Schiff E, Lai CL, Hadziyannis S, et al. Adefovir dipivoxil for wait-listed and post-liver transplantation patients with lamivudine-resistant hepatitis B: final long-term results. Liver Transpl 2007;13:349–60.

53. Schiff ER, Lai CL, Hadziyannis S, et al. Adefovir dipivoxil therapy for lamivudine-resistant hepatitis B in pre- and post-liver transplantation patients. Hepatology 2003;38:1419–27.

54. Liaw YF, Sheen IS, Lee CM, et al. Tenofovir disoproxil fumarate (TDF), emtricitabine/TDF, and entecavir in patients with decompensated chronic hepatitis B liver disease. Hepatology 2011;53:62–72.

55. Campsen J, Zimmerman M, Trotter J, et al. Liver transplantation for hepatitis B liver disease and concomitant hepatocellular carcinoma in the United States With hepatitis B immunoglobulin and nucleoside/nucleotide analogues. Liver Transpl 2013;19:1020–9.

56. Samuel D, Bismuth A, Mathieu D, et al. Passive immunoprophylaxis after liver transplantation in HBsAg-positive patients. Lancet 1991;337:813–5.

57. Terrault NA, Zhou S, Combs C, et al. Prophylaxis in liver transplant recipients using a fixed dosing schedule of hepatitis B immunoglobulin. Hepatology 1996;24:1327–33.

58. McGory RW, Ishitani MB, Oliveira WM, et al. Improved outcome of orthotopic liver transplantation for chronic hepatitis B cirrhosis with aggressive passive immunization. Transplantation 1996;61:1358–64.

59. Konig V, Hopf U, Neuhaus P, et al. Long-term follow-up of hepatitis B virus-infected recipients after orthotopic liver transplantation. Transplantation 1994;58:553–9.

60. Muller R, Gubernatis G, Farle M, et al. Liver transplantation in HBs antigen (HBsAg) carriers. Prevention of hepatitis B virus (HBV) recurrence by passive immunization. J Hepatol 1991;13:90–6.

61. Sawyer RG, McGory RW, Gaffey MJ, et al. Improved clinical outcomes with liver transplantation for hepatitis B-induced chronic liver failure using passive immunization. Ann Surg 1998;227:841–50.

62. Cholongitas E, Papatheodoridis GV. High genetic barrier nucleos(t)ide analogue(s) for prophylaxis from hepatitis B virus recurrence after liver transplantation: a systematic review. Am J Transplant 2013;13:353–62.
63. Fox AN, Terrault NA. The option of HBIG-free prophylaxis against recurrent HBV. J Hepatol 2012;56:1189–97.
64. Loomba R, Rowley AK, Wesley R, et al. Hepatitis B immunoglobulin and Lamivudine improve hepatitis B-related outcomes after liver transplantation: meta-analysis. Clin Gastroenterol Hepatol 2008;6:696–700.
65. Perrillo R, Buti M, Durand F, et al. Entecavir and hepatitis B immune globulin in patients undergoing liver transplantation for chronic hepatitis B. Liver Transpl 2013;19:887–95.
66. Wesdorp DJ, Knoester M, Braat AE, et al. Nucleoside plus nucleotide analogs and cessation of hepatitis B immunoglobulin after liver transplantation in chronic hepatitis B is safe and effective. J Clin Virol 2013;58:67–73.
67. Na GH, Kim DG, Han JH, et al. Prevention and risk factors of hepatitis B recurrence after living donor liver transplantation. J Gastroenterol Hepatol 2014;29: 151–6.
68. Gao YJ, Zhang M, Jin B, et al. A clinical-pathological analysis of hepatitis B virus recurrence after liver transplantation in Chinese patients. J Gastroenterol Hepatol 2014;29(3):554–60.
69. Tanaka T, Renner EL, Selzner N, et al. One year of hepatitis B immunoglobulin plus tenofovir therapy is safe and effective in preventing recurrent hepatitis B post-liver transplantation. Can J Gastroenterol 2014;28:41–4.
70. Gane EJ, Angus PW, Strasser S, et al. Lamivudine plus low-dose hepatitis B immunoglobulin to prevent recurrent hepatitis B following liver transplantation. Gastroenterology 2007;132:931–7.
71. Angus PW, Patterson SJ, Strasser SI, et al. A randomized study of adefovir dipivoxil in place of HBIG in combination with lamivudine as post-liver transplantation hepatitis B prophylaxis. Hepatology 2008;48:1460–6.
72. Degertekin B, Han SH, Keeffe EB, et al. Impact of virologic breakthrough and HBIG regimen on hepatitis B recurrence after liver transplantation. Am J Transplant 2010;10:1823–33.
73. Teperman LW, Poordad F, Bzowej N, et al. Randomized trial of emtricitabine/tenofovir disoproxil fumarate after hepatitis B immunoglobulin withdrawal after liver transplantation. Liver Transpl 2013;19:594–601.
74. Angelico M, Di Paolo D, Trinito MO, et al. Failure of a reinforced triple course of hepatitis B vaccination in patients transplanted for HBV-related cirrhosis. Hepatology 2002;35:176–81.
75. Sanchez-Fueyo A, Rimola A, Grande L, et al. Hepatitis B immunoglobulin discontinuation followed by hepatitis B virus vaccination: a new strategy in the prophylaxis of hepatitis B virus recurrence after liver transplantation. Hepatology 2000;31:496–501.
76. Rosenau J, Hooman N, Hadem J, et al. Failure of hepatitis B vaccination with conventional HBsAg vaccine in patients with continuous HBIG prophylaxis after liver transplantation. Liver Transpl 2007;13:367–73.
77. Klein CG, Cicinnati V, Schmidt H, et al. Compliance and tolerability of subcutaneous hepatitis B immunoglobulin self-administration in liver transplant patients: a prospective, observational, multicenter study. Ann Transplant 2013;18:677–84.
78. Wadhawan M, Gupta S, Goyal N, et al. Living related liver transplantation for hepatitis B-related liver disease without hepatitis B immune globulin prophylaxis. Liver Transpl 2013;19:1030–5.

79. Fung J, Chan SC, Cheung C, et al. Oral nucleoside/nucleotide analogs without hepatitis B immune globulin after liver transplantation for hepatitis B. Am J Gastroenterol 2013;108:942–8.
80. Terrault N. Prophylaxis in HBV-infected liver transplant patients: end of the HBIG era? Am J Gastroenterol 2013;108:949–51.
81. Marzano A, Gaia S, Ghisetti V, et al. Viral load at the time of liver transplantation and risk of hepatitis B virus recurrence. Liver Transpl 2005;11:402–9.
82. Chazouilleres O, Mamish D, Kim M, et al. "Occult" hepatitis B virus as source of infection in liver transplant recipients. Lancet 1994;343:142–6.
83. Dickson RC, Everhart JE, Lake JR, et al. Transmission of hepatitis B by transplantation of livers from donors positive for antibody to hepatitis B core antigen. The National Institute of Diabetes and Digestive and Kidney Diseases Liver Transplantation Database. Gastroenterology 1997;113:1668–74.
84. Bohorquez HE, Cohen AJ, Girgrah N, et al. Liver transplantation in hepatitis B core-negative recipients using livers from hepatitis B core-positive donors: a 13-year experience. Liver Transpl 2013;19:611–8.
85. Wachs ME, Amend WJ, Ascher NL, et al. The risk of transmission of hepatitis B from HBsAg(-), HBcAb(+), HBIgM(-) organ donors. Transplantation 1995;59: 230–4.
86. Prieto M, Gomez MD, Berenguer M, et al. De novo hepatitis B after liver transplantation from hepatitis B core antibody-positive donors in an area with high prevalence of anti-HBc positivity in the donor population. Liver Transpl 2001; 7:51–8.
87. Munoz SJ. Use of hepatitis B core antibody-positive donors for liver transplantation. Liver Transpl 2002;8:S82–7.
88. Manzarbeitia C, Reich DJ, Ortiz JA, et al. Safe use of livers from donors with positive hepatitis B core antibody. Liver Transpl 2002;8:556–61.
89. Barcena R, Moraleda G, Moreno J, et al. Prevention of de novo HBV infection by the presence of anti-HBs in transplanted patients receiving core antibody-positive livers. World J Gastroenterol 2006;12:2070–4.
90. Yu AS, Vierling JM, Colquhoun SD, et al. Transmission of hepatitis B infection from hepatitis B core antibody–positive liver allografts is prevented by lamivudine therapy. Liver Transpl 2001;7:513–7.
91. Chang MS, Olsen SK, Pichardo EM, et al. Prevention of de novo hepatitis B with adefovir dipivoxil in recipients of liver grafts from hepatitis B core antibody-positive donors. Liver Transpl 2012;18:834–8.
92. Abdelmalek MF, Pasha TM, Zein NN, et al. Subclinical reactivation of hepatitis B virus in liver transplant recipients with past exposure. Liver Transpl 2003;9: 1253–7.
93. Thomas DL, Yarbough PO, Vlahov D, et al. Seroreactivity to hepatitis E virus in areas where the disease is not endemic. J Clin Microbiol 1997;35:1244–7.
94. Kuniholm MH, Purcell RH, McQuillan GM, et al. Epidemiology of hepatitis E virus in the United States: results from the Third National Health and Nutrition Examination Survey, 1988-1994. J Infect Dis 2009;200:48–56.
95. Kamar N, Rostaing L, Legrand-Abravanel F, et al. How should hepatitis E virus infection be defined in organ-transplant recipients? Am J Transplant 2013;13: 1935–6.
96. Pischke S, Wedemeyer H. Chronic hepatitis E in liver transplant recipients: a significant clinical problem? Minerva Gastroenterol Dietol 2010;56:121–8.
97. Kamar N, Weclawiak H, Guilbeau-Frugier C, et al. Hepatitis E virus and the kidney in solid-organ transplant patients. Transplantation 2012;93:617–23.

98. Lhomme S, Abravanel F, Dubois M, et al. Hepatitis E virus quasispecies and the outcome of acute hepatitis E in solid-organ transplant patients. J Virol 2012;86: 10006–14.
99. Kamar N, Garrouste C, Haagsma EB, et al. Factors associated with chronic hepatitis in patients with hepatitis E virus infection who have received solid organ transplants. Gastroenterology 2011;140:1481–9.
100. Pischke S, Suneetha PV, Baechlein C, et al. Hepatitis E virus infection as a cause of graft hepatitis in liver transplant recipients. Liver Transpl 2010;16: 74–82.
101. Kamar N, Mansuy JM, Cointault O, et al. Hepatitis E virus-related cirrhosis in kidney- and kidney-pancreas-transplant recipients. Am J Transplant 2008;8: 1744–8.
102. Kamar N, Selves J, Mansuy JM, et al. Hepatitis E virus and chronic hepatitis in organ-transplant recipients. N Engl J Med 2008;358:811–7.
103. Gerolami R, Moal V, Colson P. Chronic hepatitis E with cirrhosis in a kidney-transplant recipient. N Engl J Med 2008;358:859–60.
104. Hering T, Passos AM, Perez RM, et al. Past and current hepatitis E virus infection in renal transplant patients. J Med Virol 2014;86(6):948–53.
105. Kenfak-Foguena A, Schoni-Affolter F, Burgisser P, et al. Hepatitis E Virus seroprevalence and chronic infections in patients with HIV, Switzerland. Emerg Infect Dis 2011;17:1074–8.
106. Kaba M, Richet H, Ravaux I, et al. Hepatitis E virus infection in patients infected with the human immunodeficiency virus. J Med Virol 2011;83:1704–16.
107. Jagjit Singh GK, Ijaz S, Rockwood N, et al. Chronic Hepatitis E as a cause for cryptogenic cirrhosis in HIV. J Infect 2013;66:103–6.
108. Mateos-Lindemann ML, Diez-Aguilar M, Galdamez AL, et al. Patients infected with HIV are at high-risk for hepatitis E virus infection in Spain. J Med Virol 2014;86:71–4.
109. Colson P, Dhiver C, Poizot-Martin I, et al. Acute and chronic hepatitis E in patients infected with human immunodeficiency virus. J Viral Hepat 2011;18: 227–8.
110. Motte A, Roquelaure B, Galambrun C, et al. Hepatitis E in three immunocompromized children in southeastern France. J Clin Virol 2012;53:162–6.
111. le Coutre P, Meisel H, Hofmann J, et al. Reactivation of hepatitis E infection in a patient with acute lymphoblastic leukaemia after allogeneic stem cell transplantation. Gut 2009;58:699–702.
112. Abravanel F, Mansuy JM, Huynh A, et al. Low risk of hepatitis E virus reactivation after haematopoietic stem cell transplantation. J Clin Virol 2012;54:152–5.
113. Haagsma EB, Riezebos-Brilman A, van den Berg AP, et al. Treatment of chronic hepatitis E in liver transplant recipients with pegylated interferon alpha-2b. Liver Transpl 2010;16:474–7.
114. Kamar N, Rostaing L, Izopet J. Hepatitis E virus infection in immunosuppressed patients: natural history and therapy. Semin Liver Dis 2013;33:62–70.
115. Kamar N, Rostaing L, Abravanel F, et al. Ribavirin therapy inhibits viral replication on patients with chronic hepatitis e virus infection. Gastroenterology 2010; 139:1612–8.
116. Chaillon A, Sirinelli A, De Muret A, et al. Sustained virologic response with ribavirin in chronic hepatitis E virus infection in heart transplantation. J Heart Lung Transplant 2011;30:841–3.
117. Mallet V, Nicand E, Sultanik P, et al. Brief communication: case reports of ribavirin treatment for chronic hepatitis E. Ann Intern Med 2010;153:85–9.

118. Kamar N, Rostaing L, Abravanel F, et al. Pegylated interferon-alpha for treating chronic hepatitis E virus infection after liver transplantation. Clin Infect Dis 2010; 50:e30–3.

119. Pischke S, Hardtke S, Bode U, et al. Ribavirin treatment of acute and chronic hepatitis E: a single-centre experience. Liver Int 2013;33:722–6.

120. Kamar N, Izopet J, Tripon S, et al. Ribavirin for chronic hepatitis E virus infection in transplant recipients. N Engl J Med 2014;370:1111–20.

121. Kamar N, Abravanel F, Selves J, et al. Influence of immunosuppressive therapy on the natural history of genotype 3 hepatitis-E virus infection after organ transplantation. Transplantation 2010;89:353–60.

122. Aggarwal R. Diagnosis of hepatitis E. Nat Rev Gastroenterol Hepatol 2013;10: 24–33.

123. Abravanel F, Chapuy-Regaud S, Lhomme S, et al. Performance of anti-HEV assays for diagnosing acute hepatitis E in immunocompromised patients. J Clin Virol 2013;58:624–8.

124. Bendall R, Ellis V, Ijaz S, et al. A comparison of two commercially available anti-HEV IgG kits and a re-evaluation of anti-HEV IgG seroprevalence data in developed countries. J Med Virol 2010;82:799–805.

125. Mast EE, Alter MJ, Holland PV, et al. Evaluation of assays for antibody to hepatitis E virus by a serum panel. Hepatitis E Virus Antibody Serum Panel Evaluation Group. Hepatology 1998;27:857–61.

126. Rossi-Tamisier M, Moal V, Gerolami R, et al. Discrepancy between anti-hepatitis E virus immunoglobulin G prevalence assessed by two assays in kidney and liver transplant recipients. J Clin Virol 2013;56:62–4.

127. Baylis SA, Hanschmann KM, Blumel J, et al. Standardization of hepatitis E virus (HEV) nucleic acid amplification technique-based assays: an initial study to evaluate a panel of HEV strains and investigate laboratory performance. J Clin Microbiol 2011;49:1234–9.

128. Baylis SA, Blumel J, Mizusawa S, et al. World Health Organization International Standard to harmonize assays for detection of hepatitis E virus RNA. Emerg Infect Dis 2013;19:729–35.

129. Haagsma EB, Niesters HG, van den Berg AP, et al. Prevalence of hepatitis E virus infection in liver transplant recipients. Liver Transpl 2009;15:1225–8.

130. Hoerning A, Hegen B, Wingen AM, et al. Prevalence of hepatitis E virus infection in pediatric solid organ transplant recipients–a single-center experience. Pediatr Transplant 2012;16:742–7.

131. Legrand-Abravanel F, Kamar N, Sandres-Saune K, et al. Hepatitis E virus infection without reactivation in solid-organ transplant recipients, France. Emerg Infect Dis 2011;17:30–7.

132. Pas SD, de Man RA, Mulders C, et al. Hepatitis E virus infection among solid organ transplant recipients, the Netherlands. Emerg Infect Dis 2012;18:869–72.

133. Buti M, Cabrera C, Jardi R, et al. Are recipients of solid organ transplantation a high-risk population for hepatitis E virus infection? Liver Transpl 2010;16:106–7 [author reply: 108].

134. Kamar N, Bendall RP, Peron JM, et al. Hepatitis E virus and neurologic disorders. Emerg Infect Dis 2011;17:173–9.

135. Del Bello A, Arne-Bes MC, Lavayssiere L, et al. Hepatitis E virus-induced severe myositis. J Hepatol 2012;57:1152–3.

136. Taton B, Moreau K, Lepreux S, et al. Hepatitis E virus infection as a new probable cause of de novo membranous nephropathy after kidney transplantation. Transpl Infect Dis 2013;15:E211–5.

137. Wang Y, Zhou X, Debing Y, et al. Calcineurin inhibitors stimulate and mycophenolic acid inhibits replication of hepatitis E virus. Gastroenterology 2014;146(7): 1775–83.
138. Kamar N, Legrand-Abravanel F, Izopet J, et al. Hepatitis E virus: what transplant physicians should know. Am J Transplant 2012;12:2281–7.
139. Unzueta A, Rakela J. Hepatitis E infection in liver transplant recipients. Liver Transpl 2014;20(1):15–24.
140. Schlosser B, Stein A, Neuhaus R, et al. Liver transplant from a donor with occult HEV infection induced chronic hepatitis and cirrhosis in the recipient. J Hepatol 2012;56:500–2.
141. Thomas RM, Brems JJ, Guzman-Hartman G, et al. Infection with chronic hepatitis C virus and liver transplantation: a role for interferon therapy before transplantation. Liver Transpl 2003;9:905–15.
142. Forns X, Garcia-Retortillo M, Serrano T, et al. Antiviral therapy of patients with decompensated cirrhosis to prevent recurrence of hepatitis C after liver transplantation. J Hepatol 2003;39:389–96.
143. Carrion JA, Martinez-Bauer E, Crespo G, et al. Antiviral therapy increases the risk of bacterial infections in HCV-infected cirrhotic patients awaiting liver transplantation: a retrospective study. J Hepatol 2009;50:719–28.
144. Mathias A, Cornpropst M, Clemons D. No clinically significant pharmacokinetic drug-drug interactions between sofosbuvir (CG-7977) and the immunosuppressants, cyclosporine a or tacrolimus in healthy volunteers. Hepatology 2012; 56(Suppl 1):1063A–4A.
145. Ouwerkerk-Mahadevan S, Sinmion A, Mortier S. No clinically significant interaction between the Investigational HCV protease Inhibitor TMC435 and the immunosuppressives cyclosporine and tacrolimus. Hepatology 2012;56(Suppl 1): 231A.
146. Kwo P, Mantry P, Coakley E, et al. Results of the phase 2 study M12-999: interferon-free regimen of ABT-450/R/ABT-267 + ABT-333 + ribavirin in liver transplant recipients with recurrent HCV genotype 1 infection. J Hepatol 2014;60:S47.
147. Haagsma EB, van den Berg AP, Porte RJ, et al. Chronic hepatitis E virus infection in liver transplant recipients. Liver Transpl 2008;14:547–53.
148. Halac U, Beland K, Lapierre P, et al. Chronic hepatitis E infection in children with liver transplantation. Gut 2012;61:597–603.
149. Junge N, Pischke S, Baumann U, et al. Results of single-center screening for chronic hepatitis E in children after liver transplantation and report on successful treatment with ribavirin. Pediatr Transplant 2013;17:343–7.

Liver Transplant for Hepatocellular Cancer

Very Small Tumors, Very Large Tumors, and Waiting Time

Kayvan Roayaie, MD, PhD[a], Sasan Roayaie, MD[b],*

KEYWORDS

• UNOS stage 1 • Resection • Drop out • Expansion • Milan criteria • Recurrence

KEY POINTS

- There is uncertainty as to the best initial approach for patients with hepatocellular cancer (HCC) less than 2 cm in size: watchful waiting until tumor reaches 2 cm, immediate ablation, or resection.
- There continues to be significant debate regarding the expansion of criteria for Model for End-Stage Liver Disease (MELD) exception for HCC beyond Milan criteria despite conflicting data on outcomes.
- Awarding of MELD exception for patients with HCC is resulting in the need for a higher score to reach transplant for all patients.
- More data are emerging regarding the benefits of observation time on the waiting list.

VERY SMALL TUMORS

With the implementation of MELD in 2002, patients with United Network for Organ Sharing (UNOS) stage 1 HCC ($\leq$2 cm) were afforded priority on the waiting list with 24 points. Consequently, 86% of patients with stage 1 HCC underwent transplant within 3 months.[1] However, it was eventually discovered that 31% of these patients actually had no HCC present in the explanted liver.[2] This dramatic discovery eventually led to revocation of priority for UNOS stage 1 HCC, and currently, clinicians are left with a substantial dilemma with regards to the best approach for HCC between 1 and 2 cm in size (**Fig. 1**).

A publication by Livraghi and colleagues[3] has generated a significant amount of debate regarding the best first-line treatment of HCC less than or equal to 2 cm.

Disclosure: None.
^a Division of Abdominal Organ Transplantation, Department of Surgery, Oregon Health and Sciences University, 3181 SW Sam Jackson Park Road, L-590, Portland, OR 97239, USA; ^b Liver Cancer Program, Hofstra-North Shore LIJ School of Medicine, Lenox Hill Hospital, New York, NY, USA
* Corresponding author. 110 East 59th Street, Suite 10B, New York, NY 10022.
E-mail address: sasan.roayaie@gmail.com

http://dx.doi.org/10.1016/j.cld.2014.05.013
1089-3261/14/$ – see front matter © 2014 Elsevier Inc. All rights reserved.

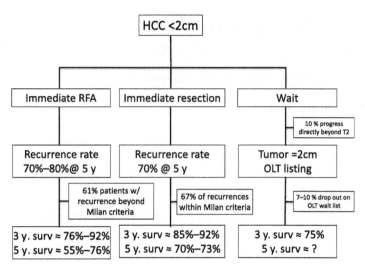

Fig. 1. Choices of treatment available for HCC less than 2 cm with approximated outcomes with each strategy. OLT, liver transplantation.

The researchers showed a 5-year survival of 55% for all patients with a single HCC less than or equal to 2 cm treated initially with radiofrequency ablation (RFA) and a 5-year survival of 65% in the subgroup that could potentially have been candidates for resection. These and similar findings have led the Barcelona Clinic Liver Cancer (BCLC) group to amend their staging system so that for patients with a single HCC less than or equal to 2 cm who are not candidates for liver transplant, RFA is now the recommended first-line treatment.[4]

RFA is associated with a high recurrence rate, 80% at 5 years, even when treating such early tumors.[3] A study by Tsuchiya and colleagues,[5] despite demonstrating a 5-year survival of 70% for patients with HCC within Milan criteria treated with RFA, found that more than 60% of the cohort experienced recurrence beyond Milan criteria after 5 years of follow-up. This has raised speculation that the strategy of ablate and wait may result in a significant percentage of these patients presenting with recurrence that renders them no longer eligible for transplant.[6] However, one must keep in mind that patients with a single HCC less than 2 cm represented the earliest of the tumors included in the analysis by Tsuchiya and colleagues and that ablation of tumors greater than 2 cm was an independent predictor of recurrence beyond Milan criteria. Therefore, the likelihood of untransplantable recurrence after ablation of an HCC less than 2 cm still remains unknown.

Another proposed approach has been to wait and not ablate and allow the tumor to reach 2 cm, at which point the patient would become eligible for MELD exception. At the 2013 American Association for the Study of Liver Diseases (AASLD) meeting, 114 patients with T1 (<2 cm) HCC who were treated using this approach[7] were described, with 9% of patients progressing directly from T1 to beyond T2. The authors found that the 3-year survival rate with transplant for this approach was 75%. For the sake of comparison, 3-year survival after ablation was 84% in the Tsuchiya study and 92% in a review of the Liver Cancer Study Group of Japan, with both studies including more advanced tumors larger than 2 cm.[5,8]

Finally, for patients with HCC less than 2 cm and well preserved liver function, resection continues to be an attractive treatment approach. Japanese and Western series have shown 3-year survival rates of 92% and 85%, respectively.[8,9] Like ablation, recurrence continues to be a significant problem after hepatic resection with rates reported at 70% at 5 years even for HCC less than 2 cm. However, a study from the Beaujon group found that, unlike ablation, most recurrences after resection are within Milan criteria and that information gained from the resected tumor can be useful in selection of patients for eventual salvage transplant.[10]

As with many areas of HCC management, there is a lack of sufficient data to come to a robust conclusion regarding the best approach to HCC less than 2 cm. Intermediate survival outcome at 3 years seems to favor immediate treatment with ablation or, if liver function permits, resection. Although the overall rate of recurrence is high with either of these interventions, it is not known what percentage of those with recurrence are amenable to salvage transplant when specifically studying primary tumors that were less than 2 cm. Likewise, one lacks long-term data on the wait and do not ablate approach. Given the current shortage of organs and the availability of alternatives to transplant that offer such outstanding results, it seems logical to avoid transplant until a clear and compelling benefit is established for patients with HCC less than 2 cm.

VERY LARGE TUMORS

The concept of expanding indication for transplanting HCC beyond Milan criteria first gained momentum with a publication from the University of San Francisco (UCSF) group in 2001.[11] Since then, numerous studies have been published on this topic. However, most of them were performed in a retrospective manner using pathologic data thereby making intention-to-treat analyses impossible and limiting their value. In addition, most of the reports included only a small number of patients beyond Milan criteria who were "diluted" in a much larger pool of patients within Milan criteria. Consequently, most studies showing no difference in outcome using their expanded criteria can likely attribute their findings to a lack of statistical power rather than to a true similarity in outcomes when compared with patients within Milan criteria. In a recent review, assuming 5-year survival of 64% for patients within Milan criteria and 50% for those beyond with an alpha level of 5%, Silva and Sherman calculated that a properly powered study would require 139 patients per arm.[12]

This article does not review all the studies in the literature on expansion of criteria but focuses on a few recent and interesting publications on expansion based on tumor size/number, tumor biology, and downstaging.

Extended Criteria—Tumor Size and Number

The original UCSF paper on expansion generated controversy because it was performed retrospectively, based on pathology and included only 14 patients with HCC beyond Milan criteria.[11] In 2007, the group prospectively validated their criteria using preoperative imaging by comparing 130 patients within Milan criteria to 38 patients beyond Milan but within UCSF criteria.[13] Recurrence-free survival at 5 years was 90% for the group within Milan criteria and 93% for the group beyond Milan criteria but within the UCSF criteria. Overall survival was not reported.

Another study performed in a prospective manner using radiological assessment came from the group in Navarra.[14] The investigators compared 47 patients within Milan criteria to 26 patients beyond and reported a 5-year intention-to-treat survival of 73% and 72%, respectively.

Perhaps the most interesting data regarding expansion of criteria have come as a result of the decision among centers in UNOS Region 4 to extend MELD exception to patients within the R4T3 criteria. An initial review of the outcomes showed no difference in survival between the 363 patients who underwent transplant within Milan criteria and the 82 patients beyond Milan criteria but within R4T3 at 3 years.[15]

However, a more mature analysis of the subgroup that underwent transplant at Simmons Transplant Institute (formerly Baylor) found a significantly lower 5-year survival of 69% for the R4T3 patients compared with 79% for those within Milan (**Table 1**).[16]

Finally, a multinational study including more than 1000 patients who underwent transplant for HCC published by Mazzaferro and colleagues[17] clearly showed that there is no magic cutoff in terms of tumor size and number below which survival is equivalent to tumors within Milan criteria. Rather, the relationship between tumor characteristics and survival is a continuous spectrum with increasing tumor size and number diminishing survival (**Fig. 2**).

Downstaging

Downstaging studies address tumors beyond Milan criteria, with the additional requirement that the tumors display a response to a neoadjuvant treatment and that the remaining viable tumor fits a prespecified criteria before transplant. Downstaging studies often suffer from many of the same shortcomings found with the extended criteria reports. The more recent prospective studies are listed in **Table 2**.[18–20] A quick glance reveals the small sample size and short follow-up that plague all the studies and make reaching any robust conclusion clearly impossible.

Tumor Biology

Tumor size and number are clearly crude surrogates for the biologic aggressiveness of HCC. Several centers have evaluated expansion of criteria based on tumor differentiation, genetic profile, and alpha fetoprotein (AFP) levels.

The group from Padua updated their original series of patients with HCC who were selected for transplant based on preoperative liver biopsy.[21,22] This study was a prospective one of 100 patients listed for transplant that excluded patients with extrahepatic disease, vascular invasion, and poorly differentiated tumors based on pretransplant biopsy; 40 were beyond Milan criteria. Eventually, 68 patients underwent transplant without a single incident of recurrent HCC.

These findings have been corroborated by a retrospective review from the University of Toronto.[23] The series consisted of 105 patients who were outside Milan criteria at the time of transplant. In addition to the traditional parameters of size and number of tumors, the group studied the utility of a pretransplant biopsy. They found that poorly differentiated tumor grade on the biopsy of the dominant lesion used as an exclusion criteria resulted in an increase in the 5-year survival of patients that exceeded the Milan criteria from 61% to 77%. However, selecting out poorly differentiated tumors made no difference in outcome for patients who were within the Milan criteria.

Although the use of histologic differentiation seems appealing, one has to keep in mind the heterogeneity of large HCC, which may limit the accuracy of a preoperative biopsy.[24] In addition, there are concerns over the risk of tumor seeding by biopsy, which has been reported as having an incidence as high as 2.7%.[25]

In 2008, the group at Mount Sinai reported the identification of 9 microsatellites, which could potentially identify patients with large but biologically favorable tumors[26] from the tumors of 70 patients, half within and the other half outside Milan criteria. They studied the number of copies of microsatellites near known oncogenes and tumor suppressor genes by a technique known as allelic imbalance. They then used a univariate analysis to determine instability of which of the microsatellites was associated with recurrence. They found that in the cohort that exceeded the Milan criteria, a low fraction of significant alleles imbalanced was associated with only a 10% 5-year probability of HCC recurrence, with an accuracy of 89%. Although their source

Table 1
Selected prospective studies on expanded criteria for transplant for HCC

Author	Criteria	Within Milan Criteria (n)	Outside Milan Criteria (n)	5-y Survival (%) Within Milan Criteria	5-y Survival (%) Outside Milan Criteria	Median Follow-up (mo)
Yao et al,[13] 2007	UCSF 1 lesion ≤6.5 cm 2–3 lesions ≤4.5 cm Total diameter ≤8 cm	130	38	90	93[a]	26
Kim et al,[16] 2013	R4T3 1 lesion ≤6 cm 2–3 lesions ≤5 cm Total diameter ≤9 cm	176	49	79	69	56
Herrero et al,[14] 2008	Navarra 1 lesion ≤6 cm 2–3 lesions ≤5 cm	59	26	66	68	Not reported

[a] Recurrence-free probability.

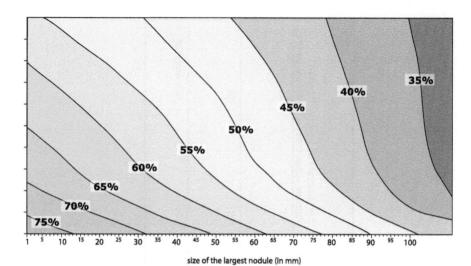

Fig. 2. Estimated survival at 5 years according to tumor size and number, not taking into account the presence or absence of vascular invasion. (*Adapted from* Mazzaferro V, Llovet JM, Miceli R, et al. Predicting survival after liver transplantation in patients with hepatocellular carcinoma beyond the Milan criteria: a retrospective, exploratory analysis. Lancet Oncol 2009;10(1):39; with permission.)

material was the explanted liver, this technique could potentially be applied to preoperative biopsy specimens, with the sample bias caveat mentioned earlier.

Finally, investigators have studied the use of AFP as a marker of biologic aggressiveness of HCC in the transplant setting. In 2009, the group at the University of Alberta studied using total tumor volume (TTV) and AFP as possible combined predictors of disease recurrence post–liver transplant.[27] The researchers retrospectively reviewed the results of 6478 patients, who had received a liver transplant with a diagnosis of HCC, from the Scientific Registry of Transplant Recipients database. They calculated the volume of each lesion using its maximal diameter and the formula for the volume of a sphere. The volumes were totaled to arrive at the TTV. Their analyses indicated that patients with a TTV greater than 115 cm^3 or an AFP greater than 400 ng/mL had significantly worse survival, 50% at 3 years.

In summary, there has been a significant amount written on expansion beyond Milan criteria. Downstaging is somewhat more attractive in that it requires that tumors display a response to neoadjuvant therapy before listing for transplant thereby selecting out the more favorable candidates. At this point, the studies have too few patients and too short of a follow-up to allow any meaningful conclusions regarding the role of downstaging. Selecting patients based on tumor biology is perhaps the most appealing of the strategies discussed but continues to be in its infancy.

WAITING TIME

Perhaps the difficulty in establishing selection criteria that accurately determine the risk of recurrent HCC after transplant has arisen from the fact that most attempts have been based on a static assessment of the tumors based on either tumor number and size or biopsy at a single point in time. Some have argued that perhaps the best assessment of a tumor's aggressiveness is achieved by observing its behavior over a certain period of time.

Table 2
Prospective trials on downstaging of HCC before transplant

Author	Criteria for Enrollment	Downstaged Criteria	Enrolled N	Successfully Downstaged N (%)	Waiting Period	Liver transplantation N (%)	5-y Survival (%)	5-y Survival (%) Intent to Treat	Median Follow-up (mo)
Yao et al,[18] 2008	1 lesion ≤8 cm 2–3 lesions ≤5 cm 4–5 lesions ≤3 cm Total diameter ≤8 cm No macrovascular invasion	Milan	61	43 (71)	3 mo	35 (57)	92 (4 y)	69 (4 y)	25
Ravaioli et al,[19] 2008	1 lesion ≤6 cm 2 lesions ≤5 cm 5 nodules ≤3 cm Total diameter ≤12 cm No macrovascular invasion	Milan + AFP<400	386	160 (42)	None	37 (10)	72 (3 y)	56	30
Chapman et al,[20] 2008	Any tumor size or number Intrahepatic portal or hepatic vein invasion OK No extrahepatic disease Child A, B Bilirubin <4	Milan	76	18 (24)	None	17 (22)	94	Not reported	20

This concept was first introduced by the Northwestern group in 2004 when they proposed that fast-tracking of patients with HCC toward transplant with the use of live donors resulted in higher rates of recurrence.[28] Initially, a small series from San Francisco seemed to contradict these findings.[29] However, a more recent review of UNOS data presented at the 2013 AASLD Meeting showed that longer time on the waiting list was independently associated with better posttransplant survival for patients receiving MELD exception for HCC.[30]

Along similar lines, a study from the Cleveland Clinic found that tumor growth rate greater than 1.6 cm^3/mo was an independent predictor of recurrence in the cohort.[31] The same cutoff was also able to select patients beyond Milan criteria who had a recurrence rate of only 11%. Although not explicitly described in the article, clearly a certain period of observation on the waiting list is required to assess the rate of tumor growth.

With a longer wait, patients with aggressive tumors will likely progress beyond transplant criteria and drop out. The remaining patients with more indolent tumors will likely have a lower incidence of recurrence. The problem with measuring posttransplant survival as the end point is that lengthening the wait time not only results in better and better outcomes but also translates into a higher number of drop outs. With a long enough wait time, one would eventually begin to remove patients with relatively indolent tumors who would likely have done well after transplant. Thus, the key is an approach that maximizes intention-to-treat survival for patients with HCC on the waiting list.

An intriguing presentation by the transplant team at Columbia University at the 2013 American Transplant Congress was exactly on this issue.[32] The team was able to demonstrate that listing in a region with short wait time was associated not only with a worse posttransplant survival when compared with listing in a region with long wait time but also with a worse intention-to-treat survival for patients with HCC receiving MELD exception. If their findings are validated, it would make a compelling argument for a mandatory waiting time for all patients with HCC. Clearly, an ideal waiting period that optimizes intention-to-treat survival would need to be calculated.

Although additional time on the waiting list may turn out to be beneficial for patients with HCC, the same is clearly not true for patients without tumors. Another presentation at the 2013 AASLD meeting demonstrated that the granting of priority to patients with HCC has led to MELD inflation, resulting in higher scores needed to reach transplant for all patients in all regions.[33]

SUMMARY

We have certainly come a long way since the original publication of the Milan criteria in 1996 in terms of understanding the role of transplant for HCC. With very small tumors, it is fortunate to have several therapies with excellent outcomes at our disposal and the dilemma rests in which to choose. With very large tumors, it is being discovered that there is no perfect formula in terms of number and size of tumors that results in a good outcome. A better understanding of the tumor's biology is necessary to select out the favorable patients. Finally, a period of observation may help one to better select HCC cases for transplant.

REFERENCES

1. Sharma P, Balan V, Hernandez JL, et al. Liver transplantation for hepatocellular carcinoma: the MELD impact. Liver Transpl 2004;10(1):36–41.
2. Wiesner RH, Freeman RB, Mulligan DC. Liver transplantation for hepatocellular cancer: the impact of the MELD allocation policy. Gastroenterology 2004; 127(5 Suppl 1):S261–7.

3. Livraghi T, Meloni F, Di Stasi M, et al. Sustained complete response and complications rates after radiofrequency ablation of very early hepatocellular carcinoma in cirrhosis: Is resection still the treatment of choice? Hepatology 2008;47(1):82–9.

4. Forner A, Llovet JM, Bruix J. Hepatocellular carcinoma. Lancet 2012;379(9822):1245–55.

5. Tsuchiya K, Asahina Y, Tamaki N, et al. Risk factors for exceeding the Milan criteria after successful radiofrequency ablation in patients with early-stage hepatocellular carcinoma. Liver Transpl 2014;20(3):291–7.

6. Yao FY. Conundrum of treatment for early-stage hepatocellular carcinoma: radiofrequency ablation instead of liver transplantation as the first-line treatment? Liver Transpl 2014;20(3):257–60.

7. Mehta N, Dodge JL, Fidelman N, et al. Intention-to-treat outcome of T1 hepatocellular carcinoma using the approach of "wait and not ablate" until meeting T2 criteria for liver transplant listing. Hepatology 2013;58(SI):212A.

8. Hasegawa K, Kokudo N, Makuuchi M, et al. Comparison of resection and ablation for hepatocellular carcinoma: a cohort study based on a Japanese nationwide survey. J Hepatol 2013;58(4):724–9.

9. Roayaie S, Obeidat K, Sposito C, et al. Resection of hepatocellular cancer ≤ 2 cm: results from two Western centers. Hepatology 2013;57(4):1426–35.

10. Fuks D, Dokmak S, Paradis V, et al. Benefit of initial resection of hepatocellular carcinoma followed by transplantation in case of recurrence: an intention-to-treat analysis. Hepatology 2012;55(1):132–40.

11. Yao FY, Ferrell L, Bass NM, et al. Liver transplantation for hepatocellular carcinoma: expansion of the tumor size limits does not adversely impact survival. Hepatology 2001;33(6):1394–403.

12. Silva MF, Sherman M. Criteria for liver transplantation for HCC: what should the limits be? J Hepatol 2011;55(5):1137–47.

13. Yao FY, Xiao L, Bass NM, et al. Liver transplantation for hepatocellular carcinoma: validation of the UCSF-expanded criteria based on preoperative imaging. Am J Transplant 2007;7(11):2587–96.

14. Herrero JI, Sangro B, Pardo F, et al. Liver transplantation in patients with hepatocellular carcinoma across Milan criteria. Liver Transpl 2008;14(3):272–8.

15. Guiteau JJ, Cotton RT, Washburn WK, et al. An early regional experience with expansion of Milan criteria for liver transplant recipients. Am J Transplant 2010;10(9):2092–8.

16. Kim PT, Onaca N, Chinnakotla S, et al. Tumor biology and pre-transplant locoregional treatments determine outcomes in patients with T3 hepatocellular carcinoma undergoing liver transplantation. Clin Transplant 2013;27(2):311–8.

17. Mazzaferro V, Llovet JM, Miceli R, et al. Predicting survival after liver transplantation in patients with hepatocellular carcinoma beyond the Milan criteria: a retrospective, exploratory analysis. Lancet Oncol 2009;10(1):35–43.

18. Yao FY, Kerlan RK Jr, Hirose R, et al. Excellent outcome following down-staging of hepatocellular carcinoma prior to liver transplantation: an intention-to-treat analysis. Hepatology 2008;48(3):819–27.

19. Ravaioli M, Grazi GL, Piscaglia F, et al. Liver transplantation for hepatocellular carcinoma: results of down-staging in patients initially outside the Milan selection criteria. Am J Transplant 2008;8(12):2547–57.

20. Chapman WC, Majella Doyle MB, Stuart JE, et al. Outcomes of neoadjuvant transarterial chemoembolization to downstage hepatocellular carcinoma before liver transplantation. Ann Surg 2008;248(4):617–25.

21. Cillo U, Vitale A, Bassanello M, et al. Liver transplantation for the treatment of moderately or well-differentiated hepatocellular carcinoma. Ann Surg 2004; 239(2):150–9.

22. Cillo U, Vitale A, Grigoletto F, et al. Intention-to-treat analysis of liver transplantation in selected, aggressively treated HCC patients exceeding the Milan criteria. Am J Transplant 2007;7(4):972–81.

23. DuBay D, Sandroussi C, Sandhu L, et al. Liver transplantation for advanced hepatocellular carcinoma using poor tumor differentiation on biopsy as an exclusion criterion. Ann Surg 2011;253(1):166–72.

24. Pawlik TM, Gleisner AL, Anders RA, et al. Preoperative assessment of hepatocellular carcinoma tumor grade using needle biopsy: implications for transplant eligibility. Ann Surg 2007;245(3):435–42.

25. Silva MA, Hegab B, Hyde C, et al. Needle track seeding following biopsy of liver lesions in the diagnosis of hepatocellular cancer: a systematic review and meta-analysis. Gut 2008;57(11):1592–6.

26. Schwartz M, Dvorchik I, Roayaie S, et al. Liver transplantation for hepatocellular carcinoma: extension of indications based on molecular markers. J Hepatol 2008; 49(4):581–8.

27. Toso C, Asthana S, Bigam DL, et al. Reassessing selection criteria prior to liver transplantation for hepatocellular carcinoma utilizing the Scientific Registry of Transplant Recipients database. Hepatology 2009;49(3):832–8.

28. Fisher RA, Kulik LM, Freise CE, et al. Hepatocellular carcinoma recurrence and death following living and deceased donor liver transplantation. Am J Transplant 2007;7(6):1601–8.

29. Chao SD, Roberts JP, Farr M, et al. Short waitlist time does not adversely impact outcome following liver transplantation for hepatocellular carcinoma. Am J Transplant 2007;7(6):1594–600.

30. Schlansky B, Chen Y, Austin D, et al. Wait list time predicts survival after liver transplantation for hepatocellular carcinoma: a cohort study in the UNOS Registry. Hepatology 2013;58(SI):208A.

31. Hanouneh IA, Macaron C, Lopez R, et al. Rate of tumor growth predicts recurrence of hepatocellular carcinoma after liver transplantation in patients beyond Milan or UCSF criteria. Transplant Proc 2011;43(10):3813–8.

32. Halazun K, Verna E, Samstein B, et al. A priority pass to death - prioritization of liver transplant for HCC worsens survival. Am J Transplant 2013;13(SI):46.

33. Northup PG, Intagliata NM, Shah NL, et al. MELD inflation: the current hepatocellular carcinoma exception policy is primarily responsible for steadily increasing MELD scores at the time of liver transplant in all regions of the US. Hepatology 2013;58(SI):208A.

The Adolescent Liver Transplant Patient

Deirdre Kelly, FRCPCH, FRCP, FRCPI, MD[a,b],*, Jo Wray, PhD, C Psychol[c]

KEYWORDS

- Pediatric • Liver transplantation • Adolescent • Adherence

KEY POINTS

- Advances in medical and surgical therapy mean that significant numbers of children with previously fatal liver disease survive into adolescence and adult life with or without transplantation.
- Eighty percent of transplant recipients, irrespective of time of transplant, are expected to survive for more than 20 years.
- Survivors of childhood liver disease require a different approach than other young adults. Physicians need to consider their emotional, social, and sexual health and be aware of the high rate of nonadherence both for clinic appointments and medication and the implications for graft loss/progress of liver disease.
- Physicians need to be familiar with the long-term consequences of liver transplantation in childhood and adolescence (eg, renal failure, recurrent disease, osteoporosis, and post-transplant malignancies, especially post-transplant lymphoproliferative disease).
- Developing adequate transitional care for these young people is based on effective collaboration at the pediatric–adult interface and is a major challenge for pediatric and adult providers alike in the 21st century.

INTRODUCTION

Over the last 25 years, there have been significant advances in medical technology and therapy, improving diagnosis and management of pediatric liver disease. Children with previously fatal diseases now survive into adult life in increasing numbers, but some require transplantation in adolescence.

Improvements in operative techniques, preoperative and postoperative management, organ preservation, donor management, and the availability of more potent and less toxic immunosuppressive drugs have contributed to better outcome in

Disclosure: None.
[a] The Liver Unit, Birmingham Children's Hospital, Steelhouse Lane, Birmingham B4 6NH, UK; [b] University of Birmingham, Edgbaston, Birmingham B15 2TT, UK; [c] Critical Care and Cardiorespiratory Division, Great Ormond Street Hospital for Children NHS Foundation Trust, London, United Kingdom
* Corresponding author. The Liver Unit, Birmingham Children's Hospital, Steelhouse Lane, Birmingham B4 6NH, UK.
E-mail address: Deirdre.Kelly@bch.nhs.uk

Clin Liver Dis 18 (2014) 613–632
http://dx.doi.org/10.1016/j.cld.2014.05.006
1089-3261/14/$ – see front matter © 2014 Elsevier Inc. All rights reserved.

pediatric and adolescent liver transplantation (LT). These improvements have led to 1-year survival rates of more than 90% and 5- and 10-year survival rates of 80%.[1–3]

The success of liver transplantation means that the long-term survival rate for child and adolescent recipients of LT is 80% over 20 years; thus most children with liver disease can expect to become adults.

DEFINITION OF ADOLESCENCE

The World Health Organization defines adolescence as the period of growth and development occurring between childhood and adulthood, from 10 to 19 years of age.[4] Adolescents are developmentally, psychologically, and medically distinct from both adults and children.[5]

Adolescence is a challenging time for any young person as adolescents need to

- Achieve autonomy and independence while maintaining supportive links with their family
- Develop a sense of identity, particularly through social relationships

Chronic illness and transplantation in adolescence exaggerate these challenges and place the young person at risk of social isolation, delayed development of peer support networks, and enforced dependency on family members.

SPECIFIC ISSUES IN ADOLESCENCE

Adolescence is a time of egocentrism, a change from concrete to more abstract thinking, and a time for experimenting with risk taking, which is the same for all adolescents including those with liver disease. Although the brain continues to develop through adolescence, it does not do so evenly; the areas controlling physical coordination, emotion, and motivation develop first, and the prefrontal cortex, which is responsible for executive functioning (eg, planning, problem solving, impulse control), does not mature until about 25 years old. The result is a young person who is likely to seek high excitement and indulge in risky behaviors (drugs, alcohol, sex), demonstrating poor planning and judgment without considering negative consequences. Assuming responsibility for managing treatment protocols and adhering to medications can therefore be genuinely challenging for the adolescent with liver disease.

INDICATIONS FOR TRANSPLANTATION

LT is standard therapy for acute or chronic liver failure at any age (**Box 1**).

Chronic Liver Failure

The main reasons for transplantation for chronic liver failure are

- Decompensated cirrhosis
- Portal hypertension unresponsive to therapy
- Intractable variceal bleeding
- Ascites
- Encephalopathy
- Malnutrition

In adolescents, growth failure and delayed puberty with amenorrhea in girls are additional issues.

Box 1
Indications for LT in adolescents

Chronic liver failure

  Biliary atresia

  Autoimmune hepatitis I and II

  Fibropolycystic liver disease +/– Caroli syndrome

  Immunodeficiency

Inborn errors of metabolism

  Alagille syndrome

  Progressive familial intrahepatic cholestasis (PFIC-3)

  a_1-Antitrypsin deficiency

  Cystic fibrosis

  Glycogen storage type IV

  Tyrosinemia type I

  Wilson disease

Acute liver failure

  Acetaminophen poisoning

  Autoimmune hepatitis I and II

  Viral hepatitis (A, B, C, E, or indeterminate)

  Wilson disease

Inborn errors of metabolism with extrahepatic disease

  Crigler–Najjar type I

  Primary oxalosis

Liver tumors

  Benign tumors

  Unresectable malignant tumors

Biliary Atresia

Extrahepatic biliary atresia (EHBA) is a disease of unknown etiology in which there is obstruction or destruction of the extrahepatic biliary tree. It occurs in approximately 1 out of every 15,000 live births.[6] Initial management is based on early diagnosis and palliative surgery, the Kasai portoenterostomy in which the biliary tree is excised to expose biliary channels, and a Roux loop is created for drainage. The operation is successful if there is restoration of biliary flow within 6 months, but is dependent on the age of surgery, the expertise of the surgeon, and the extent of fibrosis at operation.[7]

Biliary atresia is the main indication for LT worldwide and accounts for 76% transplants in children younger than 2 years; 80% of children who have a successful operation do not require transplantation before adolescence.[7]

Inherited Metabolic Liver Disease

a_1-Antitrypsin deficiency

a_1-Antitrypsin deficiency is the most common form of inherited metabolic liver disease in childhood in Europe. Although 50% to 70% of children develop persistent liver disease progressing to cirrhosis, only 20% to 30% require transplantation in childhood or adolescence.[8,9]

Alagille syndrome

This autosomal dominant condition has an incidence of 1 case per 100,000 live births.[10] It is a multisystem disorder with cardiac, facial, renal, ocular, and skeletal abnormalities. The condition is caused by mutations in the *Jagged 1* gene (*JAG1*), which encodes a ligand of *Notch 1*.[11] The main clinical issues are cholestasis, malnutrition, and cardiac or renal disease. The development of liver failure is unusual, and with adequate support, about 50% of children regain normal liver function without significant cholestasis by adolescence, while approximately 30% require liver transplantation.[12]

Progressive Familial Intrahepatic Cholestasis

This group of inherited cholestatic diseases is caused by mutations in the hepatocellular transport system genes involved in bile synthesis. They are rare, with an incidence of 1 case per 50,000 population to 1 case per 100,000 population worldwide occurrence and equal sex distribution.

Progressive familial intrahepatic cholestasis 1 (PFIC1) is caused by mutations in *ATP8B1*[13] and presents in the first months of life with episodes of jaundice and severe pruritus and very high serum bile acid levels. Due to the extrahepatic expression of *ATP8B1*, other clinical features include pancreatitis, diarrhea (loss of the ileal transporter), sensorineural deafness, and short stature.

PFIC2 is caused by mutations in *ABCB11*[14] and presents with persistent cholestasis from birth, coagulopathy secondary to fat-soluble vitamin K deficiency, and pruritus. Hepatocellular carcinoma has been reported in infancy.

PFIC3 is caused by mutations in *ABCB4*[15] and presents anytime during childhood or adult life with complications of chronic liver disease or liver failure. Pruritus is often mild.

PFIC1 and PFIC2 both have low-normal gamma glutamyl transferase (GGT) despite marked cholestasis in contrast to the elevated GGT in PFIC3. Cholesterol tends to be low. Synthetic function is maintained until liver failure develops.

Most patients require LT in childhood, although those with a milder phenotype require transplantation in adolescence for biliary cirrhosis and portal hypertension.

Tyrosinemia Type I

Tyrosinemia type I is an autosomal recessive disorder caused by a defect of fumaryl acetoacetase (FAA).[16] There is a lifetime risk of developing hepatocellular carcinoma (HCC).[17]

Clinical features are heterogeneous, even within the same family. Acute liver failure is a common presentation in infants, while older children or adolescents present with chronic liver disease, rickets, a hypertrophic cardiomyopathy, renal failure or a porphyria-like syndrome with self-mutilation. Renal tubular dysfunction and hypophosphatemic rickets may occur at any age.

Management is with a phenylalanine and tyrosine-restricted diet and nitisone, which prevents the formation of toxic metabolites and allows normal growth and development.[18] The long-term outcome has significantly improved with nitisone therapy and transplantation is now only indicated in those adolescents who do not respond to nitisone, or develop HCC[19] delaying.

Cystic Fibrosis

Cystic fibrosis (CF) occurs in 1 in every 3000 live births worldwide.[20] The gene defect is an abnormality in the cystic fibrosis transmembrane conductance regulator (CFTR) located on chromosome 7 q31. It is a multiorgan disease mainly affecting the lungs and pancreas. Cystic fibrosis associated liver disease (CFLD) occurs in 27% to 35% of patients and usually presents before the age of 18 years.[21] Approximately 5% to 10 % of patients develop cirrhosis and portal hypertension during the first decade of life and present with complications in adolescence or early adult life.[22]

The indications for LT include malnutrition unresponsive to nutritional support, intractable portal hypertension, and hepatic dysfunction. It is essential that transplantation is carried out before pulmonary disease becomes irreversible,[23] especially as there is stabilization of pulmonary function and nutrition, but deaths from respiratory failure in adult life should be anticipated.[24]

Wilson Disease

Wilson disease is an autosomal recessive disorder with an incidence of 1 case per 30,000 live births. The defective gene is on chromosome 13 and encodes a copper transporting P-type adenosinetriphosphatase (ATPase) (ATP7B).[25]

Clinical features in adolescence include hepatic dysfunction (40%) fulminant hepatitis, chronic hepatitis or cirrhosis, and psychiatric symptoms (35%). Neurologic symptoms may be nonspecific, but deteriorating school performance, abnormal behavior, lack of coordination, and dysarthria are common. Renal tubular abnormalities, renal calculi, and hemolytic anemia are associated features.

LT is indicated for those with advanced liver disease (Wilson score >6), fulminant liver failure or progressive hepatic disease despite therapy.[26,27]

Autoimmune liver disease types I and II

Most adolescents with autoimmune liver disease types I or II respond to immunosuppression with prednisolone or azathioprine. LT is indicated for those who present with fulminant hepatic failure, advanced portal hypertension, or in patients who do not respond to immunosuppression despite the use of second-line drugs such as cyclosporine A, tacrolimus, and mycophenalate mofetil.[28]

Fibropolycystic Liver Disease

Fibropolycystic liver disease is a rare indication for LT in adolescence, as liver function remains normal for many years even with severe portal hypertension. Liver replacement is only indicated if hepatic decompensation develops or hepatic enlargement interferes with quality of life. The disease may be associated with polycystic kidney disease, and both liver and kidney replacement may be required at the time of renal replacement.[29]

Primary Immunodeficiency

Young people with CD40 ligand deficiency (hyper IgM syndrome) have recurrent cryptosporidial infection of the gut and biliary tree leading to sclerosing cholangitis. It is important to carry out bone marrow transplantation before the development of significant liver disease or to consider combined liver and bone marrow transplantation.[30]

Timing of Transplantation for Adolescents with Chronic Liver Failure

As many adolescents with cirrhosis and portal hypertension have well-compensated liver function, the timing of LT may be difficult to predict and is based on

- Deterioration in hepatic function
- Failure of nutrition and growth
- Difficulty in maintaining normal life and education

In practice, the need for liver transplantation is indicated by

- Persistent rise in total bilirubin greater than 150 mmol/L

- Prolongation of prothrombin ratio (international normalized ratio [INR] >1.4)
- Fall in serum albumin less than 35 g/L.[1]

These parameters are used in the pediatric end-stage liver disease score (PELD) in order to predict death and provide prioritization on the waiting list.[31,32] There is a modified formula for children older than 12 years.[32]

It is important to consider psychosocial development. Children with chronic liver disease have lower IQ scores[33,34] and significantly impaired motor skills,[33] but some of these impairments, particularly the delay in motor skills, may be reversed following LT if it is performed early enough.[3,31] Thus, any significant delay in developmental or educational parameters is an indication for LT.

ACUTE LIVER FAILURE

The main indications for LT for acute liver failure in adolescence are drug induced, infectious hepatitis, or metabolic disease (eg, Wilson disease).[35,36]

Drug-Induced Liver Failure

Many different drugs cause acute liver failure including antibiotics, antituberculosis therapy, antiepileptic therapy, and Acetaminophen poisoning.[37]

Adolescents have a lower incidence of liver failure with acetaminophen overdose than adults, possibly because of the effect of hepatic maturation and glutathione production.[38] Transplantation is more likely to be required if the overdose was taken with another drug (eg, lysergic acid diethylamide [LSD], Ecstasy) or with alcohol.[39] Transplantation is required if there is a persistent coagulopathy (INR>4), metabolic acidosis (pH<7.3), an elevated creatinine (>300 mmol/l) or rapid progression to hepatic coma grade III. Cerebral edema may persist despite evidence of hepatic regeneration and recovery, and influence postoperative recovery.

Viral hepatitis

Hepatitis A and B are the most common causes of acute liver failure in the developing world.[40,41] However, in the United Kingdom and United States, indeterminate hepatitis is the most common cause (**Box 2**) and has the worst prognosis for spontaneous recovery.[36] Hepatitis C virus (HCV) is a rare cause for acute liver failure.[35] Hepatitis E infection occurs in travelers and is associated with acute liver failure in pregnant women.[42]

MANAGEMENT OF ADOLESCENTS WITH ACUTE LIVER FAILURE

Management includes

- Assessment of prognosis for recovery or liver transplantation
- Prevention and treatment of hepatic complications while awaiting a donor organ/regeneration of native liver
- Provision of psychosocial support and information for patients and parents

Poor prognostic factors for spontaneous recovery are

- Indeterminate hepatitis
- Rapid onset of coma with progression to grade III or IV hepatic coma
- Diminishing liver size
- Falling transaminases
- Increasing bilirubin (>300 mmol/L)
- Persistent coagulopathy (PT >40 seconds; INR >4)
- Hypoglycemia (<2.5 μmol/L)

Box 2
Pretransplant assessment

Nutritional status

  Height, weight, triceps skinfold, midarm muscle area

Identification of hepatic complications

  Ascites, hepatosplenomegaly, varices on endoscopy

Cardiac assessment

  Electrocardiogram, echo, chest radiograph (cardiac catheterization if required)

Respiratory function

  Oxygen saturation[a], ventilation perfusion scan[a], lung function tests[b]

Renal function

  Urea, creatinine, electrolytes

  Urinary protein/creatinine ratio

  Chromium EDTA (if available)

Dental assessment

Radiology

  Ultrasound of liver and spleen for vascular anatomy

  Wrist radiograph for bone age and rickets

  Magnetic resonance imaging/angiography[c]

Serology

  Cytomegalovirus

  Epstein–Barr virus

  Varicella zoster

  Herpes simplex

  Hepatitis A, B, C

  HIV

Measles

Hematology

  Full blood count, platelets, blood group

Psychosocial assessment

Patient and family knowledge and understanding of illness and treatment options, previous/current adherence to treatment, neurocognitive, psychological, and family functioning

  [a] If cyanosed.
  [b] In cystic fibrosis.
  [c] If portal vein anatomy equivocal.

INBORN ERRORS OF METABOLISM

LT is indicated for those metabolic disorders secondary to hepatic enzyme deficiencies that lead to severe extrahepatic disease such as kernicterus in Crigler–Najjar type I and systemic oxalosis in primary oxaluria. Selection and timing of transplantation depends on the quality of life on medical management and the mortality and morbidity of the primary disease compared with the risks of transplantation.[1]

Crigler–Najjar Type I

Crigler–Najjar type I is an autosomal recessive condition caused by a deficiency of bilirubin uridine diphosphate glucuronosyl transferase (UDPGT).[43] Most children require transplantation in early childhood, but those with milder forms may manage with phototherapy into adolescence. The most appropriate operation is auxiliary LT[44] or hepatocyte transplantation.[45]

Primary Hyperoxaluria

Primary hyperoxalurias is a defect of glyoxylate metabolism characterized by the overproduction of oxalate, which is deposited as calcium oxalate in various organs including the kidney.[46] Ideally, liver replacement should be prior to the development of irreversible renal failure. If this is not possible, liver and kidney replacement may be required simultaneously.[47] Children with milder phenotypes will not require intervention until adolescence.

LIVER TUMORS

Liver tumors are an unusual indication for transplantation in adolescence, but occasionally LT is required for unresectable benign tumors causing hepatic dysfunction and unresectable HCC without evidence of extrahepatic metastases.[48,49]

PRETRANSPLANT EVALUATION

This should include

1. Assessment of the severity of the liver disease and complications (see **Box 2**)
2. Establishing the urgency for transplantation
3. Assessment of whether the operation is technically feasible
4. Exclusion of contraindications to successful transplantation
5. Psychological assessment and preparation of the adolescent and family

Renal Function

Careful assessment of renal function is required to modify the potentially nephrotoxic effects of post-transplant immunosuppression and to assess the need for perioperative renal support. Adolescents with pretransplant exposure to nephrotoxic drugs (eg, cystic fibrosis and HCC) are particularly at risk.

Cardiac Assessment

Particular attention should be paid to adolescents with congenital cardiac disease (eg, peripheral pulmonary stenosis in Alagille syndrome). Cardiomyopathy may develop secondary to tyrosinema type I or as a result of chemotherapy of malignant tumors. Cardiac catheterization may be necessary to determine whether: (1) cardiac function is adequate to withstand the hemodynamic changes during the operation; (2) corrective surgery is required preoperatively; or (3) the cardiac defect is inoperable, and LT is contraindicated.[1]

Respiratory Assessment

Few adolescents with end-stage liver disease develop intrapulmonary shunts (hepatopulmonary syndrome) and require pulmonary function studies, ventilation–perfusion scans, bubble echocardiography, and/or cardiac catheterization.[50,51]

Neuropsychological Assessment

The aim of LT is to improve quality of life after the transplant. Thus, it is important to identify any existing neurologic or psychological deficits that may not be reversible after transplantation. The neuropsychological assessment of adolescents may be undertaken using validated tests such as the Wechsler Abbreviated Scale of Intelligence,[52] the Stanford-Binet intelligence scales,[53] and the NEPSY(r)-II.[54]

CONTRAINDICATIONS FOR TRANSPLANTATION

The few contraindications include

1. Severe systemic sepsis, particularly fungal sepsis, at the time of operation
2. Malignant hepatic tumors with extrahepatic spread, because of rapid recurrence
3. Severe extrahepatic disease that is not reversible following LT (eg, severe cardiopulmonary disease for which corrective surgery is not possible), or severe structural brain damage.[1]

PREPARATION FOR TRANSPLANTATION
Immunization

Most adolescents should have been fully immunized in childhood.

Management of Hepatic Complications

Optimum management of hepatic complications is essential.

Nutritional Support

Adequate nutrition is important. In the adolescent, this involves high-calorie supplements to normal diet, but nocturnal nasogastric enteral feeding or continuous feeding may be required. If enteral feeding is not tolerated, due to ascites, variceal bleeding or recurrent hepatic complications, parenteral nutrition is required.

Psychological Preparation

A skilled multidisciplinary team, including a psychologist, is essential for counseling and preparation of the adolescent and family. Young people need to be involved in the decision making wherever possible, and previous experience of illness, knowledge about their condition and treatment, previous/current adherence to prescribed medical regimens, and self-management behaviors need to be explored. Parents and appropriate relatives must be fully informed of the necessity for LT in their child and of the risks, complications, and the long-term implications of the operation.

Particularly careful counseling is necessary for parents and children being considered for transplantation because of extrahepatic disease due to an inborn error of metabolism. As these young people are not dying from liver disease, they may find it difficult to accept the risks and complications and the necessity for compliance with long-term immunosuppression.

Parents of adolescents who require transplantation for acute liver failure may be too distressed to fully appreciate the implications of LT, and the young people themselves may be too ill to be involved in the discussions and decision making. Ongoing counseling and education should be provided postoperatively to help this particular group.

Liver Transplant Surgery

LT is a complex procedure. Grafts are obtained from heart-beating cadavers, non-heart beating donors, or live donors and may be whole, reduced, or split grafts depending on the size of the patient. Grafts are matched by ABO compatibility and if possible by cytomegalovirus (CMV) status.

Post-Transplant Management

The main causes of graft loss in the first week include primary nonfunction (PNF), hepatic artery or portal vein thrombosis, systemic sepsis, and multiorgan failure (<10%). Other significant early complications are acute (50%) or chronic rejection (10%), biliary leaks/strictures (5%–25%), viral infections (especially CMV and Epstein Barr virus), acute kidney injury and fluid imbalance.[2,3,55–58]

Current immunosuppression regimes are based on low-dose calcineurin inhibitors (eg, tacrolimus or cyclosporine) with corticosteroids or mycophenolate mofetil (MMF).[59–61] Induction therapy with the interleukin (IL)-2 receptor antibody basiliximab has improved rejection rates.[62] Addition of MMF or mammalian target of rapamycin (mTOR) inhibitors such as sirolimus allows reduction in steroid and calcineurin inhibitor use.[63]

Survival and Quality of Life

Patient survival rates are 90% at 1 to 5 years[64,65] and 75% at 15 to 20 years with good quality of life.[2,3,66] Survival following transplantation for acute liver failure has improved from 1-year survival from 70% to 87%, with 5-year survival of improved to 67% to 80%.[67–69]

Nutrition, growth, and endocrine development

Most studies demonstrate the beneficial effect of transplantation on improving nutrition and growth, although this depends on the extent of malnutrition preoperatively and the prolonged use of steroids postoperatively. Preoperative weight and height z scores predict catch-up growth, as those who have lower weight percentiles have less growth acceleration, while those with lower height percentiles have accelerated growth.[70]

Chronic liver disease delays the onset of puberty or menarche, but both occur following successful transplantation.[71]

Psychosocial development

Child and adolescent LT patients perform less well on tests of physical and psychosocial functioning compared with healthy norms, although their performance is similar to that of other chronically ill young people. A study of more than 800 recipients found psychosocial function was more affected than physical function, particularly if there was cognitive impairment or significant school absence.[66] In a further study, 16% of adolescents reported symptoms consistent with post-traumatic stress disorder (PTSD),[72] and parents also reported symptoms of PTSD and significant stress and anxiety.[73]

Neurocognitive function

Chronic liver disease from childhood may affect neurodevelopment, possibly because of malnutrition or encephalopathy. Studies evaluating neurocognitive function before and after LT have noted that neurocognitive delay persists after physical rehabilitation.[74] Ten percent to 15% of recipients may have severely impaired intellectual ability, while 30% require special education after transplant.[75] In addition to significant delays in global intelligence, some adolescents have impairments in visuospatial functioning,[76] language, and verbal skills.[77]

In contrast, long-term data from Birmingham (UK) on 117 survivors more than 15 years old demonstrated that 32% had been to university and 50% to college.

Eighteen percent were still at school, and 35% were employed in full-time work, demonstrating that good outcomes are possible.[66]

Quality of life

Quality of life data measured with validated questionnaires suggest that scores are lower in transplant survivors compared with healthy norms,[78–81] although comparable to or better than young people with chronic liver disease, chronic heart failure, diabetes, or those undergoing cancer treatment. In contrast, 1 recent study reported better scores in adolescents after LT than healthy norms.[82]

Emotional functioning is similar to healthy peers, but there is a higher incidence of behavior problems in LT recipients, Those who were transplanted at a young age had higher self-esteem and better family functioning were more likely to have better health-related quality of life.[83,84]

Risk Factors Affecting Survival

Long-term survival and quality of life are affected by late technical complications, graft function, adverse effects of immunosuppression, recurrent disease, adherence, and transition to adult care.[70]

Late technical complications

Late technical complications include hepatic artery thrombosis (3%–10%), late portal vein thrombosis (2%–10%), and biliary strictures (5%–25%). Portal vein anastomotic strictures may develop in reduced or split grafts.

Treatment for hepatic artery thrombosis or portal vein thrombosis may not be required if there is adequate blood flow through collaterals. Thrombolysis is not effective, and surgical reconstruction is contraindicated, so retransplantation may be required, particularly if portal hypertension develops.

Radiological treatment of biliary strictures is indicated if necessary, and drainage of intrahepatic abscesses/bilomas is required.

Maintaining graft function

Immunosuppression Effective immunosuppression is essential to maintain graft function but must be balanced against the risks of adverse effects and overimmunosuppression. The use of calcineurin inhibitor (CNI) regimens, currently based on tacrolimus, has transformed outcomes, as episodes of rejection are less common.[60]

Acute and chronic rejection Acute rejection (AR) usually occurs within 7 to 10 days after transplant but may occur at any time after transplant if immunosuppression is inadequate.[70] Chronic rejection (CR) is a major cause of long-term graft dysfunction and fibrosis and the main indication for retransplantation. It is related to nonadherence in adolescents, particularly after transfer to adult services.[85] The use of the new drugs such as sirolimus may reduce the rate of CR and the need for retransplantation, except in nonadherent adolescents.[63]

Graft hepatitis The use of serial protocol liver biopsies after transplantation has demonstrated the presence of graft or indeterminate hepatitis and fibrosis despite normal biochemistry at 5 and 10 years with a 15% progression to cirrhosis,[86–88] suggesting that this may be a cause for graft failure and retransplantation. Data from Birmingham on 117 pediatric survivors more than 15 years old showed that the main causes of graft dysfunction were CR (33%) and graft fibrosis (33%), but none required transplantation.[66]

No clear etiology for graft hepatitis has been identified, but it may reflect early immunosuppression regimes, especially as graft hepatitis has improved with increased immunosuppression. De novo autoimmune or otherwise unexplained hepatitis occurs in 5% to 10% of children after transplantation but has not been reported to require retransplantation.[89]

Recurrent disease

In contrast to adults, few adolescents are transplanted for diseases that recur after transplant such as hepatitis C, primary sclerosing cholangitis, or autoimmune hepatitis. Recurrence rates and management are similar to adults. However, recurrence may occur following transplantation for the genetic disease PFIC 2 (BSEP; ABCB11), which is related to the development of anti-BSEP antibodies against the BSEP receptor and may need retransplantation.[90]

In young people transplanted for PFIC 1, management focuses on the extrahepatic manifestations, especially diarrhea, which is worse after transplantation and requires bile salt resins for control. Graft steatosis leading to cirrhosis and the need for retransplant may occur.[91]

Adverse effects of immunosuppression

Two-thirds of late post-transplant mortality is associated with the complications of immunosuppression, infection, or malignancy.[70,92] Immunosuppression drugs are associated with an increased risk of renal dysfunction, diabetes, hyperlipidemia, hypertension, obesity, and metabolic syndrome.[93-96]

Renal function

Calcineurin inhibitors contribute to both acute and chronic post-transplant renal dysfunction in 24% to 70% of reported series.[94] Renal function falls by about 30% immediately after transplant and remains stable for 1 to 5 years after transplantation.[96] In the Birmingham study of 117 pediatric survivors more than 15 years old, renal dysfunction occurred in 15% of patients, and 5 patients required a renal transplant.[66]

Diabetes mellitus

The incidence of post-transplant diabetes (PTDM) is much less than observed in adults, and only 10% of primary LT recipients developed new-onset diabetes after transplantation, with cumulative incidences of reaching 11.2% at 5 years. The risk was higher in children with cystic fibrosis, older age at transplant, and African-American race, although the increase in obesity in the population may affect this incidence in the future.[97]

Cardiovascular disease

Cardiovascular disease is a significant comorbidity in adults, and it is likely to affect long-term pediatric survivors on CNI inhibitors, particularly if they become obese or develop metabolic syndrome.[93] Studies in Pediatric Liver and Intestinal Transplant (SPLIT) data on 461 survivors documented obesity in 12% and hypercholesterolemia in 7% at 5 years, while 19% and 23% of 10-year survivors had increased cholesterol and triglycerides.[95] In addition, 20% of 5- to 10-year survivors had blood pressure greater than the 95th percentile or were taking antihypertensive medication.

Sexual health

Contraception and pregnancy Providing appropriate advice to adolescent females about contraception and pregnancy is extremely important, particularly to newly transplanted patients. Most patients are able to safely use hormonal methods of contraception.[98] Many women have had successful pregnancies after LT,[99] but 12 months after transplant is the minimum time before conception. Patients need to be counseled about immunosuppression during pregnancy an the potential for birth complications due to the increased likelihood of pregnancy-induced hypertension and pre-eclampsia.[100] However, mortality is no higher than in the general population, and the rates of AR and graft loss are similar to other LT recipients.[101]

In a Finnish study, adult survivors of pediatric LT reported similar sexual health to controls, although LT recipients had problems with their orgasm strength.[102]

Sexually transmitted diseases Sexually transmitted diseases may be more serious inn immunosuppressed adolescents, so sexual health education should be provided, and the use of barrier contraception encouraged.[103]

Risk-taking behaviors

Risk taking is one of the normal adaptive behaviors used by adolescents to achieve the developmental tasks of identity formation, establishing relationships outside the family, and separation–individuation.[104] Risk-taking behaviors range from age-appropriate benign activities to high-risk substance abuse. Although transplanted adolescents may not be different to their healthy peers with risk-taking behaviors, the consequences may be more serious, particularly if they are nonadherent. Alcohol and drug abuse may damage the transplanted liver, and counseling is needed. Sexual promiscuity may result in unwanted pregnancies, while teenage pregnancies may result in poorer physical health.[105]

Adherence

Non-adherence to the medical regimen is part of the risk-taking spectrum of behavior,[106] and approximately 33% to 50% of adolescents with a chronic illness are nonadherent in some way with their treatment protocol.[107,108] In a recent study, 75% of post-LT adolescents were nonadherent and reported poorer health perceptions, lower self-esteem, more limitations in social and school activities, and poorer mental health than those who were adherent.[79] Factors such as history of substance abuse, previous psychiatric problems, older age, female gender, and living in a 1-parent household have been associated with poorer adherence.[109,110]

Nonadherence to medication is associated with increased medical complications and higher rates of rejection and graft loss.[111–113] In addition, other aspects of nonadherence include clinic nonattendance, missing routine blood tests, and inconsistent timing of medications. The desire to be like their friends can result in nonadherence to different aspects of the treatment regimen. The monitoring and management of nonadherence can be challenging, necessitating a nonjudgmental approach, with a focus on individual adherence plans, improved education, behavioral strategies to encourage self-management and self-motivation and a recognition of the role of treatment burden for patients and their families.[114]

Transition to Adult Care

Increasing survival rates have led to greater numbers of young people transferring to adult care and a growing awareness of the importance of transitional care. Transition can be a risky time for young people because of their complex medical and psychosocial needs, and several studies have identified an increase in nonadherence to medication and hospital visits following transfer to adult clinics, resulting in graft loss and the need for retransplantation in transplant survivors.[115,116] The causes are complex and include the difficulties young people experience in the psychosocial journey from children to adults, their need to become self-reliant, the different approaches adopted in adult and pediatric care, and the loss of psychosocial support as young people move to the adult care system.[117–120]

It is essential to establish a transition team with key workers and trained personnel to manage the process. Several key strategies have been identified to improve the success of transition:

- Use of an individualized transition plan for each young person
- Identified key worker for each young person and family
- Preparation from 11 years onwards
- Regular assessment of patient knowledge of LT and follow-up care, using tools such as a health passport
- Individualized education program addressing medical, educational, vocational and psychosocial aspects
- Guidance on how to shift responsibility for self-management from the parent to the young person
- Strategies for improving a young person's self-management skills
- Assessment of transition readiness
- Not transitioning in a crisis (medical) or during other adolescent transitions (eg, educational)
- Ongoing support from the multidisciplinary team
- Joint adult and pediatric clinics

SUMMARY

The increasing numbers of young people surviving LT and contributing to society are a testament to the advances in both medical and surgical innovation over the last 20 years. Important lessons have been learned about how best to prevent the long-term complications and to preserve graft function, including the need to prepare the adolescent and his or her future adult providers for transfer to adult care.

REFERENCES

1. Kelly DA. Current results and evolving indications for liver transplantation in children. J Pediatr Gastroenterol Nutr 1998;27:214–21.
2. Duffy JP, Kao K, Ko CY, et al. Long-term patient outcome and quality of life after liver transplantation: analysis of 20-year survivors. Ann Surg 2010;252(4):652–61.
3. Kamath BM, Olthoff KM. Liver transplantation in children: update 2010. Pediatr Clin North Am 2010;57(2):401–14.
4. WHO. Maternal, newborn, child and adolescent health: Adolescent development. 2014. Available at: www.who.int/maternal_child_adolescent/topics/adolescence/dev/en/. Accessed January 31, 2014.
5. Radzik M, Sherer S, Neinstein LS. Psychosocial development in normal adolescents. In: Neinstein LS, Gordon C, Katzman D, et al, editors. Adolescent health care: a practical guide. Philadelphia: Lippincott Williams & Wilkins; 2007. p. 27–31.
6. McKiernan PJ, Baker AJ, Kelly DA. The frequency and outcome of biliary atresia in the UK and Ireland. Lancet 2000;355:25.
7. Hartley JL, Davenport M, Kelly DA. Biliary atresia. Lancet 2009;374(9702):1704–13.
8. Francavilla R, Castellaneta SP, Hadzic N, et al. Prognosis of alpha-a-antitrypsin deficiency-related liver disease in the era of paediatric liver transplantation. J Hepatol 2000;32:986–92.
9. Kayler LK, Rasmussen CS, Dykstra DM, et al. Liver transplantation in children with metabolic disorders in the United States. Am J Transplant 2003;3(3):334–9.

10. Li L, Krantz ID, Deng Y, et al. Alagille syndrome is caused by mutations in human Jagged1, which encodes a ligand for NOTCH1. Nat Genet 1997;16(3): 243–51.
11. McDaniell R, Warthen DM, Sanchez-Lara PA, et al. NOTCH2 mutations cause Alagille syndrome, a heterogeneous disorder of the notch signaling pathway. Am J Hum Genet 2006;79(1):169–73.
12. Lykavieris P, Hadchouel M, Chardot C, et al. Outcome of liver disease in children with Alagille syndrome: a study of 163 patients. Gut 2001;49:431–5.
13. Bull LN, van Eijk MJ, Pawlikowska L, et al. A gene encoding a P-type ATPase mutated in two forms of hereditary cholestasis. Nat Genet 1998;18:219–24.
14. Strautnieks SS, Bull LN, Knisely AS, et al. A gene encoding a liver- specific ABC transporter is mutated in progressive familial intrahepatic cholestasis. Nat Genet 1998;20:233–8.
15. Crawford AR, Smith AJ, Hatch VC, et al. Hepatic secretion of phospholipid vesicles in the mouse critically depends on mdr2 or MDR3 P-glycoprotein expression. Visualization by electron microscopy. J Clin Invest 1997;100(10): 2562–7.
16. Heath SK, Gray RG, McKiernan P, et al. Mutation screening for tyrosinaemia type I. J Inherit Metab Dis 2002;25:523–4.
17. Weinberg AG, Mize CE, Worthen HG. The occurrence of hepatoma in the chronic form of hereditary tyrosinemia. J Pediatr 1976;88:434–8.
18. Lindstedt S, Holme E, Lock EA, et al. Treatment of hereditary tyrosinaemia type I by inhibition of 4-hydroxyphenylpyruvate dioxygenase. Lancet 1992;340:813–7.
19. McKiernan PJ. Nitisinone in the treatment of hereditary tyrosinaemia type 1. Drugs 2006;66:743–50.
20. Rowe SM, Miller S, Sorscher EJ. Mechanisms of disease, cystic fibrosis. N Engl J Med 2005;352:1992–2001.
21. Colombo C, Battezzati PM, Crosignani A, et al. Liver disease in cystic fibrosis: a prospective study on incidence, risk factors and outcome. Hepatology 2002;36: 1374–82.
22. Debray D, Lykavieris P, Gauthier F, et al. Outcome of cystic fibrosis-associated liver cirrhosis: management of portal hypertension. J Hepatol 1999;31:77–83.
23. Milkiewicz P, Skiba G, Kelly D, et al. Transplantation for cystic fibrosis: outcome following early liver transplantation. J Gastroenterol Hepatol 2002;17:208.
24. Dowman JK, Watson D, Loganathan S, et al. Long term impact of liver transplantation on respiratory function and nutritional status in children and adults with cystic fibrosis. Am J Transplant 2012;12(4):954–64.
25. Frydman M, Bonne-Tamir B, Farrer LA, et al. Assignment of the gene for Wilson disease to chromosome 13: linkage to the esterase D locus. Proc Natl Acad Sci U S A 1985;82:1819–21.
26. Dhawan A, Taylor RM, Cheeseman P, et al. Wilson's disease in children: 37-year experience and revised King's score for liver transplantation. Liver Transpl 2005; 11:441–8.
27. Rela M, Heaton ND, Vougas V, et al. Orthotopic liver transplantation for hepatic complications of Wilson's disease. Br J Surg 1993;80:909–11.
28. Chai PF, Lee WS, Brown RM, et al. Childhood autoimmune liver disease: indications and outcome of liver transplantation. J Pediatr Gastroenterol Nutr 2010; 50(3):295–302.
29. Rawat D, Kelly D, Milford DV, et al. Phenotypic variation and long-term outcome of children with congenital hepatic fibrosis. J Pediatr Gastroenterol Nutr 2013; 57(2):161–6.

30. Hadzic N. Paediatric sclerosing cholangitis associated with primary immunode-ficiency. J Pediatr Gastroenterol Nutr 1999;28:579.
31. McDiarmid SV, Anand R, Lindblad A, et al. Development of a pediatric end stage liver disease score to predict poor outcome in children awaiting liver transplantation. Transplantation 2002;74:173–81.
32. Shneider BL, Suchy FJ, Emre S. National and regional analysis of exceptions to the Pediatric End-Stage Liver Disease scoring system (2003-2004). Liver Transpl 2006;12(1):40–5.
33. Stewart SM, Uauy R, Waller DA, et al. Mental and motor development correlates in patients with end-stage biliary atresia awaiting liver transplantation. Pediatrics 1987;79:882–8.
34. Moser JJ, Veale PM, McAllister DL, et al. A systematic review and quantitative analysis of neurocognitive outcomes in children with four chronic illnesses. Paediatr Anaesth 2013;23:1084–96.
35. Lee WS, McKiernan P, Kelly DA. Etiology, outcome and prognostic indicators of childhood fulminant hepatic failure in the United Kingdom. J Pediatr Gastroenterol Nutr 2005;40:575–81.
36. Squires RH Jr, Shneider BL, Bucuvalas J, et al. Acute liver failure in children: the first 348 patients in the pediatric acute liver failure study group. J Pediatr 2006; 148:652–8.
37. Murray KF, Hadzic N, Wirth S, et al. Drug-related hepatotoxicity and acute liver failure. J Pediatr Gastroenterol Nutr 2008;47:395–405.
38. Lauterberg BH, Vaishnar Y, Stillwell WB, et al. The effects of age and glutathione depletion on hepatic glutathione turnover in vivo determined by acetaminophen probe analysis. J Pharmacol Exp Ther 1980;213:54–8.
39. Mahadevan SB, McKiernan PJ, Davies P, et al. Paracetamol induced hepatotoxicity. Arch Dis Child 2006;91(7):598–603.
40. Bravo LC, Gregorio GV, Shafi F, et al. Etiology, incidence and outcomes of acute hepatic failure in 0-18 year old Filipino children. Southeast Asian J Trop Med Public Health 2012;43(3):764–72.
41. Barış Z, Saltik Temızel IN, Uslu N, et al. Acute liver failure in children: 20-year experience. Turk J Gastroenterol 2012;23(2):127–34.
42. Ijaz S, Vyse AJ, Morgan D, et al. Indigenous hepatitis E virus infection in England: more common than it seems. J Clin Virol 2009;44(4):272–6.
43. Labrune P, Myara A, Hadchouel M, et al. Genetic heterogeneity of Crigler-Najjar syndrome type I: a study of 14 cases. Hum Genet 1994;94(6):693–7.
44. Rela M, Muiesan P, Vilca-Melendez H, et al. Auxiliary partial orthotopic liver transplantation for Crigler- Najjar syndrome type I. Ann Surg 1999;229(4):565–9.
45. Lysy PA, Najimi M, Stephenne X, et al. Liver cell transplantation for Crigler-Najjar syndrome type I: update and perspectives. World J Gastroenterol 2008;14(22): 3464–70.
46. Rezvani I, Auerbach VH. Primary hyperoxaluria. N Engl J Med 2013;369(22):2162–3.
47. Strobele B, Loveland J, Britz R, et al. Combined paediatric liver-kidney transplantation: analysis of our experience and literature review. S Afr Med J 2013; 103(12):925–9.
48. Romano F, Stroppa P, Bravi M, et al. Favorable outcome of primary liver transplantation in children with cirrhosis and hepatocellular carcinoma. Pediatr Transplant 2011;15(6):573–9.
49. Malek MM, Shah SR, Atri P, et al. Review of outcomes of primary liver cancers in children: our institutional experience with resection and transplantation. Surgery 2010;148(4):778–82 [discussion: 782–4].

50. Hobeika J, Houssain D, Bernard O, et al. Orthotopic liver transplantation in children with chronic liver disease and severe hypoxaemia. Transplantation 1995; 57:224–8.
51. Uemoto S, Vinomarta Y, Tanarka A, et al. Living related liver transplantation in children with hypoxaemia related to intrapulmonary shunting. Transpl Int 1996; 9(Suppl 1):S157–9.
52. Wechsler D. Wechsler abbreviated scale of intelligence. New York: The Psychological Corporation: Harcourt Brace & Company; 1999.
53. Roid GH. Stanford-Binet intelligence scales. 5th edition. Itasca (IL): Riverside Publishing; 2003.
54. Korkman M, Kirk U, Kemp S. NEPSY: a developmental neuropsychological assessment. San Antonio (TX): The Psychological Corporation; 1998.
55. Duffy JP, Hong JC, Farmer DG, et al. Vascular complications of orthotopic liver transplantation: experience in more than 4,200 patients. J Am Coll Surg 2009; 208(5):896–903 [discussion: 903–5].
56. Anderson CD, Turmelle YP, Darcy M, et al. Biliary strictures in pediatric liver transplant recipients - early diagnosis and treatment results in excellent graft outcomes. Pediatr Transplant 2010;14(3):358–63.
57. Martin SR, Atkison P, Anand R, et al. Studies of pediatric liver transplantation 2002: patient and graft survival and rejection in pediatric recipients of a first liver transplant in the United States and Canada. Pediatr Transplant 2004;8(3):273–83.
58. Heffron TG, Pillen T, Smallwood G, et al. Incidence, impact, and treatment of portal and hepatic venous complications following pediatric liver transplantation: a single-center 12-year experience. Pediatr Transplant 2010;14(6):722–9.
59. Kelly D, Jara P, Rodeck B, et al. Tacrolimus and steroids versus ciclosporin microemulsion, steroids, and azathioprine in children undergoing liver transplantation: randomised European multicentre trial. Lancet 2004;364(9439):1054–61.
60. Kelly D. Safety and efficacy of tacrolimus in pediatric liver recipients. Pediatr Transplant 2011;15(1):19–24.
61. Spada M, Petz W, Bertani A, et al. Randomized trial of basimiliximab induction versus steroid therapy in pediatric liver allograft recipients under tacrolimus immunosuppression. Am J Transplant 2006;6:1913–21.
62. Beckebaum S, Klein CG, Sotiropoulos GC, et al. Combined mycophenolate mofetil and minimal dose calcineurin inhibitor therapy in liver transplant patients: clinical results of a prospective randomized study. Transplant Proc 2009; 41(6):2567–9.
63. Casas-Melley AT, Falkenstein KP, Flynn LM, et al. Improvement in renal function and rejection control in pediatric liver transplant recipients with the introduction of sirolimus. Pediatr Transplant 2004;8(4):362–6.
64. Utterson EC, Shepherd RW, Sokol RJ, et al. Biliary atresia: clinical profiles, risk factors, and outcomes of 755 patients listed for liver transplantation. J Pediatr 2005;147(2):180–5.
65. Arnon R, Annunziato R, Miloh T, et al. Orthotopic liver transplantation for children with Alagille syndrome. Pediatr Transplant 2010;14(5):622–8.
66. Legarda M, Smith M, Lewis P, et al. Long term outcome of children following liver transplantation. Pediatr Transplant 2013;17(1):40.
67. Miloh T, Kerkar N, Parkar S, et al. Improved outcomes in pediatric liver transplantation for acute liver failure. Pediatr Transplant 2010;14(7):863–9.
68. Mohamed El Moghazy W, Ogura Y, Mutsuko M, et al. Pediatric living-donor liver transplantation for acute liver failure: analysis of 57 cases. Transpl Int 2010; 23(8):823–30.

69. Farmer DG, Venick RS, McDiarmid SV, et al. Fulminant hepatic failure in children: superior and durable outcomes with liver transplantation over 25 years at a single center. Ann Surg 2009;250(3):484–93.
70. Kelly DA, Bucuvalas JC, Alonso M, et al. Long-term medical management of the pediatric patient after liver transplantation: 2013 Practice Guideline by the American Association for the Study of Liver Diseases and the American Society of Transplantation. Liver Transpl 2013;19:796–825.
71. Codoner-Franch P, Bernard O, Alvarez F. Long-term follow-up of growth in height after successful Liver Transpl. J Pediatr 1994;124:368–73.
72. Mintzer LL, Stuber ML, Seacord D, et al. Traumatic stress symptoms in adolescent organ transplant recipients. Pediatrics 2005;115:1640–4.
73. Young GS, Mintzer LL, Seacord D, et al. Symptoms of posttraumatic stress disorder in parents of transplant recipients: incidence, severity, and related factors. Pediatrics 2003;111:e725–31.
74. Gilmour S, Adkins R, Liddell GA, et al. Assessment of psychoeducational outcomes after pediatric liver transplant. Am J Transplant 2009;9(2):294–300.
75. Gilmour SM, Sorensen LG, Anand R, et al. School outcomes in children registered in the Studies for Pediatric Liver Transplant (SPLIT) consortium. Liver Transpl 2010;16(9):1041–8.
76. Haavisto A, Korkman M, Tormanen J, et al. Visuospatial impairment in children and adolescents after liver transplantation. Pediatr Transplant 2011;15:184–92.
77. Krull K, Fuchs C, Yurk H, et al. Neurocognitive outcome in pediatric liver transplant recipients. Pediatr Transplant 2003;7:111–8.
78. Sanchez C, Eymann A, De Cunto C, et al. Quality of life in pediatric liver transplantation in a single center in South America. Pediatr Transplant 2010;14:332–6.
79. Fredericks EM, Magee JC, Opipari-Arrigan L, et al. Adherence and health-related quality of life in adolescent liver transplant recipients. Pediatr Transplant 2008;12:289–99.
80. Bucuvalas JC, Britto M, Krug S, et al. Health-related quality of life in pediatric liver transplant recipients: a single-center study. Liver Transpl 2003;9:62–71.
81. Kaller T, Boeck A, Sander K, et al. Cognitive abilities, behaviour and quality of life in children after liver transplantation. Pediatr Transplant 2010;14:496–503.
82. Roblin E, Audhuy F, Boillot O, et al. Long-term quality of life after pediatric liver transplantation. Arch Pediatr 2012;19:1039–52.
83. Ng VL, Alonso EM, Bucuvalas JC, et al. Health status of children alive 10 years after pediatric liver transplantation performed in the US and Canada: report of the studies of pediatric liver transplantation experience. J Pediatr 2012;160:820–6.
84. Taylor RM, Franck LS, Gibson F, et al. Study of the factors affecting health-related quality of life in adolescents after liver transplantation. Am J Transplant 2009;9:1179–88.
85. Watson AR. Problems and pitfalls of transition from paediatric to adult renal care. Pediatr Nephrol 2005;20(2):113–7.
86. Evans HM, Kelly DA, McKiernan PJ, et al. Progressive histological damage in liver allografts following pediatric liver transplantation. Hepatology 2006;43(5):1109–17.
87. Scheenstra R, Peeters PM, Verkade HJ, et al. Graft fibrosis after pediatric liver transplant recipients: ten years of follow up. Hepatology 2009;49(3):880–6.
88. Hubscher S. What does the long-term liver allograft look like for the pediatric recipient? Liver Transpl 2009;15(Suppl 2):S19–24.

89. Gupta P, Hart J, Millis JM, et al. De novo hepatitis with autoimmune antibodies and atypical histology: a rare cause of late graft dysfunction after pediatric liver transplantation. Transplantation 2001;71(5):664–8.
90. Keitel V, Burdelski M, Vojnisek Z, et al. De novo bile salt transporter antibodies as a possible cause of recurrent graft failure after liver transplantation: a novel mechanism of cholestasis. Hepatology 2009;50(2):510–7.
91. Lykavieris P, van Mil S, Cresteil D, et al. Progressive familial intrahepatic chole-stasis type 1 and extrahepatic features: no catch-up of stature growth, exacer-bation of diarrhea and appearance of liver steatosis after liver transplantation. J Hepatol 2003;39:447–52.
92. Wallot MA, Mathot M, Janssen M, et al. Long-term survival and late graft loss in pediatric liver transplant recipients– a15-year single-center experience. Liver Transpl 2002;8(7):615–22.
93. Nobili V, de Ville de Goyet J. Pediatric post-transplant metabolic syndrome: new clouds on the horizon. Pediatr Transplant 2013;17:216–23.
94. Bartosh SM, Alonso EM, Whitington PF. Renal outcomes in pediatric liver trans-plantation. Clin Transplant 1997;11(5 Pt 1):354–60.
95. McLin VA, Anand R, Daniels SR, et al, SPLIT Research Group. Blood pressure elevation in long-term survivors of pediatric liver transplantation. Am J Trans-plant 2012;12(1):183–90.
96. Arora-Gupta N, Davies P, McKiernan P, et al. The effect of long-term calcineurin inhibitor therapy on renal function in children after liver transplantation. Pediatr Transplant 2004;8(2):145–50.
97. Kuo HT, Lau C, Sampaio MS, et al. Pretransplant risk factors for new-onset dia-betes mellitus after transplant in pediatric liver transplant recipients. Liver Transpl 2010;16(11):1249–56.
98. Sucato GS, Murray PJ. Developmental and reproductive health issues in adoles-cent solid organ transplant recipients. Semin Pediatr Surg 2006;15:170–8.
99. Armenti VT, Daller JA, Constantinescu S, et al. Report from the National Trans-plantation Pregnancy Registry: outcomes of pregnancy after transplantation. Clin Transplant 2006;57–70.
100. Coscia LA, Constantinescu S, Moritz MJ, et al. Report from the National Trans-plantation Pregnancy Registry (NTPR): outcomes of pregnancy after transplan-tation. Clin Transplant 2008;89–105.
101. Kelly DA, Bucuvalas JC, Alonso EM, et al. Long-term medical management of the pediatric patient after liver transplantation: 2013 practice guideline by the American Association for the Study of Liver Diseases and the American Society of Transplantation. Liver Transpl 2013;19:798–825.
102. Kosola S, Lampela H, Lauronen J, et al. General health, health-related quality of life and sexual health after pediatric liver transplantation: a nationwide study. Am J Transplant 2012;12:420–7.
103. Surti B, Tan J, Saab S. Pregnancy and liver transplantation. Liver Int 2008;28: 1200–6.
104. Ponton LE. The romance of risk. New York: Basic Books; 1997.
105. Patel PH, Sen B. Teen motherhood and long-term health consequences. Matern Child Health J 2012;16:1063–71.
106. Shaw RJ. Treatment adherence in adolescents: development and psychopathol-ogy. Clinical Child Psychology Psychiatry 2001;6:137–50.
107. La Greca AM, Schuman WB. Adherence to prescribed medical regimens. In: Roberts MC, editor. Handbook of pediatric psychology. 2nd edition. New York: Guilford; 1995. p. 55–83.

108. Smith BA, Shuchman M. Problem of nonadherence in chronically ill adolescents: strategies for assessment and intervention. Curr Opin Pediatr 2005;17:613–8.

109. Berquist Berquist RK, Berquist WE, Esquivel CO, et al. Non-adherence to post-transplant care: prevalence, risk factors and outcomes in adolescent liver transplant recipients. Pediatr Transplant 2008;12:194–200.

110. Lurie S, Shemesh E, Sheiner PA, et al. Non-adherence in pediatric liver transplant recipients–an assessment of risk factors and natural history. Pediatr Transplant 2000;4:200–6.

111. Dew MA, Dabbs AD, Myaskovsky L, et al. Meta-analysis of medical regimen adherence outcomes in pediatric solid organ transplantation. Transplantation 2009;88:736–46.

112. Burra P. The adolescent and liver transplantation. J Hepatol 2012;56:714–22.

113. Stuber ML, Shemesh E, Seacord D, et al. Evaluating non-adherence to immunosuppressant medications in pediatric liver transplant recipients. Pediatr Transplant 2008;12:284–8.

114. O'Grady JG, Asderakis A, Bradley R, et al. Multidisciplinary insights into optimizing adherence after solid organ transplantation. Transplantation 2010;89:627–32.

115. Annunziato RA, Emre S, Shneider B, et al. Adherence and medical outcomes in pediatric liver transplant recipients who transition to adult services. Pediatr Transplant 2007;11(6):608–14.

116. Viner R. Transition from paediatric to adult care. Bridging the gaps or passing the buck? Arch Dis Child 1999;81(3):271–5.

117. Soanes C, Timmons S. Improving transition: a qualitative study examining the attitudes of young people with chronic illness transferring to adult care. J Child Health Care 2004;8(2):102–12.

118. McDonagh JE, Kelly DA. Transitioning care of the paediatric recipient to adult caregivers. Pediatr Clin North Am 2003;50(6):1561–83.

119. Viner RM. Transition of care from paediatric to adult services: one part of improved health services for adolescents. Arch Dis Child 2008;93:160–3.

120. Shemesh E, Shneider BL, Savitzky JK, et al. Medication adherence in pediatric and adolescent liver transplant recipients. Pediatrics 2004;113:825–32.

Expanded Criteria Donors

Sandy Feng, MD, PhD[a],*, Jennifer C. Lai, MD, MBA[b]

KEYWORDS

- Deceased donor • Surgery • Outcomes • Steatosis • Donor age

KEY POINTS

- The expanded criteria donor graft connotes an organ with characteristics associated with suboptimal transplant outcomes that fall into 2 categories of risk: (1) graft dysfunction and (2) disease transmission.
- Graft characteristics associated with increased risk of graft dysfunction include older donor age, donation after cardiac death, large droplet steatosis, prolonged cold ischemia time.
- Donor characteristics associated with increased risk of disease transmission include positive hepatitis B core antibody, positive hepatitis C antibody, behaviors known to be associated with increased risk of human immunodeficiency virus, hepatitis B or C infection, and known history of malignancy.

THE SPECTRUM OF DONOR QUALITY: IDEAL, STANDARD, AND EXPANDED

The ideal deceased donor liver, a whole liver from a brain dead donor less than 40 years of age who died of trauma, is well defined. The standard graft and the expanded liver graft are, in contrast, relative concepts that may evolve with time. A standard liver connotes an organ of average quality relative to the spectrum currently utilized for transplantation, while an expanded liver connotes an organ of lower than average quality, coming from a donor with characteristics known to be associated with suboptimal transplant outcomes. There is general consensus that the criteria fall into 2 categories of risk: (1) graft dysfunction and (2) disease transmission.

Donor Risk Factors for Graft Dysfunction

Older donor age

Although the young adult donor is widely recognized as ideal, utilization of livers from older donors represents a logical means to expand the donor pool. In the nontransplant setting, the liver's physiologic function remains well preserved throughout life, likely a result of its unique regenerative capacity.[1] However, in the transplant setting,

Disclosure Statement: The authors have nothing to disclose.
[a] Division of Abdominal Transplantation, Department of Surgery, University of California, 505 Parnassus Avenue, UCSF Box 0780, San Francisco, San Francisco, CA 94143, USA; [b] Division of Gastroenterology/Hepatology, Department of Medicine, University of California, San Francisco, San Francisco, CA, USA
* Corresponding author.
E-mail address: Sandy.feng@ucsfmedctr.org

Clin Liver Dis 18 (2014) 633–649
http://dx.doi.org/10.1016/j.cld.2014.05.005
1089-3261/14/$ – see front matter © 2014 Elsevier Inc. All rights reserved.

liver grafts from older donors are associated with a higher risk of graft failure and mortality.[2–11] Although there is marked heterogeneity in the age cut-offs used to define an older donor, decreased patient and graft survival rates have been reported regardless of the age cut-off used: 50, 60, or 70 years.[4–7] From 2008 to 2012, 1-year unadjusted graft survival for recipients of grafts from donors younger than 40 years, 40 to 49 years, 50 to 59 years, 60 to 69 years, and 70 years and older was 88%, 86%, 84%, 85%, and 82%, respectively ($P<.001$).[12]

There are at least 2 probable mechanisms for this age-related increased risk of liver allograft failure. First, older hepatic parenchyma has increased vulnerability to ischemia/reperfusion injury owing to relatively fewer hepatocytes and decreased regenerative capacity.[1] In mouse models, older livers demonstrate significantly more necrosis and neutrophil accumulation[13] and lower hepatic expression of heat shock proteins that protect hepatocytes from cellular injury.[14] A second, and potentially synergistic, mechanism is the increased burden of medical comorbidities in older donors. Obesity, diabetes, hypertension, and dyslipidemia may lead to hepatic steatosis and atherosclerotic disease,[8,15,16] further increasing susceptibility to injury.

The vulnerability of livers from older deceased donors manifests in multiple pathways of allograft dysfunction or failure. Several studies have shown that older donor livers are associated with primary nonfunction (PNF), defined as initial poor function requiring retransplantation or causing death within 7 days of transplantation.[11,17–19] Recipients of older livers have increased rates of hepatic artery thrombosis[16,20,21] and more severe ischemia reperfusion injury.[9,13,14] Higher rates of biliary complications and cholestasis have also been reported among recipients of livers from donors at least 60 years of age.[5,7] Finally, longer transplant hospitalization length of stay, higher transplant costs, and increased resource utilization are strongly associated with livers with a higher donor risk index, a metric of donor quality dominated by donor age.[22–24]

Interestingly, donor age exerts a differential impact on recipients with chronic hepatitis C virus (HCV) infection. Studies have consistently shown an interaction between older donor age and positive recipient HCV status that predisposes to fibrosing cholestatic hepatitis, more rapid fibrosis, post-transplant infections, graft failure, and mortality.[10,19,25–34] Although age cut-offs defining an older donor for HCV recipients has varied, the negative impact appears to begin at 40 years of age. In an analysis of data on all adult primary, single-organ liver transplants from 1995 to 2001, there was a statistically significant increase in graft loss for every decade increase in donor age starting at 40 years among HCV-infected recipients but not until 60 years in non-HCV-infected recipients (**Fig. 1**).[10]

Utilization of livers from deceased donors of advanced age continues to rise throughout the world,[35–38] and there is currently no consensus on an upper age limit for liver donors. One strategy to minimize risk is to have a lower biopsy threshold. A second strategy is to minimize cold ischemia time (CIT).[6,16,39] This can be accomplished through careful recipient selection, avoiding candidates expected to require protracted dissection, and through careful coordination between organ procurement and initiation of recipient surgery. In 1 Italian study of 178 patients who received livers from donors at least 60 years of age, grafts transplanted with less than 7 versus 7 or more hours of CIT demonstrated significantly higher graft survival at 1 year (84% vs 71%) and 3 years (76% vs 54%) [$P<.005$].[39] Lastly, experts have generally agreed that HCV-infected recipients are suboptimal candidates for older donor livers. This belief is likely to evolve with the availability of increasingly effective and tolerable direct-acting antiviral agents against HCV.

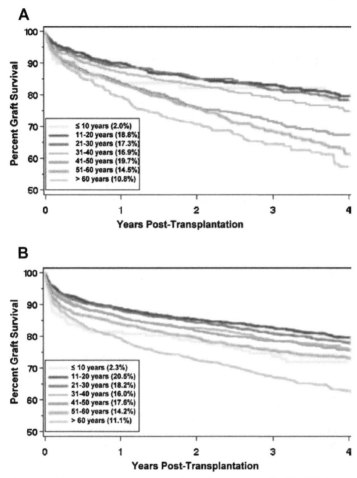

Fig. 1. Graft survival by donor age categories in patients infected with (*A*) chronic hepatitis C and (*B*) without chronic hepatitis C. The proportion of organ recipients for each donor age category is shown in parentheses. (*Adapted from* Lake JR, Shorr JS, Steffen BJ, et al. Differential effects of donor age in liver transplant recipients infected with hepatitis B, hepatitis C and without viral hepatitis. Am J Transplant 2005;5(3):549–57; with permission.)

Donation after cardiac death status

Donation after cardiac death (DCD) refers to the recovery of organs from a donor who has experienced circulatory arrest after withdrawal of life-sustaining medical interventions. Hypoperfusion during the donor's demise—a period termed warm ischemia—represents an additional injury phase that worsens post-transplant outcomes.[3,40–51] Compared with liver grafts from donors after brain death (DBD), DCD liver grafts were associated with a 51% increased risk of graft failure (95% confidence interval [CI], 19%–91%). A meta-analysis of 11 studies reported that DCD recipients (n = 489) experienced higher rates of biliary complications (odds ratio [OR] = 2.4, 95% CI = 1.8–3.4), ischemic cholangiopathy (OR = 10.8, 95% CI = 4.8–28.2), and PNF (OR = 3.6, 95% CI = 2.1–6.4), but not hepatic artery thrombosis (OR = 1.0, 95% CI = 0.6–1.8) when compared with DBD recipients (n = 4455). The odds of

1-year patient (OR = 1.6, 95% CI = 1.0–2.5) and graft (OR = 2.1, 95% CI, 1.5–2.8) survival were also significantly worse.[40]

Despite their worse outcomes, DCD utilization has steeply increased, accounting for 4.5% of all liver transplants in the United States in 2008 compared with 0.5% in 1999.[34] Several approaches have been developed to lessen the ischemic injury, both cold and warm, to improve outcomes.[52,53] Rapid surgical procurement technique and stringent thresholds of 20 to 30 minutes for organ acceptance together limit warm ischemia time, whereas selection of surgically straightforward recipients and early initiation of recipient surgery together limit CIT.[52,53] These strategies, in combination with selection of low-risk recipients (age <60 years, primary transplantation, serum creatinine <2 mg/dL, not on hemodialysis, and not on ventilator support) have yielded comparable graft survival at 1 (81% vs 80%) and 3 years (67% vs 72%) [P = .23] for DCD relative to DBD livers.[51] With careful management, DCD liver transplantation can offer survival benefit to well-selected recipients with Model for End-Stage Liver Disease (MELD) greater than 20 and patients with hepatocellular carcinoma (HCC) without MELD exception points.[54]

Steatosis

Hepatic steatosis refers to the accumulation of lipid droplets in hepatocytes and is an important risk factor for PNF and other post-transplant complications. Upon initial evaluation, aminotransferases in donors with fatty livers are generally normal or near normal but increase markedly after transplantation, suggesting that ischemia/reperfusion injury is the key to graft dysfunction in fatty livers.[55–57] In mouse models of ischemia/reperfusion injury, livers with significant fat accumulation demonstrate increased Kupffer cell activity and decreased oxidative phosphorylation, which results in severe sinusoidal lining cell damage and compromised membrane integrity relative to livers without steatosis.[57–60]

Hepatic steatosis occurs in 2 histologic patterns: macrovesicular and microvesicular (**Fig. 2**A). Traditionally, these patterns have referred to and become synonymous with the size of the fat droplet: macrovesicular for large droplet and microvesicular for small droplet fat. Distinguishing between the types of fat is critical, because the fats exert a differential impact on post-reperfusion outcomes. Compared with either lean mice or obese mice with microvesicular steatosis, obese mice with macrovesicular steatosis

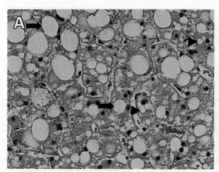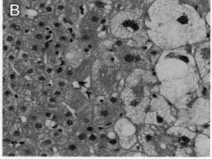

Fig. 2. (*A*) Macrovesicular fat, both large and small droplet. Large droplet (*arrows*) refers to fat globules that occupy greater than one-half of the hepatocyte, whereas small droplet (*arrowheads*) refers to fat globules that occupy less than one-half of the hepatocyte. (*B*) Microvesicular steatosis describes very small, uniform fat globules packed within hepatocytes giving the cytoplasm a characteristic foamy appearance. (*Courtesy of* L. Ferrell, MD, University of California, San Francisco, San Francisco, California.)

demonstrated significantly higher elevations of aminotransferases and more extensive necrosis following ischemia/reperfusion injury[55]; 90% of the lean or obese mice with microvesicular steatosis survived to 14 days after reperfusion compared with 0% of the obese mice with macrovesicular steatosis ($P<.05$).[55]

More recently, pathologists have increasingly recognized that microvesicular steatosis refers to the accumulation of very small, uniform lipid droplets measuring less than 1 μm (see **Fig. 2**B). Histologically, with standard light microscopy, the microvesicles themselves are difficult to discern individually but result in a characteristic foamy-appearing cytoplasm.[61] True microvesicular steatosis is rare and typically associated with conditions such as Reye syndrome, acute fatty liver of pregnancy, or drug toxicity. Macrovesicular steatosis now encompasses both large and/or small fat droplets. Large droplet fat is defined as a lipid droplet that occupies greater than one-half of the hepatocyte, and as such, displaces the cell nucleus. Factors associated with macrovesicular steatosis in the general population include obesity, alcohol intake, diabetes and/or hyperglycemia.[62–66] Unfortunately, much of the literature regarding the impact of steatosis on transplant outcomes predates these new definitions. Therefore, this article will qualify the utilization of the terms macro- and microsteatosis with the terms large and small droplet fat, as appropriate.

There is general agreement that the overall volume of large droplet fat is the key criterion to assess the suitability of a liver for transplantation since small droplet fat has not been associated with poor early graft function.[67,68] Typically, less than 30% volume of large droplet fat has been considered permissive of transplantation, while greater than 60% has been prohibitive, associated with PNF, severe acute kidney injury, longer transplant hospitalization, biliary complications, graft failure, and mortality.[67–72] In the largest study to date investigating the association between steatosis and transplant outcomes using UNOS/OPTN registry data, 5051 (23%) of the 21,777 livers transplanted from 2003 to 2008 had some degree of macrovesicular (large droplet) steatosis, but only 153 livers, or approximately 30 per year nationwide, had greater than 30%.[72] The recipients of these livers had a 71% increased adjusted risk of 1-year graft failure ($P = .007$).[72] Although most experts agree that livers with severe macrovesicular (large droplet) steatosis should be avoided, livers with macrovesicular (large droplet) steatosis between 30% and 60% may result in acceptable outcomes in select donor–recipient combinations.[68,69] Favorable donor factors include age younger than 40 years and CIT less than 6 hours; favorable recipient factors include age less than 60 years, no prior abdominal surgeries, and low MELD score.[68,69]

Historically, procurement surgeons suspect significant steatosis based on the liver's appearance and perform a biopsy to determine the overall fat content and the specific volume of large droplet fat. In situ, steatotic livers often have blunted edges and, when blanched, a yellow as opposed to a reddish-brown hue that becomes more obvious ex vivo, after exsanguination. More recently, pre-procurement liver biopsies have gained popularity as knowing that there is significant large droplet fat can initiate mitigation strategies. Pre-procurement liver biopsies are typically triggered by factors such as metabolic syndrome or alcohol intake. However, abdominal imaging — either ultrasound or cross-sectional — can also suggest hepatic steatosis. Of 492 living liver donors whose ultrasound did not suggest steatosis, 61% had none (<5%); 38% had mild (≥5–29%), and 0.8% had moderate (≥30–59%) large droplet fat on liver biopsy. No one had severe (≥60%) large droplet fat on liver biopsy.[66] In a study of unenhanced computed tomography scan and same-day percutaneous liver biopsy, both visual grading and the liver attenuation index accurately identified large droplet fat of at least 30% with area under the receiver operating characteristics curves of 0.93 (95% CI, 0.82–1.00) and 0.93 (95% CI, 0.88–0.98), respectively.[73]

Although demographics, medical history, radiographic imaging, and/or visual inspection can suggest hepatic steatosis, assessment of a fresh frozen liver biopsy remains the gold standard to determine a liver's transplantability. Histologic assessment is the only method to determine the volume of large droplet fat. Unfortunately, there are several sources of inaccuracy, including insufficient sampling, misinterpretation of freezing artifact, and inter-/intraobserver variability among pathologists who are often located at donor hospitals with little experience providing a (semi-)quantitative assessment of large and small droplet fat on frozen liver biopsies.[74,75]

Cold ischemia time

CIT is defined as the time from cardiac arrest and the initiation of in situ cold flush in the donor to removal of the organ from cold storage for implantation into the recipient. There is widespread agreement that increased CIT is associated with inferior post-transplant outcomes.[3,34,35,72,76,77] An analysis of donor and transplant-related factors using UNOS/OPTN registry data has shown that, for every hour of CIT above 8 hours, the adjusted risk of graft failure increases by 2% (95% CI = 1–3%).[35] This has been confirmed in the continental European liver transplant experience; every 15-minute increase in CIT increases 1-year graft failure risk by 0.9% (95% CI = 0.5–1.3%).[76] In addition, the risk of developing nonanastomotic biliary strictures significantly increased with every hour increase in CIT (relative risk [RR] = 1.16, 95% CI = 1.04–1.29),[78] as biliary epithelium may be particularly sensitive to ischemia-induced oxidative stress after reperfusion.[79]

Notably, CIT has significantly decreased in the United States from a median (interquartile range) of 7.1 (6.0–9.4) hours from 1998 to 2002 to 6.6 (5.0–8.3) hours from 2007 to 2010 (P<.001).[35] Europe and Canada have reported similar trends.[36,76]

Donor Risk Factors for Disease Transmission

Viral hepatitis B

Hepatitis B core antibody positive donors Utilization of organs from hepatitis B virus (HBV) surface antigen negative (HBsAg−) but hepatitis B core antibody positive (HBcAb+) donors is an accepted means of expanding the organ donor pool. This serologic profile identifies a donor who has spontaneously cleared HBV infection but who may continue to harbor covalently closed circular HBV DNA in the liver. Among 133 HBcAb+ but HBsAg− individuals in the United States, 8% had detectable HBV DNA in the liver.[80] In contrast, in a Japanese study of 22 HBcAb+ living donors with undetectable serum HBV DNA, all had detectable HBV DNA in the liver,[81] suggesting that intrahepatic HBV DNA may be more frequently present with spontaneous clearance after vertical transmission compared with adult acquisition. The prevalence of HBcAb positivity among liver donors varies widely by country: 5% in the United States,[3] 12% in Spain,[82] 7% in France,[83] 15% in Italy,[84] and upwards of 60% in East Asian countries where chronic HBV infection is endemic.[85,86]

Two clinically significant scenarios can ensue after transplantation of an HBcAb+ liver unless appropriate prophylaxis is administered: (1) de novo HBV infection, defined by detection of HBsAg in a patient without previous HBV infection or (2) recurrent HBV infection, defined as HBV viremia in a recipient with previously suppressed HBV infection. Two large meta-analyses covering studies from 2 overlapping time periods (462 transplants from 1966 to 2009 and 903 transplants from 1995 to 2010) reported that de novo HBV infection occurred in 28% to 58% of HBsAg- recipients.[87,88] Traditionally, 3 tiers of prophylaxis have substantially prevented de novo infection: (1) HBV immune globulin (HBIg) alone (19%), (2) oral nucleos(t)ide alone (2.6% for lamivudine), or (3) combination HBIg and oral nucleos(t)ide (2.8% for HBIg and lamivudine).[87] Although there is currently sparse literature regarding the efficacy of newer-generation nucleos(t)ide analogues, the high potency and resistance barriers of both entecavir and tenofovir, compared with lamivudine, telbivudine, or adefovir, predict even lower rates of de novo HBV infection.

When possible, HBcAb+ grafts should be utilized in recipients with chronic HBV who require post-transplant HBV suppressive therapy. Nine studies that evaluated this strategy of donor–recipient matching identified HBV recurrence in 11 of 80 recipients who received HBIg alone, lamivudine alone, or combination HBIg and lamivudine.[83,89–96] One instructive study of 10 recipients with HBV DNA sequencing data from pretransplant serum/explant liver samples and post-transplant liver biopsies reported that intrahepatic HBV DNA was donor derived in 2 patients, recipient derived in 4 patients, and both donor and recipient derived in 6 patients.[96]

Whether transplantation with organs from HBcAb+ versus HBcAb− donors is associated with a decrement in survival remains controversial. Among 1270 US liver transplant recipients of HBcAb+ grafts from 1994 to 2006, the adjusted hazard ratio (HR) for graft survival was 1.09 (95% CI, 0.97–1.21).[97] In contrast, a more recent analysis of all liver transplants in Italy from 2007 to 2009 revealed a significantly elevated risk of graft loss associated with livers from HBcAb+ donors (HR, 1.56; 95% CI, 1.18–2.04).[84] Interestingly, only one of these graft losses in the HBcAb+ group occurred secondary to de novo hepatitis, suggesting that HBcAb positivity may be a surrogate for suboptimal donor quality.

HBsAg+ donors

Finally and notably, there has been recent interest but limited experience in transplantation of livers without significant fibrosis from HBsAg+ donors into HBsAg+ recipients who require post-transplant HBV therapy regardless of their donor HBV status. Appropriate antiviral suppressive therapy has prevented HBV recurrence in 8 recipients at a median follow-up of approximately 2 years.[98]

Viral hepatitis C

HCVAb+ donors account for 3% of the US deceased donor pool between 2007 and 2010. Because de novo HCV infection is essentially certain with transplantation of these grafts into HCV-naïve recipients, utilization of HCVAb+ livers is limited exclusively to HCV-viremic recipients.[35] UNOS/OPTN registry analysis has shown comparable patient and graft survival for recipients of HCVAb+ versus HCVAb− grafts from 1994 to 2008.[99,100] Whether grafts from HCVAb+ donors are associated with more rapid HCV recurrence remains controversial. In 1 multicenter study of 5 US transplant centers, recipients of HCVAb+ (n = 99) compared with HCVAb− (n = 1107) liver recipients experienced a 58% increased risk of advanced fibrosis, defined as Ludwig-Batts stage 3 or 4 disease.[27] The increased risk of aggressive recurrent disease appears to be driven by HCVAb+ donors older than 45 years (HR = 1.78, 95% CI, 1.10–2.88) but not by donors 45 years old or younger (HR = 1.34; 95% CI = 0.70–2.54).[27] In a multicenter European study, the mean [± standard deviation (SD)] time to HCV recurrence was numerically faster but statistically similar between recipients of grafts from 63 HCVAb+ compared with 63 HCVAb− matched donors (8.4 ± 12.8 months versus 13.4 ± 20 months [P = .07]).[101] However, when stratified by the liver's stage of fibrosis at the time of transplant, HCV recurrence occurred more rapidly in grafts with fibrosis stage 1 or greater versus no fibrosis (P = .03).[101]

Because donor HCV genotype is typically unknown at the time of donation, and HCV genotype 1 is the most common in the United States, transplantation with HCVAb+ grafts has traditionally been restricted to recipients with genotypes 1 or 4. This strategy avoids transmitting genotypes known to have lower sustained virologic response rates with antiviral treatment (1 and 4) into recipients with the more favorable genotypes 2 or 3. The approval of more effective and more tolerable direct-acting antiviral agents against all HCV genotypes may obviate this restriction in the near future.

Human immunodeficiency virus

In 2013, the passage of the HIV Organ Policy (HOPE) Act opened the doors to allow transplantation with organs from human immunodeficiency virus (HIV)-positive donors into HIV-infected recipients.[102] This is anticipated to increase the number of organs available to HIV-infected recipients; evaluation of data from the Nationwide Inpatient Sample from 2005 to 2008 estimated that the pool of liver donors would increase by approximately 55 per year.[103] In addition, as the number of transplant centers that perform transplantation for HIV-infected recipients is currently limited, the HOPE Act may also encourage transplant centers to accept HIV-infected candidates for transplantation, thereby increasing access to HIV-infected individuals to transplant.[104]

Centers for Disease Control and Prevention classification of donors at increased risk for infection transmission

The Centers for Disease Control and Prevention (CDC) has identified that certain donor characteristics are associated with an increased risk of transmission of HIV, HCV, and/or HBV (**Box 1**).[105] Although donors who meet one or more of these criteria

---

Box 1
CDC guidelines for factors associated with an increased risk for recent HIV, HBV, or HCV infection

1. People who have had sex with a person known or suspected to have HIV, HBV, or HCV infection in the preceding 12 months

2. Men who have had sex with men (MSM) in the preceding 12 months

3. Women who have had sex with a man with a history of MSM behavior in the preceding 12 months

4. People who have had sex in exchange for money or drugs in the preceding 12 months

5. People who have had sex with a person who had sex in exchange for money or drugs in the preceding 12 months

6. People who have had sex with a person who injected drugs by intravenous, intramuscular, or subcutaneous route for nonmedical reasons in the preceding 12 months

7. A child who is less than 18 months of age and born to a mother known to be infected with, or at increased risk for, HIV, HBV, or HCV infection

8. A child who has been breastfed within the preceding 12 months, and the mother is known to be infected with, or at increased risk for, HIV infection

9. People who have injected drugs by intravenous, intramuscular, or subcutaneous route for non-medical reasons in the preceding 12 months

10. People who have been in lockup, jail, prison, or a juvenile correctional facility for more than 72 consecutive hours in the preceding 12 months

11. People who have been newly diagnosed with, or have been treated for syphilis, gonorrhea, chlamydia, or genital ulcers in the preceding 12 months

12. People who have been on hemodialysis in the preceding 12 months

Data from Seem DL, Lee I, Umscheid CA, et al. PHS guideline for reducing human immunodeficiency virus, hepatitis B virus, and hepatitis C virus transmission through organ transplantation. Public Health Rep 2013;128:247–392.

are generally younger and have fewer medical comorbidities than those who do not meet any of the criteria,[106] unintended infection transmission is a significant public health concern. The prevalence of HIV and HCV among donors classified as at increased risk for infection transmission, adjusted for false-positive antibody test results, is 0.5% and 18.2%, respectively,[107] substantially higher than the 0.1% and 3.5% baseline prevalence among donors who are not classified as at increased risk.[107] From 2005 to 2007, when all solid organ donors were required to undergo testing for HIVAb and HCVAb,[105] there were 7 cases of donor-derived HIV infection from 3 donors and 9 cases of donor-derived HCV infection from 5 donors in the United States; eight of these transmissions resulted in active infection in the recipients, and 2 transmissions resulted in death.[108,109]

In 2013, the CDC issued new guidelines recommending HCV nucleic acid testing (NAT) for all deceased donors and HIV NAT for those with at least 1 risk factor (see **Box 1**).[110] Compared with serologic testing that requires a host's immune response to generate antiviral antibodies, NAT simply requires sufficient viral replication for viral nucleic acid to be detectible in the circulation. Because it is both more sensitive and specific, NAT significantly reduces the risk of transmission when donors have recently contracted HIV or HCV or have false-negative HIVAb or HCVAb results.[111–114] The estimated risk of unintended infection transmission per 100,000 person-years from solid organ donors classified at increased risk decreases from 8.5 (95% CI, 1.5–23.4) to 2.7 (95% CI, 0.5–7.4) for HIV and from 104.9 (95% CI, 56.8–170.8) to 10.5 (95% CI, 5.6–17.2) for HCV.[107] NAT cannot eliminate transmission risk completely, as there will always remain some time immediately after infection during which there is insufficient circulating viral nucleic acid to be detected by available assays.

Cancer
Donor tumor transmission through liver transplantation has been rare. The Israel Penn International Transplant Tumor Registry has reported 38 cases in liver transplant recipients between 1965 and 2003.[115] In the United States, donor tumor transmission of neuroendocrine, pancreatic, adenocarcinoma, melanoma, and undifferentiated squamous cell carcinoma was documented in 5 liver transplant recipients between 1994 and 2000, representing 0.02% of all liver transplants[116] and resulting in 2 deaths (neuroendocrine and melanoma). Four additional cases of donor-derived tumor transmission (hepatocellular carcinoma, lymphoma, small cell lung cancer, and melanoma [possible]) were reported in 2007.[108] In the United Kingdom, 15 (0.05%) reported cases of tumor transmission among 30,765 organ transplants from 2001 to 2010 resulted in a 20% mortality rate directly attributed to the donor-derived tumor.[117]

Tumor transmission in solid organ transplantation can occur and has occurred from donors with or without a history of malignancy. Acceptance of livers from donors with a known history of cancer—either current or past—is a challenging decision for both transplant surgeons and patients who must consider the estimated risk that the tumor cells have (micro)metastasized to or are within the circulation of the donor liver. At a minimum, thorough inspection of all organs at the time of organ procurement is essential with biopsy of any suspicious lesion(s).

In 2003, a diverse group of transplant experts convened to review the current understanding of tumors in transplantation and to make specific recommendations about the organ utilization from donors with a history of malignancy. At this symposium, tumors were classified by risk of post-transplant recurrence (**Table 1**).[118] Glioblastoma multiforme, melanoma, choriocarcinoma, and lung cancer were determined to be absolute contraindications to organ donation.[118] With respect to central nervous system tumors, in addition to glioblastoma multiforme, whose aggressive

Table 1
Risk of post-transplant recurrence of pre-existing malignancy

Risk Group	Tumor Type	Patients (n)	Patents Treated >5 y Prior to Transplantation (%)	Overall Recurrence Risk (%)
Low	Incidental renal cell carcinoma (RCC)[a]	72	0	1
	Uterine	26	50	4
	Testicular	43	58	5
	Cervical	93	54	6
	Thyroid	54	38	7
Moderate	Lymphoma	37	76	11
	Wilm	78	33	13
	Prostate	33	34	18
	Colon	53	42	21
High	Breast	90	51	23
	Symptomatic RCC	222	22	27
	Bladder	55	22	29
	Sarcoma	17	24	29
	Skin	125	11	53

[a] Refers only to tumors incidentally discovered at time of bilateral nephrectomy before or concurrent with renal transplantation.

Data from Feng S, Buell JF, Chari RS, et al. Tumors and transplantation: the 2003 Third Annual ASTS State-of-the-Art Winter Symposium. Am J Transplant 2003;3(12):1481–7.

biology disrupts the blood–brain barrier, ventriculo-peritoneal shunting and invasive surgical procedures represent risk factors for tumor transmission through transplantation.[119,120] For common cancers such as breast and colon cancers, although advanced-stage disease (colon cancer stage ≥T3 or breast cancer ≥T1c) was

Table 2
Recommendations for utilization of organs from donors with a history of early stage colon and breast cancer

Cancer/Stage	Specific Characteristics	Survival	Recommended Disease-Free Interval
Colon/0 = CIS		5 y: 99%–100%	0
Colon/1 = T1/T2	Caucasian male	5 y: >95%	>1 y
Colon/1 = T1/T2	Caucasian female	5 y: 90%–95%	>5 y
Colon/1 = T1/T2	African American male	5 y: <90%	Never
Breast/0 = CIS	High risk[a] = comedo histology, extensive or high-grade disease	5 y: 99%–100%	0
Breast/1 = T1a[b] or T1b[c]		10 y: 91%	10 y
Breast/T1 = 1c[d]		10 y: 78%	Never

[a] Presence of these high-risk characteristics may increase risk of nodal disease from less than 1% to approximately 2%.
[b] 0.1 cm < Tumor < 0.5 cm.
[c] 0.5 cm < Tumor < 1.0 cm.
[d] 1.0 cm < Tumor < 2.0 cm.

Data from Feng S, Buell JF, Chari RS, et al. Tumors and transplantation: the 2003 Third Annual ASTS State-of-the-Art Winter Symposium. Am J Transplant 2003;3(12):1481–7.

considered an absolute contraindication, early stage disease may be permissible for donation, depending on the exact tumor stage and the disease-free interval **(Table 2)**.[118]

REFERENCES

1. Schmucker DL. Aging and the liver: an update. J Gerontol A Biol Sci Med Sci 1998;53(5):B315–20.
2. Kim DY, Moon J, Island ER, et al. Liver transplantation using elderly donors: a risk factor analysis. Clin Transplant 2011;25(2):270–6.
3. Feng S, Goodrich N, Bragg-Gresham J, et al. Characteristics associated with liver graft failure: the concept of a donor risk index. Am J Transplant 2006; 6(4):783–90.
4. Hoofnagle JH, Lombardero M, Zetterman RK, et al. Donor age and outcome after liver transplantation. Hepatology 1996;24(1):89–96.
5. Washburn WK, Johnson LB, Lewis WD, et al. Graft function and outcome of older (> or = 60 years) donor livers. Transplantation 1996;61(7):1062–6.
6. Singhal A, Sezginsoy B, Ghuloom AE, et al. Orthotopic liver transplant using allografts from geriatric population in the United States: is there any age limit? Exp Clin Transplant 2010;8(3):196–201.
7. Busquets J, Xiol X, Figueras J, et al. The impact of donor age on liver transplantation: influence of donor age on early liver function and on subsequent patient and graft survival. Transplantation 2001;71(12):1765–71.
8. Nardo B, Masetti M, Urbani L, et al. Liver transplantation from donors aged 80 years and over: pushing the limit. Am J Transplant 2004;4(7):1139–47.
9. Marino IR, Doyle HR, Aldrighetti L, et al. Effect of donor age and sex on the outcome of liver transplantation. Hepatology 1995;22(6):1754–62.
10. Lake JR, Shorr JS, Steffen BJ, et al. Differential effects of donor age in liver transplant recipients infected with hepatitis B, hepatitis C and without viral hepatitis. Am J Transplant 2005;5(3):549–57.
11. Moore DE, Feurer ID, Speroff T, et al. Impact of donor, technical, and recipient risk factors on survival and quality of life after liver transplantation. Arch Surg 2005;140(3):273–7.
12. Lai JC, Vittinghoff E, Feng S. The evolving face of liver donors in the United States: updating the donor risk index. Am J Transplant 2013;13(S5) [abstract: 188].
13. Park Y, Hirose R, Coatney JL, et al. Ischemia-reperfusion injury is more severe in older versus young rat livers. J Surg Res 2007;137(1):96–102.
14. Okaya T, Blanchard J, Schuster R, et al. Age-dependent responses to hepatic ischemia/reperfusion injury. Shock 2005;24(5):421–7.
15. Jiménez-Romero C, Clemares-Lama M, Manrique-Municio A, et al. Long-term results using old liver grafts for transplantation: sexagenerian versus liver donors older than 70 years. World J Surg 2013;37(9):2211–21.
16. Grazi GL, Cescon M, Ravaioli M, et al. A revised consideration on the use of very aged donors for liver transplantation. Am J Transplant 2001;1(1):61–8.
17. Ploeg RJ, D'Alessandro AM, Knechtle SJ, et al. Risk factors for primary dysfunction after liver transplantation–a multivariate analysis. Transplantation 1993; 55(4):807–13.
18. Strasberg SM, Howard TK, Molmenti EP, et al. Selecting the donor liver: risk factors for poor function after orthotopic liver transplantation. Hepatology 1994; 20(4 Pt 1):829–38.

19. Uemura T, Nikkel LE, Hollenbeak CS, et al. How can we utilize livers from advanced aged donors for liver transplantation for hepatitis C? Transpl Int 2012;25(6):671–9.

20. Wall WJ, Mimeault R, Grant DR, et al. The use of older donor livers for hepatic transplantation. Transplantation 1990;49(2):377–81.

21. DeBakey ME, Lawrie GM, Glaeser DH. Patterns of atherosclerosis and their surgical significance. Ann Surg 1985;201(2):115–31.

22. Showstack J, Katz PP, Lake JR, et al. Resource utilization in liver transplantation: effects of patient characteristics and clinical practice. NIDDK Liver Transplantation Database Group. JAMA 1999;281(15):1381–6.

23. Salvalaggio PR, Dzebisashvili N, MacLeod KE, et al. The interaction among donor characteristics, severity of liver disease, and the cost of liver transplantation. Liver Transpl 2011;17(3):233–42.

24. Axelrod DA, Gheorghian A, Schnitzler MA, et al. The economic implications of broader sharing of liver allografts. Am J Transplant 2011;11(4):798–807.

25. Cescon M, Grazi GL, Ercolani G, et al. Long-term survival of recipients of liver grafts from donors older than 80 years: is it achievable? Liver Transpl 2003; 9(11):1174–80.

26. Ghobrial RM, Gornbein J, Steadman R, et al. Pretransplant model to predict posttransplant survival in liver transplant patients. Ann Surg 2002;236(3): 315–22 [discussion: 322–3].

27. Lai JC, O'Leary JG, Trotter JF, et al. Risk of advanced fibrosis with grafts from hepatitis C antibody-positive donors: a multicenter cohort study. Liver Transpl 2012;18(5):532–8.

28. Shores NJ, Dodge JL, Feng S, et al. Donor risk index for African American liver transplant recipients with hepatitis C virus. Hepatology 2013;58(4):1263–9.

29. Lai JC, Verna EC, Brown RS, et al. Hepatitis C virus-infected women have a higher risk of advanced fibrosis and graft loss after liver transplantation than men. Hepatology 2011;54(2):418–24.

30. Wali M, Harrison RF, Gow PJ, et al. Advancing donor liver age and rapid fibrosis progression following transplantation for hepatitis C. Gut 2002;51(2): 248–52.

31. Khapra AP, Agarwal K, Fiel MI, et al. Impact of donor age on survival and fibrosis progression in patients with hepatitis C undergoing liver transplantation using HCV+ allografts. Liver Transpl 2006;12(10):1496–503.

32. Alonso O, Loinaz C, Moreno E, et al. Advanced donor age increases the risk of severe recurrent hepatitis C after liver transplantation. Transpl Int 2005;18(8): 902–7.

33. Samonakis DN, Triantos CK, Thalheimer U, et al. Immunosuppression and donor age with respect to severity of HCV recurrence after liver transplantation. Liver Transpl 2005;11(4):386–95.

34. Thuluvath PJ, Guidinger MK, Fung JJ, et al. Liver transplantation in the United States, 1999-2008. Am J Transplant 2010;10(4 Pt 2):1003–19.

35. Lai JC, Vittinghoff E, Feng S. The evolving face of the liver donor: updating the donor risk index [abstract]. Am J Transplant 2013;13(S5):4–589.

36. Sela N, Croome KP, Chandok N, et al. Changing donor characteristics in liver transplantation over the last 10 years in Canada. Liver Transpl 2013;19(11): 1236–44.

37. Adam R, Karam V, Delvart V, et al. Evolution of indications and results of liver transplantation in Europe. A report from the European Liver Transplant Registry(ELTR). J Hepatol 2012;57(3):675–88.

38. Halldorson J, Roberts JP. Decadal analysis of deceased organ donation in Spain and the United States linking an increased donation rate and the utilization of older donors. Liver Transpl 2013;19(9):981–6.
39. Ravaioli M, Grazi GL, Cescon M, et al. Liver transplantations with donors aged 60 years and above: the low liver damage strategy. Transpl Int 2009;22(4): 423–33.
40. Jay CL, Lyuksemburg V, Ladner DP, et al. Ischemic cholangiopathy after controlled donation after cardiac death liver transplantation. Ann Surg 2011; 253(2):259–64.
41. Abt PL, Desai NM, Crawford MD, et al. Survival following liver transplantation from non-heart-beating donors. Ann Surg 2004;239(1):87–92.
42. Chan EY, Olson LC, Kisthard JA, et al. Ischemic cholangiopathy following liver transplantation from donation after cardiac death donors. Liver Transpl 2008; 14(5):604–10.
43. de Vera ME, Lopez-Solis R, Dvorchik I, et al. Liver transplantation using donation after cardiac death donors: long-term follow-up from a single center. Am J Transplant 2009;9(4):773–81.
44. Foley DP, Fernandez LA, Leverson G, et al. Donation after cardiac death. Ann Surg 2005;242(5):724–31.
45. Fujita S, Mizuno S, Fujikawa T, et al. Liver transplantation from donation after cardiac death: a single center experience. Transplantation 2007; 84(1):46–9.
46. Manzarbeitia CY, Ortiz JA, Jeon H, et al. Long-term outcome of controlled, non-heart-beating donor liver transplantation. Transplantation 2004;78(2):211 5.
47. Grewal HP, Willingham DL, Nguyen J, et al. Liver transplantation using controlled donation after cardiac death donors: an analysis of a large single-center experience. Liver Transpl 2009;15(9):1028–35.
48. Pine JK, Aldouri A, Young AL, et al. Liver transplantation following donation after cardiac death: an analysis using matched pairs. Liver Transpl 2009;15(9): 1072–82.
49. Skaro AI, Jay CL, Baker TB, et al. The impact of ischemic cholangiopathy in liver transplantation using donors after cardiac death: the untold story. Surgery 2009; 146(4):543–53.
50. Merion RM, Pelletier SJ, Goodrich N, et al. Donation after cardiac death as a strategy to increase deceased donor liver availability. Trans Meet Am Surg Assoc Am Surg Assoc 2006;124:220–7.
51. Mateo R, Cho Y, Singh G, et al. Risk factors for graft survival after liver transplantation from donation after cardiac death donors: an analysis of OPTN/UNOS data. Am J Transplant 2006;6(4):791–6.
52. Vanatta JM, Dean AG, Hathaway DK, et al. Liver transplant using donors after cardiac death: a single-center approach providing outcomes comparable to donation after brain death. Exp Clin Transplant 2013;11(2):154–63.
53. Hong JC, Yersiz H, Kositamongkol P, et al. Liver transplantation using organ donation after cardiac death: a clinical predictive index for graft failure-free survival. Arch Surg 2011;146(9):1017–23.
54. Jay CL, Skaro AI, Ladner DP, et al. Comparative effectiveness of donation after cardiac death versus donation after brain death liver transplantation: recognizing who can benefit. Liver Transpl 2012;18(6):630–40.
55. Selzner N, Selzner M, Jochum W, et al. Mouse livers with macrosteatosis are more susceptible to normothermic ischemic injury than those with microsteatosis. J Hepatol 2006;44(4):694–701.

56. Berthiaume F, Barbe L, Mokuno Y, et al. Steatosis reversibly increases hepato-cyte sensitivity to hypoxia-reoxygenation injury. J Surg Res 2009;152(1):54–60.
57. Taneja C, Prescott L, Koneru B. Critical preservation injury in rat fatty liver is to hepatocytes, not sinusoidal lining cells. Transplantation 1998;65(2):167–72.
58. Teramoto K, Bowers JL, Kruskal JB, et al. Hepatic microcirculatory changes after reperfusion in fatty and normal liver transplantation in the rat. Transplantation 1993;56(5):1076–82.
59. Fukumori T, Ohkohchi N, Tsukamoto S, et al. The mechanism of injury in a stea-totic liver graft during cold preservation. Transplantation 1999;67(2):195–200.
60. Caraceni P, Bianchi C, Domenicali M, et al. Impairment of mitochondrial oxida-tive phosphorylation in rat fatty liver exposed to preservation-reperfusion injury. J Hepatol 2004;41(1):82–8.
61. Chalasani N, Younossi Z, Lavine JE, et al. The diagnosis and management of non-alcoholic fatty liver disease: practice guideline by the American Association for the Study of Liver Diseases, American College of Gastroenterology, and the American Gastroenterological Association. Hepatology 2012;55(6):2005–23.
62. Marchesini G, Brizi M, Bianchi G, et al. Nonalcoholic fatty liver disease: a feature of the metabolic syndrome. Diabetes 2001;50(8):1844–50.
63. Day CP, Saksena S. Non-alcoholic steatohepatitis: definitions and pathogenesis. J Gastroenterol Hepatol 2002;17(Suppl 3):S377–84.
64. Sanyal AJ. AGA technical review on nonalcoholic fatty liver disease. Gastroen-terology 2002;123(5):1705–25.
65. Marchesini G. Nonalcoholic fatty liver, steatohepatitis, and the metabolic syndrome. Hepatology 2003;37(4):917–23.
66. Ahn JS, Sinn DH, Gwak GY, et al. Steatosis among living liver donors without evidence of fatty liver on ultrasonography. Transplantation 2013;95(11):1404–9.
67. de Graaf EL, Kench J, Dilworth P, et al. Grade of deceased donor liver macro-vesicular steatosis impacts graft and recipient outcomes more than the donor risk index. J Gastroenterol Hepatol 2012;27(3):540–6.
68. Dutkowski P, Schlegel A, Slankamenac K, et al. The use of fatty liver grafts in modern allocation systems. Ann Surg 2012;256(5):861–9.
69. Chavin KD, Taber DJ, Norcross M, et al. Safe use of highly steatotic livers by utilizing a donor/recipient clinical algorithm. Clin Transplant 2013;27:732–41.
70. Gabrielli M, Moisan F, Vidal M, et al. Steatotic livers. Can we use them in OLTX? Outcome data from a prospective baseline liver biopsy study. Ann Hepatol 2012;11(6):891–8.
71. McCormack L, Petrowsky H, Jochum W, et al. Use of severely steatotic grafts in liver transplantation. Ann Surg 2007;246(6):940–8.
72. Spitzer AL, Lao OB, Dick AA, et al. The biopsied donor liver: incorporating mac-rosteatosis into high-risk donor assessment. Liver Transpl 2010;16(7):874–84.
73. Lee SW, Park SH, Kim KW, et al. Unenhanced CT for assessment of macrovesic-ular hepatic steatosis in living liver donors: comparison of visual grading with liver attenuation index 1. Radiology 2007;244(2):479–85.
74. Franzén LE, Ekstedt M, Kechagias S, et al. Semiquantitative evaluation overes-timates the degree of steatosis in liver biopsies: a comparison to stereological point counting. Mod Pathol 2005;18(7):912–6.
75. Brunt EM. Histopathology of nonalcoholic fatty liver disease. World J Gastroen-terol 2010;16(42):5286.
76. Silberhumer GR, Rahmel A, Karam V, et al. The difficulty in defining extended donor criteria for liver grafts: the Eurotransplant experience. Transpl Int 2013; 26(10):990–8.

77. Burroughs AK, Sabin CA, Rolles K, et al. 3-month and 12-month mortality after first liver transplant in adults in Europe: predictive models for outcome. Lancet 2006;367(9506):225–32.
78. Guichelaar MM, Benson JT, Malinchoc M, et al. Risk factors for and clinical course of non-anastomotic biliary strictures after liver transplantation. Am J Transplant 2003;3(7):885–90.
79. Brunner SM, Junger H, Ruemmele P, et al. Bile duct damage after cold storage of deceased donor livers predicts biliary complications after liver transplantation. J Hepatol 2013;58(6):1133–9.
80. Van Thiel DH, De Maria N, Colantoni A, et al. Can hepatitis B core antibody positive livers be used safely for transplantation: hepatitis B virus detection in the liver of individuals who are hepatitis B core antibody positive. Transplantation 1999;68(4):519–22.
81. Suehiro T, Shimada M, Kishikawa K, et al. Prevention of hepatitis B virus infection from hepatitis B core antibody-positive donor graft using hepatitis B immune globulin and lamivudine in living donor liver transplantation. Liver Int 2005; 25(6):1169–74.
82. Prieto M, Gomez MD, Berenguer M, et al. De novo hepatitis B after liver transplantation from hepatitis B core antibody-positive donors in an area with high prevalence of anti-HBc positivity in the donor population. Liver Transpl 2001; 7(1):51–8.
83. Roque-Afonso AM, Feray C, Samuel D, et al. Antibodies to hepatitis B surface antigen prevent viral reactivation in recipients of liver grafts from anti-HBC positive donors. Gut 2002;50(1):95–9.
84. Angelico M, Nardi A, Marianelli T, et al. Hepatitis B-core antibody positive donors in liver transplantation and their impact on graft survival: evidence from the LiverMatch cohort study. J Hepatol 2013;58(4):715–23.
85. Lee KH, Wai CT, Lim SG, et al. Risk for de novo hepatitis B from antibody to hepatitis B core antigen-positive donors in liver transplantation in Singapore. Liver Transpl 2001;7(5):469–70.
86. Chen YS, Wang CC, de Villa VH, et al. Prevention of de novo hepatitis B virus infection in living donor liver transplantation using hepatitis B core antibody positive donors. Clin Transplant 2002;16(6):405–9.
87. Cholongitas E, Papatheodoridis GV, Burroughs AK. Liver grafts from anti-hepatitis B core positive donors: a systematic review. J Hepatol 2010;52(2):272–9.
88. Skagen CL, Jou JH, Said A. Risk of de novo hepatitis in liver recipients from hepatitis-B core antibody-positive grafts - a systematic analysis. Clinical Transplantation 2011;25(3):E243–9.
89. Manzarbeitia C. Safe use of livers from donors with positive hepatitis B core antibody. Liver Transpl 2002;8(6):556–61.
90. Yu AS, Vierling JM, Colquhoun SD, et al. Transmission of hepatitis B infection from hepatitis B core antibody–positive liver allografts is prevented by lamivudine therapy. Liver Transpl 2001;7(6):513–7.
91. Joya-Vazquez PP, Dodson FS, Dvorchik I, et al. Impact of anti-hepatitis Bc-positive grafts on the outcome of liver transplantation for HBV-related cirrhosis. Transplantation 2002;73(10):1598–602.
92. Nery JR, Nery-Avila C, Reddy KR, et al. Use of liver grafts from donors positive for antihepatitis B-core antibody (anti-HBc) in the era of prophylaxis with hepatitis-B immunoglobulin and lamivudine. Transplantation 2003;75(8):1179–86.
93. Montalti R, Nardo B, Bertelli R, et al. Donor pool expansion in liver transplantation. Transplant Proc 2004;36(3):520–2.

94. Donataccio D, Roggen F, Reyck C, et al. Use of anti-HBc positive allografts in adult liver transplantation: toward a safer way to expand the donor pool. Transpl Int 2006;19(1):38–43.

95. Prakoso E, Strasser SI, Koorey DJ, et al. Long-term lamivudine monotherapy prevents development of hepatitis B virus infection in hepatitis B surface-antigen negative liver transplant recipients from hepatitis B core-antibody-positive donors. Clin Transplant 2006;20(3):369–73.

96. Cheung CKY, Lo CM, Man K, et al. Occult hepatitis B virus infection of donor and recipient origin after liver transplantation despite nucleoside analogue prophylaxis. Liver Transpl 2010;16(11):1314–23.

97. Yu L, Koepsell T, Manhart L, et al. Survival after orthotopic liver transplantation: the impact of antibody against hepatitis B core antigen in the donor. Liver Transpl 2009;15(10):1343–50.

98. Choi Y, Choi JY, Yi NJ, et al. Liver transplantation for HBsAg-positive recipients using grafts from HBsAg-positive deceased donors. Transpl Int 2013;26(12): 1173–83.

99. Northup PG, Argo CK, Nguyen DT, et al. Liver allografts from hepatitis C positive donors can offer good outcomes in hepatitis C positive recipients: a US National Transplant Registry analysis. Transpl Int 2010;23(10):1038–44.

100. Burr AT, Li Y, Tseng JF, et al. Survival after liver transplantation using hepatitis C virus-positive donor allografts: case-controlled analysis of the UNOS database. World J Surg 2011;35(7):1590–5.

101. Ballarin R, Montalti R, Spaggiari M, et al. Liver transplantation in older adults: our point of view. J Am Geriatr Soc 2011;59(7):1359–61.

102. HIV Organ Policy Equity Act [Internet]. thomas.loc.gov. [cited May 1, 2013]. Available at: http://thomas.loc.gov/cgi-bin/query/z?c113:H.R.698. Accessed April 5, 2013.

103. Boyarsky BJ, Hall EC, Singer AL, et al. Estimating the potential pool of HIV-infected deceased organ donors in the United States. Am J Transplant 2011; 11(6):1209–17.

104. Mgbako O, Glazier A, Blumberg E, et al. Allowing HIV-positive organ donation: ethical, legal and operational considerations. Am J Transplant 2013;13(7):1636–42.

105. CDC. CDC guidelines for preventing transmission of human immunodeficiency virus through transplantation of human tissue and organs. MMWR Morb Mortal Wkly Rep 1994;43:1–26.

106. Kucirka LM, Alexander C, Namuyinga R, et al. Viral nucleic acid testing (NAT) and OPO-level disposition of high-risk donor organs. Am J Transplant 2009; 9(3):620–8.

107. Ellingson K, Seem D, Nowicki M, et al, for the Organ Procurement Organization Nucleic Acid Testing Yield Project Team. Estimated risk of human immunodeficiency virus and hepatitis C virus infection among potential organ donors from 17 organ procurement organizations in the United States. Am J Transplant 2011;11(6):1201–8.

108. Ison MG, Hager J, Blumberg E, et al. Donor-derived disease transmission events in the United States: data reviewed by the OPTN/UNOS Disease Transmission Advisory Committee. Am J Transplant 2009;9(8):1929–35.

109. Ison MG, Llata E, Conover CS, et al. Transmission of human immunodeficiency virus and hepatitis C virus from an organ donor to four transplant recipients. Am J Transplant 2011;11(6):1218–25.

110. Seem DL, Lee I, Umscheid GA, et al. Guideline for reducing transmission of human immunodeficiency virus, hepatitis B virus, and hepatitis C virus

through organ transplantation. 2011. Available at: www.cdc.gov. Accessed January 2, 2013.

111. Yao F, Seed C, Farrugia A, et al. The risk of HIV, HBV, HCV and HTLV infection among musculoskeletal tissue donors in Australia. Am J Transplant 2007; 7(12):2723–6.

112. Biswas R, Tabor E, Hsia CC, et al. Comparative sensitivity of HBV NATs and HBsAg assays for detection of acute HBV infection. Transfusion 2003;43:788–98.

113. Busch MP, Glynn SA, Wright DJ, et al. Relative sensitivities of licensed nucleic acid amplification tests for detection of viremia in early human immunodeficiency virus and hepatitis C virus infection. Transfusion 2005;45(12):1853–63.

114. Giachetti C, Linnen JM, Kolk DP, et al. Highly sensitive multiplex assay for detection of human immunodeficiency virus type 1 and hepatitis C virus RNA. J Clin Microbiol 2002;40(7):2408–19.

115. Buell JF, Beebe TM, Trofe J, et al. Donor transmitted malignancies. Ann Transplant 2004;9(1):53–6.

116. Kauffman HM, McBride MA, Cherikh WS, et al. Transplant tumor registry: donor related malignancies. Transplantation 2002;74(3):358–62.

117. Desai R, Collett D, Watson CJ, et al. Cancer transmission from organ donors—unavoidable but low risk. Transplantation 2012;94(12):1200–7.

118. Feng S, Buell JF, Chari RS, et al. Tumors and transplantation: the 2003 third annual ASTS State-of-the-Art Winter Symposium. Am J Transplant 2003;3(12): 1481–7.

119. Collignon FP, Holland EC, Feng S. Organ donors with malignant gliomas: an update. Am J Transplant 2004;4(1):15–21.

120. Finger EB, Feng S. Central nervous system tumors and organ donation: an update. Curr Opin Organ Transplant 2006;11(2):146–50.

Challenges in Living Donor Liver Transplantation

James F. Trotter, MD

KEYWORDS

- Living donor liver transplantation • Hepatocellular carcinoma
- ABO-incompatible transplant • Living donor

KEY POINTS

- Living donor liver transplantation (LDLT) is a procedure that accounts for approximately 3% of adult liver transplants in the United States. The enthusiasm toward this operation has waned in recent years.
- Although there is no apparent survival advantage for LDLT recipients with hepatocellular carcinoma, properly selected candidates may benefit from the shorter waiting time compared with deceased donor liver transplantation (DDLT).
- The publication of recent protocols with ABO-incompatible LDLT suggests that this barrier may be successfully overcome to expand the potential living donor pool.

INTRODUCTION

Adult-to-adult LDLT is a procedure that has evolved over the past 2 decades. First introduced in the United States in the 1990s, LDLT was primarily relegated to pediatric recipients until late in the decade. Then, a combination of factors contributed to a proliferation of cases. Waiting times for liver transplant increased in the late 1990s as the number of patients listed for transplant far exceeded the modest gain in deceased donors. In addition, important changes in the operative technique improved LDLT recipient outcomes. The initial experience with LDLT used the smaller left hepatic lobe. Although this small graft was adequate for diminutive (pediatric) recipients, initial results in adults were poor. In the late 1990s, selected centers demonstrated favorable recipient outcomes by transplanting the larger right hepatic lobe.[1,2] As the advantage of right hepatic lobe LDLT became apparent, the popularity of the procedure increased and the annual number of LDLTs increased from fewer than 100 to more than 500 in 2002, accounting for approximately 10% of adult liver transplants in the United States.[3] The application of LDLT over the past decade, however, has dropped substantially to fewer than 200 adult cases per year, representing only approximately

Disclosure: None.
Department of Medicine, Baylor University Medical Center, 3410 Worth Street, #860, Dallas, TX 75246, USA
E-mail address: james.trotter@baylorhealth.edu

3% of all liver transplants. The reasons for the decline of LDLT are not entirely understood but are likely due to a combination of forces.[4] As with any novel procedure, there is initial enthusiasm leading to rapid growth followed by a more measured approach as the full spectrum of risks and complications becomes apparent over time. Such is the case with LDLT. Over the past decade, there have been several publications highlighting complications in donors and recipients (discussed later), which has tempered interest in the procedure. The most important complication of LDLT, donor death, has received widespread media attention, although its occurrence is rare, at just over 1/500. Finally, federal regulators have placed transplant centers under increasing scrutiny for favorable outcomes. Consequently, transplant centers have become more risk averse and this may have had an impact on their decision to offer LDLT to their patients. The trend toward limited application of LDLT in the United States is largely reflective of the European experience, where living liver donor rates are approximately 1 donor per million (dpm) population. In some parts of the world, however, the procedure is thriving; most notable is South Korea, with 17 dpm, the highest rate worldwide, followed by Turkey (8 dpm), Egypt (5 dpm), and Japan (4 dpm). The Asan Medical Center in Seoul, South Korea, performs approximately 300 LDLTs per year surpassing the entire US volume by approximately 2-fold. This review focuses on 3 of the most important developments in LDLT in recent years: hepatocellular carcinoma (HCC), ABO-incompatible transplant, and donor risk and its management.

LDLT FOR HEPATOCELLULAR CARCINOMA

Compared with DDLT, LDLT offers the potential advantages of speed and timing, which can be particularly important for patients with HCC. The average living donor evaluation takes approximately 6 to 8 weeks; so, LDLT can often be performed faster than DDLT, where waiting times are months to a few years for HCC patients. Prolonged pretransplant waiting times increase the risk of tumor progression, which, in turn, increases the risk of removal from the DDLT list and posttransplant recurrence. Up to 20% of HCC patients are removed from the list due to disease progression while awaiting a transplant.[5–7] Therefore, rapid procession to transplantation potentially offers a therapeutic advantage in the treatment of HCC. Despite the theoretic advantage of LDLT for HCC patients, however, 3 separate reports have each concluded that there is no survival advantage for LDLT patients. A study from Toronto, which has a robust LDLT program, reported no survival advantage with LDLT.[8] It compared survival and HCC recurrence rates for 345 transplant recipients after LDLT, 58 (17%), and DDLT, 287 (83%), over a 16-year period. As expected, the LDLT recipients had significantly shorter waiting times compared with DDLT (3.1 vs 5.3 months; $P = .003$). There was no difference in 5-year HCC recurrence rates for LDLT (15%) and DDLT (17%) for the DDLT group ($P = $ not significant [NS]). There was also no difference in 5-year survival rates for LDLT (75%) and DDLT (75%) ($P = $ NS). Similar results were reported from a French group in 183 patients with HCC, with LDLT (n = 36) and DDLT (n = 147).[9] At listing, patient and tumor characteristics were comparable in the 2 groups, whereas the mean waiting time was shorter with LDLT (2.6 months) compared with DDLT (7.9 months) ($P = .001$). All of the 27 (18%) of patients who dropped off the list, primarily for tumor progression, prior to transplant were listed for DDLT. There was no difference in posttransplant recurrence rates, however, between the 2 groups, at 13% each ($P = $ NS). More important, there was no difference in survival on an intention-to-treat basis. Finally, the Adult-to-Adult Living Donor Liver Transplantation Cohort Study Group (A2ALL) has published a large (n = 229) intention-to-treat analysis evaluating LDLT and DDLT in HCC patients who had at least 1 potential donor evaluated.[10] The LDLT cohort included patients undergoing this procedure, whereas the remainder comprised the DDLT cohort and included patients whose donor was rejected or those receiving DDLT before completion of donor evaluation. Predictably, the LDLT patients had a shorter time to transplant, were more likely to have tumors exceeding Milan criteria, and had higher α-fetoprotein (AFP) levels. As a result, the unadjusted risk of HCC recurrence was more than 3-fold higher with LDLT (38%) compared with DDLT (11%, $P = 0.0004$), as was the adjusted risk (hazard ratio [HR] 2.35; 95% CI, 1.04–5.35; $P = .04$). Perhaps the most important finding is the lack of a survival advantage with LDLT; the adjusted risk of death from the time of donor evaluation was similar for patients who received LDLT compared with other patients (HR 0.73; 95% CI, 0.36–1.45; $P = .36$). Two meta-analyses that evaluated the efficacy of LDLT compared with DDLT in HCC patients reiterated these results.[11,12]

How can these data be interpreted related to the selection of LDLT candidates?[13] For advocates of LDLT, these data provide a basis for its continued application; the outcomes for LDLT recipients are as good as for DDLT. For selected HCC patients, LDLT could be their best option. Small patients (who have inherent difficulty securing a size-appropriate deceased donor) in high–Model for End-Stage Liver Disease (MELD) regions (with long waiting times for HCC patients) may benefit from the predictably shorter waiting times associated with LDLT. An additional consideration with LDLT, however, is the impact on the donor, who undergoes a major operation with no medical benefit. Therefore, a more critical assessment is that LDLT could be worse than DDLT for HCC patients. With equivalent recipient survival and potential harm to the donor, LDLT has more potential for medical harm with no apparent additional benefit. There is likely a middle ground, however, between these 2 extremes. One of the reasons for the absence of benefit with LDLT is the high priority awarded to DDLT candidates with HCC under MELD-based liver allocation, which was implemented in 2002. As a result, HCC patients could initially be transplanted in less than 90 days with a DDLT, often faster than an LDLT can even be arranged. Over the past decade, however, the waiting times for HCC patients have increased, even with additional MELD points awarded over time. At many US centers, the waiting times for DDLT exceed 1 year for HCC patients. Therefore, the lack of benefit for LDLT found in these studies (which evaluated patients transplanted from years ago) may not be applicable to current liver transplant candidates. Another reason for the lack of benefit with LDLT could be that HCC patients who are selected for LDLT have worse tumor biology than DDLT patients. The diagnosis of HCC creates understandable anxiety for patients, their families (of potential donors), and the transplant team. The possibility of offering an expedited LDLT places the transplant team under pressure to "make the transplant happen." These powerful forces may have an impact on the selection of donors and recipients for LDLT. Data from the A2ALL study provide clear evidence that LDLT recipients have worse tumor biology than DDLT patients. LDLT recipients have significantly higher AFP, more advanced tumor stage, large tumor size, and higher percentage over Milan and University of California San Francisco criteria.[10] Therefore, LDLT recipients may be fundamentally different from DDLT patients, thereby explaining their worse outcomes after transplant. In summary, transplant physicians need to be cautious in offering LDLT to HCC patients. In particular, patients with poor tumor biology (higher AFP and advanced stage disease) may be poor candidates for LDLT, despite the opportunity to offer a desperate patient a potentially life-saving operation. LDLT may be effective, however, in patients with a long anticipated waiting time, in particular, small recipients with favorable tumor characteristics listed in donor service areas with high MELD scores.

ABO-INCOMPATIBLE LDLT

There have been several recent developments to overcome donation barriers related to ABO incompatiblity, including medical treatment protocols as well as innovative strategies of matching donors and recipients. Historically, liver transplantation with ABO incompatibility between the donor and recipient has been associated with poor outcomes.[14] Recipients of ABO-incompatible donor livers have antibodies directed against ABO antigens that are expressed on many cells, including the endothelium of blood vessels in the donor liver. As a result, such recipients are prone to developing diffuse hepatic vasculitis leading to biliary complications and graft loss.[15] Until recently, attempts to reduce the circulating antibodies with plasmapheresis, splenectomy, and infusional prostacyclin (to prevent hepatic inflammation with) have largely been unsuccessful.[16,17] ABO-incompatible recipients have lower patient and graft survival rates with significantly higher biliary complications compared with ABO-identical or -compatible recipients. There have been several publications, however, of successful implementation of innovative treatments to reduce circulating antibodies.[17–28] These protocols have all used Rituximab, which is an antibody directed against the cell surface marker, CD20, expressed on plasma cells, the source of the destructive antibodies. These novel therapies for ABO-incompatible LDLT have largely been pioneered in Japan, where DDLT is rarely performed. The Japanese are willing to pursue a more aggressive approach toward LDLT because it is the only transplant option for most patients. One of the most comprehensive reports is a multi-center experience from Japan, which underscored several important findings.[29] First, the number of ABO-incompatible LDLT has increased by approximately 10-fold from before 2000, when fewer than 5 yearly cases were done, to approximately 50 cases per year in 2011. The increased number of cases is likely due to the newfound success of the procedure. Rituximab treatment is given between 1 and 66 days (usually 1 to 2 weeks) before the anticipated LDLT at a dose of 375 mg/m^2 to 500 mg/m^2. The administration of Rituximab was associated with a significantly lower incidence of antibody-mediated rejection (6%) than in the untreated group (23%), ($P<.001$). More important, overall survival for patients receiving Rituximab was 2-fold higher than for other patients, with an HR for mortality 0.50 ($P<.001$). There was no increased incidence of adverse events with similar rates of cytomegalovirus and bacterial infection and a significantly lower rate of fungal infection in the Rituximab patients. Although these results are encouraging, continued follow-up of this cohort is required to fully assess the impact of Rituximab on outcomes, especially as it relates to biliary complications, which are rarely reported in these studies. Whether these favorable results from Japan, where LDLT is essentially the only option for liver transplant, could be applied in the West is not clear. Most LDLT centers in the West have not considered incompatible living donors, because the option of DDLT exists. If the favorable results from Rituximab treatment are confirmed over time, however, then this approach could be considered on a selected basis.

Another important development in dealing with incompatible living donors is the use of paired donor exchange protocols. One of the first considerations in matching potential donors with living donor transplant candidates has been verification that the donor is either ABO compatible or identical with the intended recipient. Typically, incompatible donors have been rejected from further considerations for donation. With the increased need for donors, however, some innovative centers have begun complex protocols whereby a donor who is ABO incompatible with the primary recipient is matched to an unrelated, secondary recipient whose donor is compatible with the primary recipient. Such paired exchange donor protocols have been successful in living donor kidney transplantation where the large number of donors and recipients is particularly well suited for this application.[30,31] Recent publications have reported successful paired exchange LDLT on a more limited basis. Chan and colleagues[32] reported a successful donor exchange between 2 donor/recipient pairs in Hong Kong. The Asan Medical Center, the largest LDLT program in the world, instituted an active paired exchange program in 2003. They reported outcomes in 8 donor/recipient pairs who underwent LDLT through their program with a 5-year patient and graft survival rate of 94%.[33] Although this is the largest experience in the world, it represents a small number compared with kidney transplantation and less than 1% of the LDLT cases at this center. The investigators point out the difficulties in performing these cases. The patient acceptance of donor exchange was relatively low probably due to the important psychological and sociologic concerns related to this procedure. They recommend that both LDLTs in the donor exchange pair be performed simultaneously to prevent donors from not participating in the second operation. To perform 2 simultaneous LDLTs at one center requires significant resources in personnel and infrastructure that is likely only available at a few centers in the world. Therefore, although paired exchange LDLT is a novel solution to ABO incompatibility, its application in LDLT will likely remain limited.

DONOR RISK AND COMPLICATIONS

There have been recent reports documenting the risk of donor complications, the most important of which is donor death. Such data are required in counseling potential donors on the risk of their operation. Perhaps the most comprehensive study, A2ALL, noted that most complications were minor (27%) and life-threatening problems occurred in only 2% of cases.[34] The most common complications were biliary leaks (9%), bacterial infections (12%), and incisional hernia (6%). Early postoperative laboratory abnormalities resolve within a few months of surgery with the exception of low platelet counts. A small minority (approximately 10%) of donors have sustained thrombocytopenia for greater than 1 year after donation.[35] The long-term significance of the low platelet count is unknown, but the cause is likely mild portal hypertension contributing to splenomegaly. A careful study of quantitative functional hepatic tests in 12 living liver donors found evidence of a significant 68% increase in portal hypertension and shunting of portal blood flow after donor hepatectomy.[36] This is likely caused by the reduction in the overall hepatic mass, which was significantly reduced by 16% ($P<.01$) even 6 months after donation. There was a significant inverse relationship between quantitated spleen size and platelet count. Near-miss complications are another metric to measure outcomes of living donor liver surgery. A near miss is a potentially life-threatening event during which a donor's life may be in danger but after which there are no long-term sequelae. A recent survey study reported that the average near-miss rate among responding centers is 1.1% and that such complications were more likely at centers with less experience ($\leq$50 LDLTs).[37]

Donor mortality is the most significant complication as underscored in 2010 after 2 unexpected fatalities occurred within months of each other at 2 of the largest US LDLT programs. The approximate risk of donor death is less than 1%, but a more precise estimation is difficult to ascertain for several reasons. Most important, the total number of LDLTs performed in the United States is small relative to the total number of liver transplants. Between 2000 and 2010, there were 3159 living donor liver transplants, which represented only 5.1% of all liver transplantations performed in the United States.[3] In addition, unlike transplant recipients, there is no national database to register donor deaths. Consequently, reports of donor deaths are found through the media, case reports, or informal communications. Finally, there is no incentive for centers to report donor deaths owing to the negative repercussions of such disclosure. A recent article helped provide some clarity regarding mortality after donation.[38] Through the Organ Procurement and Transplantation Network, the investigators acquired the Social Security numbers of all living liver donors and cross-referenced these with the Social Security Death Master File to determine periprocedural mortality rates (within 90 days of surgery) and overall mortality rates compared with kidney donors. The 90-day mortality risk of living liver donors (1.7 per 1000 donors [0.17%]), although numerically higher, was not significantly different compared with living kidney donors (0.05%). The long-term cumulative mortality risk was comparable to that of live kidney donors and National Health and Nutrition Examination Survey participants (1.2%, 1.2%, and 1.4%, respectively) at 11 years. Because the Organ Procurement and Transplantation Network provides the full cohort of living liver donors in the United States and confirmation of mortality through the Social Security Death Master File is definitive, the results of this study are likely the best estimation of donor mortality. Although this study analyzed the largest cohort to date with the most rigorous methodology, the results are similar to previous reports. One prior analysis of publications in the medical and lay press reported donor mortality "definitely" and "definitely or possibly" related to the donor surgery at 0.15% and 0.20%, respectively.[39] Another study based on survey data estimated donor mortality risk at 0.2%.[40] An important distinction of the current article from earlier reports is the use of comparison groups.[38] The identification of an appropriate comparator group for living liver donors is difficult because of their unique characteristics. Living liver donors represent a highly selected group; up to two-thirds are rejected for the discovery of even a mild medical problem during the evaluation.[41] The finding of living liver donors who died by their own hand is notable. The current analysis discovered 2 such deaths in the early perioperative period.[38] An A2ALL study identified 2 other deaths from donor suicides or drug overdose and another attempted suicide, all of which occurred greater than 90 days after surgery.[42] Although psychiatric complications are uncommon, occurring in approximately 4% of living liver donors, they may be attributable indirectly to the operation by the stress associated with undergoing the complicated evaluation and surgery. The number of documented donor deaths by suicide and drug overdose (n = 4) rivals the total number of early perioperative deaths by other means (n = 5), highlighting the importance of the mental health of donors and prospective donors. Furthermore, the occurrence of these complications after the early postoperative period emphasizes the possibility that surgical complications may not be immediately evident. One-third of rehospitalizations for living liver donors, however, occur greater than 90 days after donation.[43]

Another area of recent interest in LDLT is mitigating the risk to the living donor. As noted previously, the total number of LDLTs in the United States has dropped significantly over the past decade, due in part to concerns over donor morbidity and mortality. Therefore, surgeons have focused on surgical techniques to improve donor outcomes. One of these is using the left hepatic (vs right hepatic) lobe for LDLT.[44] Early in the development of LDLT, almost all cases were done with the left hepatic lobe, which is typically smaller than the right lobe. Although the results were generally favorable for smaller recipients, who were primarily pediatric, most clinicians reported marginal outcomes with left hepatic lobe LDLT in larger adult recipients. The rapid growth of LDLT in the late 1990s was largely related to successful reports of right hepatic lobe adult-to-adult LDLT. There are convincing data, however, that donor complications are higher after right lobectomy compared with left lobectomy. A comparison of complications between the type of donor hepatectomy (right vs left) is compromised by (1) a low rate of serious complications, (2) inadequate data collection among centers, and (3) few left hepatic lobe donors. The best data are from Asia, which has the greatest experience in left hepatic lobe donation. An early comprehensive survey report of 1508 living liver donors reported a higher complication rate in right lobe donors (28%) than in left lateral segment (9%) or left lobe (8%) donors.[45] In particular, right lobe donors had more serious complications, such as cholestasis (7%), bile leakage (6%), biliary stricture (1%), portal vein thrombosis (0.5%), intra-abdominal bleeding (0.5%), and pulmonary embolism (0.5%). A follow-up study from Japan of 3565 donors found that complications were higher in right lobe donors (9.4%) compared with left (8.7%).[46] The proportion of right lobe donors with more serious complications (Clavien IIIa and IIIb) was also numerically higher (3.6% and 2.1%) compared with left lobe donors (2.0% and 1.5%). Because of the concerns about the safety of right hepatic lobe donation, surgical teams have increasingly begun to explore, develop, and promote left hepatic lobe LDLT. The Hong Kong group, where 95% of LDLTs have been performed using right hepatic lobe grafts, required graft weight (GW)/standard liver volume (SLV) ratio of greater than 0.4.[47] They reanalyzed their donors retrospectively, however, and found that by lowering their GW/SLV cutoff to 0.3, 29% of their cases could have been done using the left hepatic lobe, thereby exposing the donor to less risk. They concluded that the applicability of left hepatic lobe donation could be improved at their center without compromising recipient outcome. Soejima and colleagues[48] performed a retrospective review of 200 consecutive left lobe compared with 112 right lobe LDLTs. Even though the mean GW/SLV ratios were smaller with the left versus right lobes (38.7% vs 47.6%, $P<.0001$), the outcomes were identical. The 1-, 5-, and 10-year patient survival rates with left lobe LDLT were 85%, 78%, and 70%, respectively, compared with 90%, 71%, and 71%, respectively, for right lobe LDLT. Similarly, the overall donor morbidity rates were comparable between left (36%) and right lobe (34.8%), whereas postoperative liver function tests and hospital stay were significantly better ($P<.0001$) in left lobe donors. They concluded that left lobe LDLT provided favorable results and may be the preferred means of accomplishing LDLT. Similar findings have been reported in the limited US experience with 21 left hepatic lobe recipients, 16 of whom underwent portocaval shunting to reduce the risk of small-for-size syndrome.[49] Based on this experience, a position paper in support of left hepatic lobe LDLT was published in support of considering this operation over right hepatic lobe LDLT.[50] In summary, there is increasing evidence that left hepatectomy lobe LDLT may be a suitable procedure and offer sufficient hepatic mass with fewer donors problems, especially in smaller recipients where the GW/SLV ratios are favorable for this procedure.

REFERENCES

1. Yamaoka Y, Washida M, Honda K, et al. Liver transplantation using a right lobe graft from a living related donor. Transplantation 1994;57:1127–30.
2. Wachs ME, Bak TE, Karrer FM, et al. Adult living donor liver transplantation using a right hepatic lobe. Transplantation 1998;66:1313–6.
3. Available at: http://optn.transplant.hrsa.gov/latestData/rptData.asp. Accessed February 1, 2014.
4. Clavien PA, Dutkowski P, Trotter JF. Requiem for a champion? Living donor liver transplantation. J Hepatol 2009;51:635–7.
5. Park SJ, Freise CE, Hirose R, et al. Risk factors for liver transplant waitlist dropout in patients with hepatocellular carcinoma. Clin Transplant 2012;26: E359–64.

6. Washburn K, Edwards E, Harper A, et al. Hepatocellular carcinoma patients are advantaged in the current liver transplant allocation system. Am J Transplant 2010;10:1643–8.

7. Bitterman T, Niu B, Hoteit MA, et al. Waitlist priority for hepatocellular carcinoma beyond Milan criteria: a potentially appropriate decision without a structured approach. Am J Transplant 2014;14:79–87.

8. Sandhu L, Sandroussi C, Guba M, et al. Living donor liver transplantation versus deceased donor liver transplantation for hepatocellular carcinoma: comparable survival and recurrence. Liver Transpl 2012;18:315–22.

9. Bhangui P, Vibert E, Majno P, et al. Intention-to-treat analysis of liver transplantation for hepatocellular carcinoma: living versus deceased donor transplantation. Hepatology 2011;53:1570–9.

10. Kulik LM, Fisher RA, Rodrigo DR, et al. Outcomes of living and deceased donor liver transplant recipients with hepatocellular carcinoma: results of the A2ALL cohort. Am J Transplant 2012;12:2997–3007.

11. Grant RC, Sandhu L, Dixon PR, et al. Living vs. deceased donor liver transplantation for hepatocellular carcinoma: a systematic review and meta-analysis. Clin Transplant 2013;27:140–7.

12. Liang W, Wu L, Ling X, et al. Living donor liver transplantation versus deceased donor liver transplantation for hepatocellular carcinoma: a meta-analysis. Liver Transpl 2012;18:1226–36.

13. Trotter JF. Living donor liver transplantation for hepatocellular carcinoma: through the looking glass. Am J Transplant 2012;12:2873–4.

14. Gordon RD, Iwatsuki S, Esquivel CO, et al. Liver transplantation across ABO blood groups. Surgery 1986;100:342–8.

15. Demetris AJ, Jaffe R, Tzakis A, et al. Antibody-mediated rejection of human orthotopic liver allografts. A study of liver transplantation across ABO blood group barriers. Am J Pathol 1988;132:489–502.

16. Wu J, Ye S, Xu X, et al. Recipient outcomes after ABO-incompatible liver transplantation: a systematic review and meta-analysis. PLoS One 2011;6: e16521.

17. Kim JM, Kwon CH, Joh JW, et al. ABO-incompatible living donor liver transplantation is suitable in patients without ABO-matched donor. J Hepatol 2013;59: 1215–22.

18. Soejima Y, Muto J, Matono R, et al. Strategic breakthrough in adult ABO-incompatible living donor liver transplantation: preliminary results of consecutive seven cases. Clin Transplant 2013;27:227–31.

19. Raut V, Mori A, Kaido T, et al. Splenectomy does not offer immunological benefits in ABO-incompatible liver transplantation with a preoperative rituximab. Transplantation 2012;93:99–105.

20. Uchiyama H, Mano Y, Taketomi A, et al. Kinetics of anti-blood type isoagglutinin titers and B lymphocytes in ABO-incompatible living donor liver transplantation with rituximab and plasma exchange. Transplantation 2011;92:1134–9.

21. Tanabe M, Kawachi S, Obara H, et al. Current progress in ABO-incompatible liver transplantation. Eur J Clin Invest 2010;40:943–9.

22. Ikegami T, Taketomi A, Soejima Y, et al. Rituximab, IVIG, and plasma exchange without graft local infusion treatment: a new protocol in ABO incompatible living donor liver transplantation. Transplantation 2009;88:303–7.

23. Kawagishi N, Takeda I, Miyagi S, et al. Long-term outcome of ABO-incompatible living-donor liver transplantation: a single-center experience. J Hepatobiliary Pancreat Surg 2009;16:468–72.

24. Usui M, Isaji S, Mizuno S, et al. Experiences and problems pre-operative anti-CD20 monoclonal antibody infusion therapy with splenectomy and plasma exchange for ABO-incompatible living-donor liver transplantation. Clin Transplant 2007;21:24–31.

25. Usuda M, Fujimori K, Koyamada N, et al. Successful use of anti-CD20 monoclonal antibody (rituximab) for ABO-incompatible living-related liver transplantation. Transplantation 2005;79:12–6.

26. Kawagishi N, Satomi S. ABO-incompatible living donor liver transplantation: new insights into clinical relevance. Transplantation 2008;85:1523–5.

27. Egawa H, Teramukai S, Haga H, et al. Present status of ABO-incompatible living donor liver transplantation in Japan. Hepatology 2008;47:143–52.

28. Egawa H, Tanabe K, Fukushima N, et al. Current status of organ transplantation in Japan. Am J Transplant 2012;12:523–30.

29. Egawa H, Teramukai S, Haga H, et al. Impact of rituximab desensitization on blood-type-incompatible adult living donor liver transplantation: a Japanese multicenter study. Am J Transplant 2014;14:102–14.

30. Ashlagi I, Gilchrist DS, Roth AE, et al. Nonsimultaneous chains and dominos in kidney- paired donation-revisited. Am J Transplant 2011;11:984–94.

31. Rees MA, Kopke JE, Pelletier RP, et al. A nonsimultaneous, extended, altruistic-donor chain. N Engl J Med 2009;360:1096–101.

32. Chan SC, Lo CM, Yong BH, et al. Paired donor interchange to avoid ABO-incompatible living donor liver transplantation. Liver Transpl 2010;16:478–81.

33. Hwang S, Lee SG, Moon DB, et al. Exchange living donor liver transplantation to overcome ABO incompatibility in adult patients. Liver Transpl 2010;16:482–90.

34. Abecassis MM, Fisher RA, Olthoff KM, et al. Complications of living donor hepatic lobectomy–a comprehensive report. Am J Transplant 2012;12:1208–17.

35. Trotter JF, Gillespie BW, Terrault NA, et al. Laboratory test results after living liver donation in the adult-to-adult living donor liver transplantation cohort study. Liver Transpl 2011;17:409–17.

36. Everson GT, Hoefs JC, Niemann CU, et al. Functional elements associated with hepatic regeneration in living donors after right hepatic lobectomy. Liver Transpl 2013;19:292–304.

37. Cheah YL, Simpson MA, Pomposelli JJ, et al. Incidence of death and potentially life-threatening near-miss events in living donor hepatic lobectomy: a worldwide survey. Liver Transpl 2013;19:499–506.

38. Muzaale AD, Dagher NN, Montgomery RA, et al. Estimates of early death, acute liver failure, and long-term mortality among live liver donors. Gastroenterology 2012;142:273–80.

39. Trotter JF, Adam R, Lo CM, et al. Documented deaths of hepatic lobe donors for living donor liver transplantation. Liver Transpl 2006;12:1485–8.

40. Brown RS, Russo MW, Lai M, et al. A survey of liver transplantation from living adult donors in the United States. N Engl J Med 2003;348:818–25.

41. Trotter JF, Wisniewski KA, Terrault NA, et al. Outcomes of donor evaluation in adult-to-adult living donor liver transplantation. Hepatology 2007;46:1476–84.

42. Trotter JF, Hill-Callahan MM, Gillespie BW, et al. Severe psychiatric problems in right hepatic lobe donors for living donor liver transplantation. Transplantation 2007;83:1506–8.

43. Merion RM, Shearon TH, Berg CL, et al. Hospitalization rates before and after adult-to-adult living donor or deceased donor liver transplantation. Ann Surg 2010;251:542–9.

44. Greenhill C. Liver transplantation: left lobe living donor liver transplantation could improve donor outcomes. Nat Rev Gastroenterol Hepatol 2012;9:241.

45. Lo CM. Complications and long-term outcome of living liver donors: a survey of 1,508 cases in five Asian centers. Transplantation 2003;75:S12–5.

46. Hashikura Y, Ichida T, Umeshita K, et al. Donor complications associated with living donor liver transplantation in Japan. Transplantation 2009;88:110–4.

47. Chan SC, Fan ST, Chok KS, et al. Increasing the recipient benefit/donor risk ratio by lowering the graft size requirement for living donor liver transplantation. Liver Transpl 2012;18:1078–82.

48. Soejima Y, Shirabe K, Taketomi A, et al. Left lobe living donor liver transplantation in adults. Am J Transplant 2012;12:1877–85.

49. Botha JF, Langnas AN, Campos BD, et al. Left lobe adult-to-adult living donor liver transplantation: small grafts and hemiportocaval shunts in the prevention of small-for-size syndrome. Liver Transpl 2010;16:649–57.

50. Roll GR, Parekh JR, Parker WF, et al. Left hepatectomy versus right hepatectomy for living donor liver transplantation: shifting the risk from the donor to the recipient. Liver Transpl 2013;19:472–81.

Multivisceral Transplantation

Where Do We Stand?

Kalyan Ram Bhamidimarri, MD, MPH[a], Thiago Beduschi, MD[b],
Rodrigo Vianna, MD[b],*

KEYWORDS

- Liver transplantation • Intestinal transplantation • Multivisceral transplantation
- Intestinal failure

KEY POINTS

- Intestinal transplantation is the definitive therapy for patients with irreversible intestinal failure (IF) and can be combined with transplantation of other abdominal organs: multivisceral transplantation—stomach, intestine, pancreaticoduodenal complex, and liver (MVTx) or modified MVTx—without liver (MMVTx).
- There has been an increasing trend in the volume of intestinal transplantation and MVTx in the past few decades and there is also increasing trend in patient and graft survival primarily due to improved patient selection, advances in immunosuppression, and improved perioperative management.
- This review summarizes the various key elements in patient selection, types of grafts, and updates in the perioperative management involved in MVTx.

INTRODUCTION

The first human small bowel transplant was performed in humans in 1964 at the Boston Floating Hospital for Children.[1] Subsequently, the first MVTx was performed as part of a "cluster graft" by Thomas Starzl at the University of Pittsburgh in 1984.[2] The introduction of cyclosporine in the 1980s allowed a few centers around the world to perform allogeneic intestinal transplantation with improved success, but it was not until the discovery and clinical application of the then novel drug, FK506 (tacrolimus), in the early 1990s that intestinal transplantation moved from an experimental intervention to a clinical reality.[3,4] Although initially hampered by poor results, intestinal transplantation has evolved and currently stands as the only chance of cure for patients

Financial Disclosures/Conflict of Interest: None relevant to the article.
[a] Miami Transplant Institute, University of Miami, 1500 Northwest 12th Avenue, Suite 1101, Miami, FL 33136, USA; [b] Miami Transplant Institute, University of Miami, Highland Professional Building, 1801 Northwest 9th Avenue, Suite 310, Miami, FL 33136, USA
* Corresponding author.
E-mail address: rvianna@med.miami.edu

with IF who develop serious complications from parenteral nutrition (PN). Since the inception of intestinal transplantation, there have been various modifications of the graft, based on the number of organs transplanted simultaneously, which include isolated intestinal transplantation (ITx), liver-intestinal transplantation (LITx), MVTx, and MMVTx. According to the Intestinal Transplant Registry, approximately 3000 intestinal transplants and MVTxs have been performed around the world from 1985 to 2013 (**Table 1**). Because of the complexity of the intrinsic immune system of the intestine, resulting in cycles of rejection, sepsis, and graft-versus-host disease (GVHD), successful transplantation of the intestine is only now being accomplished with acceptable survival rates. In the past 10 years, graft and patient survival for ITx and MVTx have significantly improved because of advancements in the field, improved patient selection, refinement in the surgical technique, immunosuppression protocols, and improved perioperative management.[5]

INTESTINAL FAILURE

IF is characterized by the inability of the gastrointestinal tract to maintain adequate nutrition, fluid and electrolyte balance, for normal growth and development of the body.[6] Acute or chronic loss of the enteric absorptive mass beyond the critical limit can occur due to anatomic loss (congenital anomalies, surgery, or short gut syndrome) or physiologic loss (intestinal dysmotility, malabsorption, enterocyte dysfunction, or vasculopathy), which can all result in IF. Short gut syndrome may occur with a loss of 50% of the enteric mass but is certain with a loss of 70% of the enteric mass or if the remaining length of small intestine is less than 100 cm. Other variables, such as mucosal health of the intestinal remnant, presence of ileocecal valve, and remnant colon, also play an important role in the long-term prognosis of such patients. IF can be subclassified into 3 types based on the duration, severity, and prognosis:

Type 1 IF: Self-limiting, which usually follows abdominal surgery. Patients typically need short-term PN and are expected to make full recovery.

Type 2 IF: Occurs in severely ill patients who develop infectious and metabolic complications and require prolonged PN support and multidisciplinary management to ensure recovery.

Type 3 IF: Requires long-term PN combined with surgical interventions or transplantation.

The most common causes of IF in children are necrotizing enterocolitis, gastroschisis, intestinal atresia, volvulus, pseudo-obstruction, and aganglionosis. In adults, ischemia, inflammatory diseases, trauma, and tumors are the most common causes of IF. In several patients with gastrointestinal disease, a combination of massive resection and dysmotility of remnant bowel can be present.[7]

INDICATIONS

Intestinal transplantation is indicated in patients who experience life-threatening complications from the chronic use of PN. The indications for bowel transplantation

Table 1	
Global clinical activity—Intestinal Transplant Registry	
Number of Transplants	**Total Number**
Isolated intestinal	1309
Liver/intestine	898
Multivisceral	680

suggested by the American Gastroenterological Association and the American Society of Transplantation can be divided in the following categories[8]: (1) failure of PN (traditional Medicare-approved indications), (2) high risk of death due to underlying disease, and (3) nontraditional indications.

1. Failure of PN: There are 4 Medicare-approved indications for intestinal transplantation, all of which are associated with IF and complications for long-term use of TPN:
   - Impending or overt liver failure due to PN/IF-associated liver injury. The clinical manifestations include elevated serum bilirubin and/or liver enzymes, splenomegaly, thrombocytopenia, gastroesophageal varices, coagulopathy, stomal bleeding, and hepatic fibrosis/cirrhosis.
   - Thrombosis of the major central venous accesses: jugular, subclavian, and femoral veins. Thrombosis of 2 or more of these vessels is considered a life-threatening complication and failure of PN therapy. The sequelae of central venous thrombosis are lack of access for PN infusion, fatal sepsis due to infected thrombi, pulmonary embolism, superior vena cava syndrome, and chronic venous insufficiency.
   - Frequent line infection and sepsis. The development of 2 or more episodes per year of systemic sepsis secondary to line infection that requires hospitalization indicates failure of PN therapy. A single episode of line-related fungemia, septic shock, and/or acute respiratory distress syndrome is considered an indicator of PN failure.
   - Frequent episodes of severe dehydration despite intravenous fluid supplement in addition to PN. Under certain medical conditions, such as secretory diarrhea and nonconstructable gastrointestinal tract, the loss of the gastrointestinal and pancreatobiliary secretions exceeds the maximum intravenous infusion rates that can be tolerated by the cardiopulmonary system. Frequent episodes of dehydration are deleterious to all body organs, in particular kidneys and the central nervous system, with the development of multiple kidney stones, renal failure, and permanent brain damage.
2. High mortality risk due to underlying disease indications:
   - Benign/low-grade malignant tumors involving the mesenteric root, such as desmoid tumors
   - Congenital mucosal disorders
   - Ultrashort bowel syndrome (<30 cm of remnant intestine)
3. Nontraditional indications:
   - Extensive thrombosis of the portomesenteric system
   - Abdominal catastrophes
   - Intestinal dysmotility, pseudo-obstruction
   - IF with high morbidity due to recurrent hospitalizations, narcotic dependence, decreased quality of life, and low patient acceptance of PN

The type of graft used varies according with the baseline disease and possible damage to other abdominal organs. In patients with multiple abdominal surgeries or infections of the abdominal cavity, replacement of all the abdominal organs, including liver, might be necessary even without liver disease due to impossible safe dissection of the abdominal organs. If biochemical changes related to liver disease are present, a liver biopsy should be performed as part of the evaluation process. The presence of extensive fibrosis and/or cirrhosis is an indication for the replacement of the liver. In patients with mild to moderate fibrosis, liver biopsies should be obtained every 6 to 12 months and patients should have frequent examinations for the detection of possible signs of portal hypertension.

Patients with ultrashort gut syndrome (<30 cm of small bowel) and congenital enter-opathies should be considered early for transplantation to avoid IF-associated liver disease. Patients with functional disease of the digestive tract, such as chronic intestinal pseudo-obstruction, may have poor quality of life related to massive dilatation of the abdomen, nausea, vomiting, and electrolyte imbalance despite the presence of decompressive enterostomies.[8] Intestinal motility studies are required to demonstrate the type and extent of the disease.

Specific hematologic tests, including hypercoagulable studies, are frequently needed for patients with thrombotic disorders, and triple-phase CT scan or abdominal visceral angiography may be used to assess the extent of thrombosis. In these and other high-risk patients, imaging of the upper- and lower-extremity central venous system is mandatory for the safe establishment of central venous access at the time of transplant. The extent of studies required to assess the cardiopulmonary and other body organ systems is determined by patient age, complexity of the medical/surgical history, and nature of the primary disease. Because of the chronic illness and drug dependency in most of these patients, a comprehensive psychosocial evaluation is mandatory for candidacy and valuable guidance for postoperative management.[9] It is estimated that 15% to 20% of patients on chronic TPN are potential candidates for intestinal transplantation.[10] Due to lack of donor organs and surgical expertise, however, only a small fraction of these ultimately receive transplantation. Patients who are candidates for this procedure generally have a condition that is nonresponsive to standard medical or surgical therapy and are considered terminal. Because of the surgical experience required to perform this procedure, individual transplant centers are frequently dependent on 1 or 2 surgeons for the existence of a program. The complexity of this procedure, with its steep learning curve in these high-risk patients, requires meticulous attention to all medical and surgical details to ensure the best outcomes.

CONTRAINDICATIONS

The absolute contraindications for intestinal transplantation and MVTx are similar to other solid organ transplants and include

- Life-threatening illness unrelated to digestive tract (eg, significant cardiopulmonary disease)
- Severe neurologic disability
- Disseminated malignancy

The relative contraindications for ITx or MVTx are

- Severe immunologic deficiency
- Multisystem autoimmune disorder
- Inadequate vascular anatomy with questionable long-term patency
- Prematurity with lung disease

It is also important to have adequate psychological and social support because postoperative care can be quite demanding.

TYPES OF GRAFTS

The use of intestinal and multivisceral grafts is usually tailored to the specific needs of patients combined with the available expertise at the transplant center. The common element in all variants is the transplantation of the small bowel. Inclusion of the colon, pancreas, spleen, kidney, and abdominal wall is performed as appropriate to the baseline pathology and center preference. All modifications are different combinations of the cluster concept initially proposed by Starzl and colleagues.[11] In some patients, the native liver can be preserved whereas in others who have significant liver disease or have complex anatomy where the abdominal organs cannot be safely separated the liver is replaced en bloc along with the other abdominal organs.

Isolated Intestinal Transplant

Transplantation of the small intestine is performed for patients with irreversible IF in the absence of IF-associated liver disease (**Fig. 1**). One of the following criteria should also be present:

1. Recurrent catheter-related sepsis (2 or more episodes of sepsis secondary line infections per year or 1 episode of fungal infection directly related to the use of central access).
2. Thrombosis of 2 of the 6 major venous access sites (jugular, femoral, or subclavian)
3. Growth failure and developmental delay in pediatric patients

Combined Liver–Pancreas–Small Bowel Transplant

This modality of transplant is performed in patients with IF and irreversible liver disease. The native stomach, pancreaticoduodenal complex, and spleen of the recipient are preserved (**Fig. 2**). The graft is composed of the liver, pancreas, and small bowel. Even though most patients do not have evidence of pancreatic disease, the inclusion of the pancreaticoduodenal complex avoids hilar dissection by keeping intact the drainage of the common bile duct. A portacaval anastomosis is required to drain the native organs.

Multivisceral Transplantation

In MVTx, complete evisceration of the native foregut and remnant midgut is performed followed by en bloc transplantation of the stomach, pancreaticoduodenal complex, liver, and small bowel (**Fig. 3**). A variant of MVTx is the MMVTx, where the native liver is preserved and all other organs are transplanted in the manner described for MVTx (**Fig. 4**).

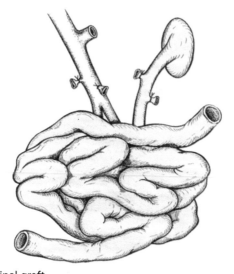

Fig. 1. Isolated intestinal graft.

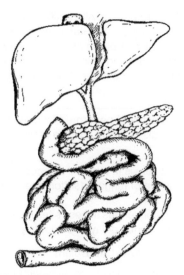

Fig. 2. Liver/pancreas/intestinal graft.

Most pediatric patients have a congenital anomaly or necrotizing enterocolitis associated with prematurity and become dependent on PN related to IF. Adults may experience the same process but are more likely to have survived some previous pathology, such as cancer, trauma, ischemia, or necrotizing pancreatitis with resultant IF or frozen abdomen complicated by liver failure. Many adult patients with cirrhosis develop severe portomesenteric thrombosis, which can be an exclusionary factor for liver transplantation. The use of MVTx in these patients can provide a surgical option for simultaneous cure of the cirrhosis and portomesenteric thrombosis in patients who otherwise have a terminal disease process.[12,13] Indications for MMVTx are more limited and include many of these conditions but with preserved liver function. Another emerging indication for MMVTx is chronic intestinal pseudo-obstruction.

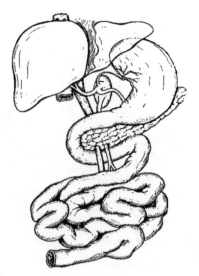

Fig. 3. Multivisceral graft.

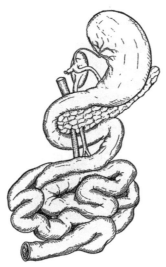

Fig. 4. Modified multivisceral graft.

SURGICAL TECHNIQUE

The surgical procedures for ITx, MVTx, and MMVTx have considerable variations. Here we only describe the surgical technique of MVTx. The donor procedure consists of mobilization of all abdominal viscera exposing the infrarenal vena cava and aorta. The celiac, superior mesenteric artery (SMA), and retrohepatic inferior vena cava (IVC) are isolated and the retrieval is performed en bloc. The recipient procedure consists of resection of native stomach, pancreaticoduodenal complex, small and large intestinal remnant, and liver with preservation of IVC. The donor procedure is usually the most challenging part of the surgery due to multiple adhesions, intrabdominal varices, and portal hypertension. Intraoperative blood loss is usually minimized by occlusion of celiac and SMA at the beginning of the surgery. Graft implantation is completed after obtaining arterial, venous, and gastrointestinal anastomoses. Vascular reconstruction techniques may differ slightly based on the anatomic complexity and the transplant surgeon's expertise. Pyloroplasty due to gastrointestinal denervation and ileostomy for easier enteral access postoperatively are performed in most cases. Graft size reduction may also be necessary, especially in pediatric and small-sized recipients to accomplish abdominal wall closure and to prevent abdominal compartment syndrome.

POSTOPERATIVE MANAGEMENT

There are several equally important components in the postoperative management of intestinal transplant and MVTx patients. A multidisciplinary team, including the transplant physicians, experienced nursing staff, dieticians, social workers, and financial and administrative personnel, are mandatory to efficiently care for these complex patients. Important aspects of patient management include graft surveillance with rejection monitoring, adequate nutrition, control of infections, malignancy surveillance, and ongoing quality-of-life assessment. In the immediate postoperative period, an early concern in small bowel transplant recipients is maintenance of adequate hydroelectrolytic balance. The transplanted small bowel can develop significant edema in the first 24 to 48 hours after surgery, which is caused mainly by ischemia-reperfusion injury. The edema can lead to massive fluid sequestration and third spacing. Edema of the graft can be deleterious for the small bowel and for the liver when included in a graft. A significant increase in intra-abdominal pressure can lead to abdominal compartment syndrome, which results in increased ventilation requirements and renal failure. Resuscitation should be balanced carefully between colloid administration and the use of vasopressors. Broad-spectrum antibiotics are typically maintained for at least a week. Patients transplanted for complex portomesenteric thrombosis usually have a higher requirement for transfusions during surgery and in general are unstable in the early postoperative period.[13] Because of the duration and magnitude of the surgery, patients develop hypothermia and all possible measures to raise the temperature should be taken. Warming the ICU, use of a thermal blanket, and infusion of warmed fluids are useful and important measures to be taken as soon as patients arrive in the surgical ICU.[14] Coagulopathy should be corrected aggressively with the appropriate use of fresh frozen plasma, platelets, and cryoprecipitate. Patients requiring massive transfusion should be monitored for hyperkalemia. Measures to manage hyperkalemia and its complications include sodium bicarbonate, calcium, insulin, diuretics, and dialysis.[15]

Patients with chronic renal failure and listed for kidney transplant should undergo dialysis during the surgery and in the early postoperative days (see **Fig. 4**). The use of the kidney perfusion machines allows the kidney transplant procedure to take place 24 to 48 hours after the MVTx. This strategy allows the kidney to be transplanted in a more favorable hemodynamic condition, reducing the rate of acute tubular necrosis in the renal graft. Abdominal drains are useful for monitoring bleeding, enteric fistulae; chylous ascites; and bile leaks, and caution should be taken to remove them as soon as the drainage decreases. Abdominal collections are a common finding after MVTx and do not require any intervention most of the times. Extubation should be performed as soon as possible and early ambulation is encouraged.

Despite the complexity of the procedure, perioperative mortality is rare in experienced hands and hospital stay has decreased drastically in the past decade, with several patients leaving the hospital in fewer than 3 weeks with complete enteral autonomy without the need for parenteral hydration or nutrition.[16]

IMMUNOSUPPRESSION

The use of induction therapy with monoclonal or polyclonal antibody preparations is a frequent practice in nearly all small bowel transplant centers.[17] The most commonly used induction agents are thymoglobulin, alemtuzumab, and basiliximab.[18–20] Tacrolimus is used in virtually all centers as the core drug for maintenance therapy. Corticosteroids are also included in the postoperative period, and they are usually weaned over variable time periods, depending on each center's preference. Sirolimus has been used in association with tacrolimus in an attempt to control early episodes of severe exfoliative rejection.[21] The use mofetil mycophenolate has also been reported, but its routine use is abandoned because of the frequent association with gastrointestinal side effects. Tacrolimus serum target levels are usually kept between 12 and 15 ng/dL in the first month after transplant and subsequently decreased to 8 to 12 ng/dL in most centers.

Nonsurgical Complications

Rejection

The intestine is the most immunogenic of all the solid transplantable organs. In the past decade, the use of induction therapy with interleukin-2 receptor blockers, antilymphocyte or antithymocyte preparations combined with a better understanding of the mechanisms of rejection has resulted in continual improvement in graft survival after intestinal transplantation. Acute cellular rejection remains the most common complication after intestinal transplantation and still occurs with higher frequency compared with transplantation of other solid abdominal organs. In 2 recent, large-center reports, the incidence of acute cellular rejection ranged between 50% and 70% in the first 90 days after transplant.[22,23] The occurrence of rejection in the first 90 days after transplant has a negative impact on long-term graft survival, as reported by the latest Intestinal Transplant Registry report.[24] The diagnosis of rejection is based on a combination of clinical signs and endoscopic findings. Confirming a theory from more than 20 years ago, the transplanted liver seems to have a protective effect on the intestinal graft, with less than 20% of patients undergoing MVTx having some degree of rejection in the first 90 days after transplantation.[24] Although high-volume stooling is the most common symptom, rejection also can manifest with fever, vomiting, ileus, cramping, severe abdominal pain, and gastrointestinal bleeding. Rejection of the small bowel causes different degrees of mucosal and intramural injuries.

Acute rejection of the small bowel can be categorized as mild, moderate, or severe depending on the severity of the following histologic features: increase in the number of apoptotic bodies, increasing space between the villae, lymphocytic infiltration of the lamina propria, crypt epithelial injury, mucosal ulceration, and intimal/transmural arteritis.[25] Several biopsies should be taken in the presence of rejection, because the injury can spare segments of the graft. Mucosal injury can lead to damage of the intestinal epithelial barrier, and life-threatening episodes of sepsis can occur with bacterial translocation. This cycle leads to high rates of morbidity and mortality in intestinal transplantation. Augmentation of baseline immunosuppression in response to rejection is generally the first step in the management of rejection, which should be cautiously weighed against the risk of infectious complications.

An ileostomy is usually constructed during the transplant, which facilitates easier endoscopic access to the intestinal graft. Protocols for graft surveillance with serial endoscopy and biopsy differ from center to center. Surveillance ileoscopy usually is performed once or twice a week for the first 2 to 3 months and then monthly for another 6 months. The ileostomy is closed 3 to 12 months after transplant. Once the normal physiologic transit is re-established, a colonoscopy is performed every 6 to 12 months or whenever clinically indicated. The use of noninvasive screening for rejection of the intestinal graft is in its infancy. Citrulline, calprotectin, perforin, and granzyme B have been used in monitoring for rejection; however, further studies are needed to confirm their applicability and prognostic importance.[26,27] Histologic evaluation continues to be the gold standard for the diagnosis of rejection. Episodes of mild rejection usually can be treated with pulsed steroids. Progression from mild to moderate or severe rejection requires the use of higher immunosuppression. Use of infliximab, an anti–tumor necrosis factor α agent, has been reported in a few patients with rejection resistant to antilymphocitic preparations.[28] Although nonspecific, all patients with high output should be investigated for acute rejection. Presence of inflammation, friability, villous blunting, edema, and vascular congestions is highly suggestive of rejection (**Fig. 5**) with correlating microscopic features.[25] Episodes of severe rejection usually take several weeks to improve. During this period, patients may experience heavy bleeding and recurrent sepsis due to loss of intestinal mucosal barrier (**Fig. 6**). Antibacterial, antifungal, and antiviral prophylaxis is mandatory at this time. Some patients may require enterectomy as a life-saving procedure. The timing to perform an enterectomy is crucial and always a difficult decision.

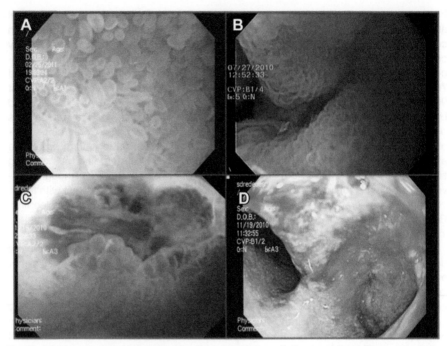

Fig. 5. (A) Normal villae. (B) Mild rejection, shortening of vilae, and hyperemia. (C) Moderate to severe rejection: presence of ulcers. (D) Severe rejection: total absence of vilae, bleeding.

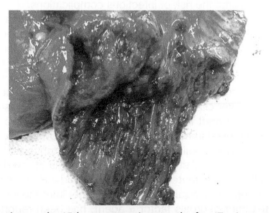

Fig. 6. Severe rejection on the 15th postoperative month after ITx. Appropriate immunosuppression was observed during all the 15 months. Patient was treated with Campath and corticosteroids bolus without reversal of the situation. After 5 weeks of treatment, the patient underwent bowel resection for refractory bleeding and sepsis. The same patient was re-transplanted 3 months after the bowel resection.

Graft-versus-host disease

GVHD typically occurs when immunocompetent donor cells damage the tissues of the recipient after transplant. The complication is feared in intestinal transplantation because of the large amount of lymphatic tissue present in the graft and its association with high mortality rates. GVHD affects between 2% and 5 % of intestinal transplant recipients. The most commonly affected areas are the skin, bone marrow, liver, lungs, and gastrointestinal tract. Skin rash is the most common presentation and all suspicious lesions should be biopsied (**Fig. 7**). Patients with severe diarrhea and negative screening for rejection should have stomach and native colon biopsies to rule out GVHD. Intense inflammatory activity and increased numbers of apoptotic bodies are common findings and are highly suspicious of GVHD in the absence of viral infection. GVHD has a high mortality rate when the bone marrow is involved. The treatment of GVHD varies widely from withdrawal of immunosuppression in mild cases to augmentation of immunosuppression with high-doses teroids and other potent immunosuppressant drugs in severe cases.[29]

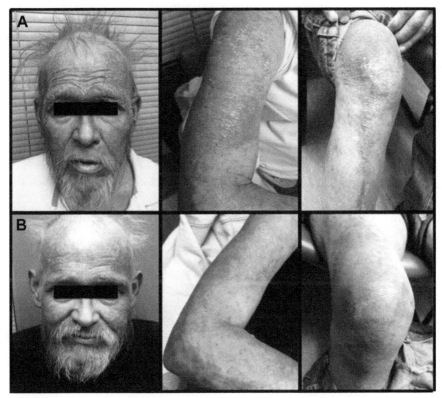

Fig. 7. GVHD. (*A*) Cutaneous involvement in a multivisceral recipient. (*B*) After 1 month of treatment.

Posttransplant lymph proliferative disorder

Posttransplant lymphoproliferative disorder (PTLD) is well defined in intestinal transplantation and remains a persistent problem. Rates of PTLD have remained stable, at 6% to 8% of all recipients, despite changes in immunosuppression regimens. PTLD has its highest incidence approximately 2 years after transplant. There is a strong association between Epstein-Barr virus infection (EBV) and PTLD. It is believed that approximately 80% of cases of PTLD are related to the EBV. Risk factors for the development of the disease are EBV-negative recipients with positive donor at the time of the transplant, pediatric recipients, and use of highly immunosuppressive induction agents.[30] Increased EBV levels in the blood should be followed by reduction of the immunosuppression and screening for PTLD with CT scan of the neck, chest, abdomen, and pelvis in search of tumors or enlarged lymph nodes. The treatment consists of 1 or more of the following strategies: reduction or withdrawal of the immunosuppression, tumor resection when indicated, rituximab for tumors positive for CD20 antibody, conventional chemotherapy, and antiviral agents.

Cytomegalovirus

Cytomegalovirus (CMV) is a common occurrence after intestinal transplantation. Recipients with negative CMV prior to transplantation who receive organs from CMV-positive donors are more likely to develop the disease. The clinical manifestations can range from diarrhea and abdominal pain to gastrointestinal bleeding and sepsis. Presence of ulcers in the transplanted intestine is a common endoscopic finding. Microscopically, there is a chronic inflammatory infiltrate composed of lymphocytes and histiocytes, with neutrophils in the lamina propria. Large inclusions of CMV in cell nuclei surrounded by a clear halo and thickening of the nuclear membrane are diagnostic. CMV infection can present clinically in various forms from an incidental finding on routine laboratory tests to severe ulceration of the intestinal mucosa. Severe infection may need enterectomy (**Fig. 8**), with some patients presenting with diffuse gastrointestinal bleeding, sepsis, and intestinal perforation. Monitoring of quantitative CMV viral load by polymerase chain reaction should be routinely performed.

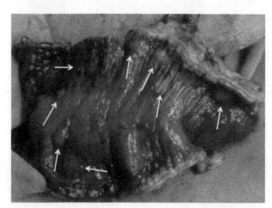

Fig. 8. Diffuse CMV in the intestine graft. Intestine is denuded, with total damage of the mucosa. Patient presented with intense gastrointestinal bleeding and intestinal perforation. Patient underwent enterectomy and was retransplanted after clinical improvement. *Arrows:* CMV colitis.

OUTCOMES

The International Small Bowel Transplant Symposium meets biannually to review current research and clinical outcomes in intestinal transplantation around the world. At the meeting, updated results are presented from the Intestinal Transplant Registry, which includes worldwide data. The XIII meeting of this association was held in 2013, and Registry data through February 2013 were presented. There have been 2887 documented intestine transplants from April 1985 through February 2013. This number is composed of 1309 isolated small bowel transplants, 898 small bowel and liver transplants, and 680 MVTxs (141 MMVTxs). Of these transplants, there are 1416 current survivors. As with other abdominal and thoracic organs, long-term transplant outcomes for intestinal transplantation were initially poor but have improved with increasing experience. Results from the 1980s included patient survival rate at 5 years of approximately 40%, with an improvement to 45% in the 1990s. Since 2000, 5-year patient survival rate is approximately 60% for all adult and pediatric recipients. Unfortunately, patients with higher risk of death include very old and very young individuals. Patients with grafts, including the liver, and those coming from home (non-hospitalized patients) have a better long-term outcome compared with other recipients.

SUMMARY

As clinical experience has increased with intestinal transplantation and MVTx, the volume of these surgeries has risen in the past decade with significantly improved outcomes. The currently reported 1-year graft and patient survival rate is 80%, which approaches that for other solid abdominal organs. Unfortunately, most of the gains in survival are seen in the first postoperative year but the long-term survival basically has remained unchanged since the early 1990s (5-year and 10-year patient survival rates approximately 60% and 40%, respectively). With improved outcomes, more centers have entered into the intestinal transplant arena. Increase in access to intestinal transplantation and more widespread awareness of this option will likely result in a consistent increase in the number of yearly transplants for the foreseeable future. Immunosuppressive regimens continue to evolve, with induction therapy the major change in the past 10 years. Although rejection rates in the first year after transplant have been reduced by induction therapy, long-term side effects of heavy immunosuppression continue to weigh negatively on transplant outcomes. Intestinal transplantation continues to be performed only in situations in which all other therapeutic modalities have failed. No randomized trials compare intestinal transplantation to long-term PN to establish guidelines for a timely referral for this treatment option. Late referral remains a crippling problem in the field of intestinal transplantation, with a great number of patients in need of simultaneous liver transplantation at the time of listing for intestinal transplantation. Early referral for ITx will reduce the need for simultaneous multiorgan transplants and increase the residual organs available for patients in need of (primarily) liver transplantation.

REFERENCES

1. Kirkman RL. Small bowel transplantation. Transplantation 1984;37(5):429–33.
2. Starzl TE, Rowe MI, Todo S, et al. Transplantation of multiple abdominal viscera. JAMA 1989;261(10):1449–57.
3. Murase N, Kim DG, Todo S, et al. Suppression of allograft rejection with FK506. I. Prolonged cardiac and liver survival in rats following short-course therapy. Transplantation 1990;50(2):186–9.
4. Murase N, Kim DG, Todo S, et al. FK506 suppression of heart and liver allograft rejection. II: the induction of graft acceptance in rats. Transplantation 1990;50(5): 739–44.
5. Abu-Elmagd KM, Costa G, Bond GJ, et al. Five hundred intestinal and multivisceral transplantations at a single center: major advances with new challenges. Ann Surg 2009;250(4):567–81.
6. Mangus RS, Subbarao GC. Intestinal transplantation in infants with intestinal failure. Clin Perinatol 2013;40(1):161–73.
7. Goulet O, Ruemmele F, Lacaille F, et al. Irreversible intestinal failure. J Pediatr Gastroenterol Nutr 2004;38(3):250–69.
8. Vianna RM, Mangus RS, Tector AJ. Current status of small bowel and multivisceral transplantation. Adv Surg 2008;42:129–50.
9. Matarese LE, Costa G, Bond G, et al. Therapeutic efficacy of intestinal and multivisceral transplantation: survival and nutrition outcome. Nutr Clin Pract 2007; 22(5):474–81.

10. Abu-Elmagd KM, Kosmach-Park B, Costa G, et al. Long-term survival, nutritional autonomy, and quality of life after intestinal and multivisceral transplantation. Ann Surg 2012;256(3):494–508.

11. Starzl TE, Todo S, Tzakis A, et al. The many faces of multivisceral transplantation. Surg Gynecol Obstet 1991;172(5):335–44.

12. Vianna R, Giovanardi RO, Fridell JA, et al. Multivisceral transplantation for diffuse portomesenteric thrombosis in a patient with life-threatening esophagogastro-duodenal bleeding. Transplantation 2005;80(4):534–5.

13. Vianna RM, Mangus RS, Kubal C, et al. Multivisceral transplantation for diffuse portomesenteric thrombosis. Ann Surg 2012;255(6):1144–50.

14. Karalapillai D, Story D. Hypothermia on arrival in the intensive care unit after surgery. Crit Care Resusc 2008;10(2):116–9.

15. Cottrell D. Managing acute hyperkalemia. Nursing 2012;42(10):68.

16. Vianna RM, Mangus RS. Present prospects and future perspectives of intestinal and multivisceral transplantation. Curr Opin Clin Nutr Metab Care 2009;12(3):281–6.

17. Grant D, Abu-Elmagd K, Reyes J, et al. 2003 report of the intestine transplant registry: a new era has dawned. Ann Surg 2005;241(4):607–13.

18. Langnas A, Chinnakotla S, Sudan D, et al. Intestinal transplantation at the University of Nebraska Medical Center: 1990 to 2001. Transplant Proc 2002;34(3):958–60.

19. Nishida S, Levi DM, Moon JI, et al. Intestinal transplantation with alemtuzumab (Campath-1H) induction for adult patients. Transplant Proc 2006;38(6):1747–9.

20. Vianna RM, Mangus RS, Fridell JA, et al. Initiation of an intestinal transplant program: the Indiana experience. Transplantation 2008;85(12):1784–90.

21. Fishbein TM, Florman S, Gondolesi G, et al. Intestinal transplantation before and after the introduction of sirolimus. Transplantation 2002;73(10):1538–42.

22. Tzakis AG, Kato T, Levi DM, et al. 100 multivisceral transplants at a single center. Ann Surg 2005;242(4):480–90 [discussion: 491–3].

23. Abu-Elmagd K, Reyes J, Bond G, et al. Clinical intestinal transplantation: a decade of experience at a single center. Ann Surg 2001;234(3):404–16 [discussion: 416–7].

24. Intestinal Transplant Registry Report. 2013. Available at: http://www.intestinal transplant.org/itr/.

25. Wu T, Abu-Elmagd K, Bond G, et al. A schema for histologic grading of small intestine allograft acute rejection. Transplantation 2003;75(8):1241–8.

26. Sudan D, Vargas L, Sun Y, et al. Calprotectin: a novel noninvasive marker for intestinal allograft monitoring. Ann Surg 2007;246(2):311–5.

27. Pappas PA, Tzakis AG, Saudubray JM, et al. Trends in serum citrulline and acute rejection among recipients of small bowel transplants. Transplant Proc 2004;36(2):345–7.

28. Pascher A, Klupp J, Langrehr JM, et al. Anti-TNF-alpha therapy for acute rejection in intestinal transplantation. Transplant Proc 2005;37(3):1635–6.

29. Wu G, Selvaggi G, Nishida S, et al. Graft-versus-host disease after intestinal and multivisceral transplantation. Transplantation 2011;91(2):219–24.

30. Abu-Elmagd KM, Mazariegos G, Costa G, et al. Lymphoproliferative disorders and de novo malignancies in intestinal and multivisceral recipients: improved outcomes with new outlooks. Transplantation 2009;88(7):926–34.

Recurrence of Nonviral Liver Diseases After Liver Transplantation

Ivo W. Graziadei, MD[a,b,*]

KEYWORDS

- Immunosuppression • Graft survival • Liver cirrhosis • Posttransplant management

KEY POINTS

- There is compelling evidence that nonviral diseases recur after liver transplantation (LT), with incidence rates ranging from 10% to 50%.
- In most patients, recurrent diseases do not negatively impact patient and graft survival.
- Recurrent alcoholism also jeopardizes the long-term outcome of LT recipients.

INTRODUCTION

Liver transplantation (LT) has become a well-accepted treatment modality for patients with acute or chronic liver failure, as well as hepatocellular carcinoma. LT does not only improve survival but also the quality of life. Mainly due to advances in surgical techniques and development of new, more potent immunosuppressive as well as anti-infective drugs, the outcome of LT recipients has dramatically improved over the past decades, leading to an increased number of long-term survivors after LT.[1,2]

Many diseases causing acute or chronic liver failure, however, may recur after LT and may negatively affect patient and graft survival. The incidence rates and the impact on patient and graft survival mainly depend on the indication for LT. In particular, recurrent hepatitis C infection is almost universal, leading to rapid fibrosis and graft loss in a significant number of patients within 5 to 10 years after LT.[3,4] With the increasing number of long-term survivors of LT recipients transplanted for nonviral diseases, in particular autoimmune hepatitis (AIH), primary biliary cirrhosis (PBC), primary sclerosing cholangitis (PSC), alcoholic liver disease (ALD), and nonalcoholic

The author has nothing to disclose.
[a] Department of Internal Medicine II (Gastroenterology and Hepatology), Medical University of Innsbruck, Anichstraße 35, A-6020 Innsbruck, Austria; [b] Department of Internal Medicine, District Hospital Hall, Milserstraße 10, A-6060 Hall, Austria
* Department of Internal Medicine, District Hospital Hall, Milserstraße 10, A-6060 Hall, Austria.
E-mail address: ivo.graziadei@i-med.ac.at

steato-hepatitis (NASH), it became evident that disease recurrence is a clinically important and prognostically relevant issue in the long-term management of these patients.

The aim of this review is to examine the current knowledge of recurrent nonviral liver diseases after LT with special emphasis on diagnosis, risk factors, therapy, and impact on patient and graft survival.

AIH, PBC, AND PSC

In contrast to patients with AIH, there is almost no effective medical treatment available for patients with PBC and PSC to cure or at least positively influence the natural history of these diseases. Consequently, LT is the only potentially curative therapeutic option for patients with liver cirrhosis secondary to PBC and PSC. End-stage liver disease due to AIH, PBC, and PSC accounts for 3% to 8% of the indications for LT according to the United Network of Organ Sharing (UNOS) and the European Liver Transplant Registry (ELTR). The long-term outcome of these patients is excellent, with actuarial 5-year and 10-year survival rates higher than 70%, 5 and 10 years after LT.[5-11] In contrast to the recurrence of viral hepatitis, which is well accepted, the recurrence of AIH, PBC, and, in particular, PSC has been a constant subject of debate with respect to diagnostic criteria and impact on long-term outcome.

AIH

Recurrence of AIH in the allograft was first described by the King's College group in 1984[12] and, subsequently, confirmed by several other reports. However, there are no standard criteria to diagnose AIH recurrence. Most investigators based their diagnosis on increased serum transaminases, positive autoantibody titers greater than 1:40, in particular antinuclear antibodies (ANAs), hyper-gamma-globulinemia, and characteristic histologic features of (peri)portal and lobular hepatitis with lymphoplasmacellular infiltration in the absence of acute cellular rejection or viral infection.[13,14] The exact differentiation between acute rejection and recurrent AIH, however, is particularly challenging. Also, markers that are helpful in the pre-LT diagnosis of AIH, such as elevated liver transaminases associated with hyper-gamma-globulinemia and the presence of autoantibodies may persist after LT without any specific diagnostic relevance for recurrent AIH.

Recurrence rates between 16% and 43% have been reported for patients transplanted for AIH-related cirrhosis. In a recent review article, including 25 publications, 23% of patients developed a recurrent disease after a median interval of 26.4 months (range: 14–55 months) after LT.[15] Pathologic findings seemed to be the most appropriate diagnostic markers. Interestingly, in one article, histologic abnormalities characteristic for recurrent AIH were found on protocol liver biopsies in the absence of elevated biochemical liver tests, demonstrating the importance for late-protocol biopsies in these patients.[16]

Results regarding possible risk factors for AIH recurrence are controversially discussed in the literature. Some investigators have shown an increased frequency of recurrent disease in HLA-DR3–positive recipients, whereas others have failed to observe this association.[7,8,17,18] HLA antigen mismatch and numbers of acute cellular rejections did not differ between patients with or without recurrent disease. In addition, no difference in AIH recurrence was found with the use of cyclosporine A or tacrolimus for immunosuppression, as well as pretransplant or posttransplant overall dose and duration of corticosteroid treatment.[15]

Most patients with recurrent AIH respond to intensified immunosuppressive therapy either in terms of higher doses of corticosteroids and/or change to more potent immunosuppressive agents, for instance tacrolimus.[9,19] Recurrent disease does not negatively influence the long-term outcome in the vast majority of patients. Fewer than 5% of patients had to undergo re-LT due to recurrent AIH.[9]

De novo AIH has been reported especially in the pediatric LT cohort, with an incidence of 1% to 5%.[20]

PBC

Recurrence of PBC was first reported in 1982 by Neuberger and colleagues.[21] The diagnosis was based on clinical features, abnormal liver tests, elevated antimitochondrial antibodies, and histologic findings compatible with features of PBC. Because of the nonspecificity of clinical, biochemical, and autoimmune parameters, strict histologic criteria for recurrent PBC were postulated in the early 1990s.[22] Although there was a constant debate about whether these findings indicate true recurrent PBC, the gold standard of the diagnosis of PBC recurrence remains liver biopsy with characteristic features for PBC (bile duct destruction caused by florid bile duct lesions) and a thorough exclusion of other diseases that can mimic recurrent PBC, such as chronic rejection or a bile flow obstruction (**Box 1**). Most studies demonstrated that antimitochondrial antibodies were not reliable markers for the assessment of recurrent disease.

A recurrence rate between 10% and 50% has been reported in the literature. Including 35 publications on PBC recurrence, Gautam and colleagues[15] showed that the prevalence was 13% after a median time of 46.5 months, with a range from 25 to 78 months post-LT. Most of the patients were women (90%) with an average

---

Box 1
Definition of primary biliary cirrhosis (PBC) recurrence after liver transplantation

- Confirmed diagnosis of PBC in the explant histology
- Positive antimitochondrial antibodies (AMA) or AMA-M2
- Characteristic histologic features:
  - Portal epitheloid granulomas
  - Mononuclear portal inflammatory infiltration
  - Portal lymphoid aggregates
  - Bile duct damage
- Exclusion of
  - Acute or chronic rejection
  - Graft versus host disease
  - Bile flow impairment or cholangitis
  - Vascular complications
  - Viral hepatitis
  - Drug-induced liver injury

Data from Hubscher SG, Elias E, Buckels JA, et al. Primary biliary cirrhosis. Histologic evidence of disease recurrence after liver transplantation. J Hepatol 1993;18:173–84.

age of approximately 52 years. Studies with protocol biopsies reported a higher incidence of PBC recurrence with rates up to 50%.

Risk factors such as an increased donor and recipient age and increased cold and warm ischemic times remain controversial because studies have produced conflicting data in this respect.[23] There is increasing evidence for a genetic predisposition for patients with PBC. In a recent article, it has been suggested that a smaller number of HLA-A, HLA-B, and HLA-DR mismatches was a significant risk factor for PBC recurrence.[24] However, further studies are needed to confirm these findings.

Several studies have argued that patients treated with tacrolimus developed PBC recurrence more often and to an earlier point of time after LT compared with patients with cyclosporine A.[5,6,25] Other groups, however, demonstrated that recurrence rates did not differ between patients receiving cyclosporine or tacrolimus.[26,27] In addition, it has to be mentioned that all these studies had a retrospective design and were not randomized. Based on the current literature, no recommendation can be given regarding the immunosuppression in patients with PBC after LT. This issue clearly needs further evaluation and a randomized controlled study is mandatory to give an answer regarding the optimal immunosuppression for patients with PBC after LT.

Although no robust data are available, most clinicians recommend initiation of ursodeoxycholic acid (UDCA) treatment once the diagnosis of PBC recurrence has been made. In a small study, patients with recurrent PBC were placed on UDCA with improvement in alkaline phosphatase in most patients.[28] An uncontrolled pilot study from the Mayo Clinic also showed that UDCA therapy for 36 months led to a normalization of alkaline phosphates levels in 52% of patients with PBC recurrence in comparison with 22% of untreated historic controls. However, UDCA did not influence patient and graft survival. Unfortunately no liver biopsies were performed in this study to provide any data on the histologic effect of UDCA on PBC recurrence.[29] There is also no evidence for the prophylactic use of UDCA.

Most studies have shown that disease recurrence does not negatively impact the long-term survival of patients with PBC after LT. In a German study, only 2% of patients with PBC developed graft dysfunction secondary to recurrent disease.[6]

PSC

The possibility of recurrent PSC was first introduced by Lerut and coworkers in 1988.[30] Thereafter, several other centers reported on this issue. Sheng and colleagues[31] reported that intrahepatic and nonanastomotic extrahepatic biliary strictures were significantly more common in patients who had undergone LT for PSC than in those who received an allograft with Roux-en-Y choledochojejunostomy for other end-stage liver diseases. Histologic evidence of PSC recurrence was provided by a study from Birmingham. The investigators demonstrated that fibro-obliterative lesions, the characteristic histologic feature for PSC, were observed only in patients who received a transplant for PSC.[32]

The diagnosis of PSC recurrence can be challenging, as biliary strictures in the allograft suggesting PSC recurrence are nonspecific and may be due to a variety of other causes, such as reperfusion injury, ischemia caused by hepatic artery thrombosis/stenosis, ABO incompatibility, biliary sepsis, or technical complications.

In different patient series, published in the past years, the diagnosis of PSC recurrence has been based on strict inclusion and exclusion criteria proposed by the Mayo Clinic.[33] These criteria are outlined in **Box 2**. A recent study has shown that magnetic resonance cholangiography (MRC) imaging is an important tool for the diagnosis of recurrent PSC.[34] Apart from its capability to diagnose biliary strictures, MRC may be of value to identify vascular complications.

Box 2
Definition of primary sclerosing cholangitis (PSC) recurrence after liver transplantation

Inclusion criteria

- Confirmed *diagnosis* of PSC before liver transplantation
- *Cholangiography:* Intrahepatic and/or extrahepatic biliary stricturing, beading, and irregularities at least more than 90 days after transplantation
- *Histology:* Fibrous cholangitis and/or fibroobliterative lesions with or without ductopenia, biliary fibrosis, or biliary cirrhosis

Exclusion criteria

- Hepatic artery thrombosis/stenosis
- Established chronic ductopenic rejection
- Anastomotic strictures alone
- Nonanastomotic strictures before posttransplantation day 90
- ABO incompatibility between donor and recipient

Data from Graziadei IW, Wiesner RH, Batts KP, et al. Recurrence of primary sclerosing cholangitis following liver transplantation. Hepatology 1999;29:1050–6.

Based on 30 publications, the PSC recurrent rate varies between 5% and 47%.[15,35,36] Information regarding timing of disease recurrence was not given in most of the studies.

Several studies, primarily from Asia, have suggested that patients with PSC undergoing live donor LT, especially with biologically related donors, may have a higher risk of developing recurrent disease compared with the deceased donor setting.[37,38] However, this fact has to be interpreted with great caution, primarily due to the rather small number of patients. Further studies analyzing pooled data of all transplant centers performing live donor LTs are needed to confirm these findings.

Numerous risk factors, including recipient age, male gender, donor-recipient gender mismatch, coexisting inflammatory bowel disease, cytomegalovirus infection, acute cellular rejection episodes, and presence of cholangiocellular carcinoma have been discussed in the literature[23]; however, all these parameters could not be confirmed by independent studies of different centers.

The treatment of biliary strictures or their complications, such as cholangitis or choledocholithiasis, either with percutaneous or endoscopic approach, is the therapy of choice for patients with recurrent PSC. Although used in most centers, the efficacy of UDCA has not yet been demonstrated in the setting of PSC recurrence. There is also no evidence for the prophylactic use of UDCA in patients transplanted for PSC so as to prevent recurrence.

Patient and graft survival do not appear to be negatively affected by disease recurrence in the intermediate term of follow-up. But, there is increasing evidence that PSC recurrence might lead to graft dysfunction and the numbers of retransplantations due to recurrent PSC seem to increase with the longer duration of patient follow-up.[35,39,40]

ALD

ALD is the second most common indication for LT in the United States and Europe.[41,42] The posttransplant survival for ALD is comparable with other indications.[42] Studies have demonstrated a higher risk for ALD recipients to develop de novo malignancies and cardiovascular diseases, especially in combination with a positive smoking history.[42,43]

Although LT effectively restores liver dysfunction, it does not treat the underlying alcoholism. Therefore, alcohol relapse after LT is common. Because of the lack of a generally accepted definition of alcohol relapse, the recurrence rates are highly variable, ranging from as low as 10% to as high as 90%. Most of these studies defined relapse as any alcohol use regardless of alcohol amount. It has been shown that most patients remain abstinent or consume only small amounts of alcohol following LT.[44,45] An "addictive," harmful pattern of drinking has been observed in 5% to 20% of patients transplanted for ALD.[45–47] Long-term studies have demonstrated that occasional or moderately heavy drinking does not impact graft function or patient survival. In contrast, based on several reports, a return to abusive drinking is associated with advanced graft fibrosis and decreased medium to long-term graft and patient survival.[46–48] In a recently published single-center study, 16% of patients transplanted for LT relapsed into alcohol use. The pattern of relapse was a single event in 3.3%, an intermittent relapse in 7.3%, and continuously heavy drinking in 5.3% of all ALD recipients. Only recurrent harmful drinking was associated with advanced fibrosis and decreased graft survival.[47]

Therefore, all patients with a positive history of ALD should be encouraged to remain completely abstinent from alcohol post-LT and to enter psychiatric therapy or counseling if they relapse into regular alcohol consumption in the postoperative course.

NONALCOHOLIC FATTY LIVER DISEASE

Nonalcoholic fatty liver disease (NAFLD) is the most common cause of chronic liver disease, affecting almost 20% to 30% of the general population in the United States and Europe. Furthermore, the prevalence is expected to further increase over the next years. NAFLD/NASH is commonly associated with type 2 diabetes, visceral obesity, hypertension, and hyperlipidemia, which are part of the increasing epidemic of the metabolic syndrome.[49,50] Several studies have shown that a proportion of patients, especially those with NASH, will develop progressive liver disease leading to cirrhosis and/or hepatocellular carcinoma.[51] Currently, NASH is the third most common indication for LT in the United States, but is on a trajectory to become the leading indication for LT.[52] In addition, there is strong evidence that NASH is the leading cause of cryptogenic cirrhosis, which accounts for 7% to 14% of LTs in the United States.[53]

Several studies have shown an excellent outcome of patients with NASH cirrhosis similar to other causes of liver disease.[52,54–56] Patients with NASH-related cirrhosis, however, are more likely to develop and die of cardiovascular complications after LT.[54,55] Risk factors for NAFLD/NASH persist or even worsen after LT,[55] placing the recipients at a high risk of recurrent disease. In fact, numerous studies have shown that NAFLD and NASH recurrence is common after LT. The first reported case of NASH recurrence was published in a patient who underwent jejuno-ileal bypass surgery before LT in 1992[57] and was subsequently confirmed by others.[58] The rates of recurrence of steatosis and steatohepatitis in these studies varied widely, ranging from 8% to 65% and 4% to 35%, respectively, mainly depending on the differences in length of follow-up periods, study population, protocol biopsies, and definition of recurrent disease.[55,58,59]

The risk factors for recurrent NAFLD/NASH include pre-LT and post-LT diabetes mellitus type 2, obesity, and hyperlipidemia.[51] In addition, patatinlike phospholipase domain–containing 3 (PNPLA3) gene polymorphisms have been linked to NAFLD, obesity, and insulin resistance, and impact disease progression.[60,61] Two recent publications have shown that LT recipients with PNPLA3 non-CC genotype have an increased risk of posttransplant obesity, insulin resistance, and development of liver steatosis.[62,63] Although progression from simple steatosis to NASH, cirrhosis, and graft failure has been demonstrated, in most patients, recurrent NASH does not lead to significant fibrosis or even liver cirrhosis; however, most of these studies are limited by short follow-up periods.[51,55,59] Therefore, the long-term outcome and natural history of post-LT NAFLD/NASH remains unclear and has to be determined in prospective studies.

No specific recommendations regarding the prevention and treatment of recurrent NASH can be made, except to avoid excessive weight gain and to control diabetes and dyslipidemia. Recurrence of NASH in LT recipients can not only be treated medically but also potentially surgically. A recent article has shown that combined bariatric surgery (sleeve resection) and LT can be performed without increased risk of peri-LT and post-LT morbidity and mortality and might be considered for selected patients with persistent obesity and metabolic syndrome before LT.[64]

OTHER RARE INDICATIONS FOR LT

Hereditary hemochromatosis and secondary hemochromatosis are rare indications for LT, ranging from 0.5% to 1% of all LT.[65] Whereas older studies demonstrated a decreased overall survival of patients who received a transplant for hemochromatosis, more recent publications have shown no difference compared with other indications.[66,67] However, patients with hemochromatosis seem to have a higher risk of dying from cardiovascular diseases and are more susceptible to bacterial and fungal infections in the post-LT course.[68,69]

There are conflicting data regarding recurrence of hemochromatosis after LT. Some studies failed to show a reaccumulation of iron in the liver allograft[70,71]; in contrast, another article demonstrated that recurrence of iron accumulation may occur after LT and may lead to reduced graft survival.[72]

LT is the only curative therapeutic option for patients with Wilson's disease who fail to respond to medical treatment and those who present with fulminant hepatic failure. Long-term results are excellent.[73–75] Removal of the liver should reverse the metabolic disorder and, so far, there have been no reports suggesting recurrent disease.

SUMMARY

There is compelling evidence that nonviral diseases recur after liver transplantation with incidence rates ranging from 10% to 50%. In most patients, recurrent diseases do not negatively impact patient and graft survival. However, current studies with a longer duration of patient follow-up have shown that PSC recurrence might lead to graft dysfunction and the number of retransplantations due to recurrent PSC seems to increase. Recurrent alcoholism also jeopardizes the long-term outcome of LT recipients.

REFERENCES

1. Busuttil RW, Farmer DG, Yersiz H, et al. Analysis of long-term outcomes of 3200 liver transplantations over two decades: a single-center experience. Ann Surg 2005;241:905–16 [discussion: 916–8].
2. Petrowsky H, Busuttil RW. Evolving surgical approaches in liver transplantation. Semin Liver Dis 2009;29:121–33.

3. Yilmaz N, Shiffman ML, Stravitz RT, et al. A prospective evaluation of fibrosis progression in patients with recurrent hepatitis C virus following liver transplantation. Liver Transpl 2007;13:975–83.
4. Berenguer M. Natural history of recurrent hepatitis C. Liver Transpl 2002;8: S14–8.
5. Liermann Garcia RF, Evangelista Garcia C, McMaster P, et al. Transplantation for primary biliary cirrhosis: retrospective analysis of 400 patients in a single center. Hepatology 2001;33:22–7.
6. Jacob DA, Neumann UP, Bahra M, et al. Long-term follow-up after recurrence of primary biliary cirrhosis after liver transplantation in 100 patients. Clin Transplant 2006;20:211–20.
7. Vogel A, Heinrich E, Bahr MJ, et al. Long-term outcome of liver transplantation for autoimmune hepatitis. Clin Transplant 2004;18:62–9.
8. Molmenti EP, Netto GJ, Murray NG, et al. Incidence and recurrence of autoimmune/alloimmune hepatitis in liver transplant recipients. Liver Transpl 2002;8: 519–26.
9. Neuberger J. Transplantation for autoimmune hepatitis. Semin Liver Dis 2002; 22:379–86.
10. Goss JA, Shackleton CR, Farmer DG, et al. Orthotopic liver transplantation for primary sclerosing cholangitis. A 12-year single center experience. Ann Surg 1997;225:472–81 [discussion: 481–3].
11. Graziadei IW, Wiesner RH, Marotta PJ, et al. Long-term results of patients undergoing liver transplantation for primary sclerosing cholangitis. Hepatology 1999; 30:1121–7.
12. Neuberger J, Portmann B, Calne R, et al. Recurrence of autoimmune chronic active hepatitis following orthotopic liver grafting. Transplantation 1984;37: 363–5.
13. Manns MP, Bahr MJ. Recurrent autoimmune hepatitis after liver transplantation—when non-self becomes self. Hepatology 2000;32:868–70.
14. Hubscher SG. Recurrent autoimmune hepatitis after liver transplantation: diagnostic criteria, risk factors, and outcome. Liver Transpl 2001;7:285–91.
15. Gautam M, Cheruvattath R, Balan V. Recurrence of autoimmune liver disease after liver transplantation: a systematic review. Liver Transpl 2006;12: 1813–24.
16. Duclos-Vallee JC, Sebagh M, Rifai K, et al. A 10 year follow up study of patients transplanted for autoimmune hepatitis: histological recurrence precedes clinical and biochemical recurrence. Gut 2003;52:893–7.
17. Narumi S, Hakamada K, Sasaki M, et al. Liver transplantation for autoimmune hepatitis: rejection and recurrence. Transplant Proc 1999;31:1955–6.
18. Gonzalez-Koch A, Czaja AJ, Carpenter HA, et al. Recurrent autoimmune hepatitis after orthotopic liver transplantation. Liver Transpl 2001;7:302–10.
19. Hurtova M, Duclos-Vallee JC, Johanet C, et al. Successful tacrolimus therapy for a severe recurrence of type 1 autoimmune hepatitis in a liver graft recipient. Liver Transpl 2001;7:556–8.
20. Kerkar N, Hadzic N, Davies ET, et al. De-novo autoimmune hepatitis after liver transplantation. Lancet 1998;351:409–13.
21. Neuberger J, Portmann B, Macdougall BR, et al. Recurrence of primary biliary cirrhosis after liver transplantation. N Engl J Med 1982;306:1–4.
22. Hubscher SG, Elias E, Buckels JA, et al. Primary biliary cirrhosis. Histological evidence of disease recurrence after liver transplantation. J Hepatol 1993;18: 173–84.

23. Duclos-Vallee JC, Sebagh M. Recurrence of autoimmune disease, primary sclerosing cholangitis, primary biliary cirrhosis, and autoimmune hepatitis after liver transplantation. Liver Transpl 2009;15(Suppl 2):S25–34.

24. Morioka D, Egawa H, Kasahara M, et al. Impact of human leukocyte antigen mismatching on outcomes of living donor liver transplantation for primary biliary cirrhosis. Liver Transpl 2007;13:80–90.

25. Neuberger J, Gunson B, Hubscher S, et al. Immunosuppression affects the rate of recurrent primary biliary cirrhosis after liver transplantation. Liver Transpl 2004;10:488–91.

26. Sanchez EQ, Levy MF, Goldstein RM, et al. The changing clinical presentation of recurrent primary biliary cirrhosis after liver transplantation. Transplantation 2003;76:1583–8.

27. Levitsky J, Hart J, Cohen SM, et al. The effect of immunosuppressive regimens on the recurrence of primary biliary cirrhosis after liver transplantation. Liver Transpl 2003;9:733–6.

28. Guy JE, Qian P, Lowell JA, et al. Recurrent primary biliary cirrhosis: peritransplant factors and ursodeoxycholic acid treatment post-liver transplant. Liver Transpl 2005;11:1252–7.

29. Charatcharoenwitthaya P, Pimentel S, Talwalkar JA, et al. Long-term survival and impact of ursodeoxycholic acid treatment for recurrent primary biliary cirrhosis after liver transplantation. Liver Transpl 2007;13:1236–45.

30. Lerut J, Demetris AJ, Stieber AC, et al. Intrahepatic bile duct strictures after human orthotopic liver transplantation. Recurrence of primary sclerosing cholangitis or unusual presentation of allograft rejection? Transpl Int 1988;1:127–30.

31. Sheng R, Campbell WL, Zajko AB, et al. Cholangiographic features of biliary strictures after liver transplantation for primary sclerosing cholangitis: evidence of recurrent disease. AJR Am J Roentgenol 1996;166:1109–13.

32. Harrison RF, Davies MH, Neuberger JM, et al. Fibrous and obliterative cholangitis in liver allografts: evidence of recurrent primary sclerosing cholangitis? Hepatology 1994;20:356–61.

33. Graziadei IW, Wiesner RH, Batts KP, et al. Recurrence of primary sclerosing cholangitis following liver transplantation. Hepatology 1999;29:1050–6.

34. Brandsaeter B, Schrumpf E, Bentdal O, et al. Recurrent primary sclerosing cholangitis after liver transplantation: a magnetic resonance cholangiography study with analyses of predictive factors. Liver Transpl 2005;11:1361–9.

35. Graziadei IW. Recurrence of primary sclerosing cholangitis after liver transplantation. Liver Transpl 2002;8:575–81.

36. Kotlyar DS, Campbell MS, Reddy KR. Recurrence of diseases following orthotopic liver transplantation. Am J Gastroenterol 2006;101:1370–8.

37. Tamura S, Sugawara Y, Kaneko J, et al. Recurrence of primary sclerosing cholangitis after living donor liver transplantation. Liver Int 2007;27:86–94.

38. Graziadei IW. Live donor liver transplantation for primary sclerosing cholangitis: is disease recurrence increased? Curr Opin Gastroenterol 2011;27:301–5.

39. Maheshwari A, Yoo HY, Thuluvath PJ. Long-term outcome of liver transplantation in patients with PSC: a comparative analysis with PBC. Am J Gastroenterol 2004;99:538–42.

40. Fosby B, Karlsen TH, Melum E. Recurrence and rejection in liver transplantation for primary sclerosing cholangitis. World J Gastroenterol 2012;18:1–15.

41. Lucey MR. Liver transplantation in patients with alcoholic liver disease. Liver Transpl 2011;17:751–9.

42. Burra P, Senzolo M, Adam R, et al. Liver transplantation for alcoholic liver disease in Europe: a study from the ELTR (European Liver Transplant Registry). Am J Transplant 2010;10:138–48.

43. Finkenstedt A, Graziadei IW, Oberaigner W, et al. Extensive surveillance promotes early diagnosis and improved survival of de novo malignancies in liver transplant recipients. Am J Transplant 2009;9:2355–61.

44. DiMartini A, Crone C, Dew MA. Alcohol and substance use in liver transplant patients. Clin Liver Dis 2011;15:727–51.

45. DiMartini A, Dew MA, Chaiffetz D, et al. Early trajectories of depressive symptoms after liver transplantation for alcoholic liver disease predicts long-term survival. Am J Transplant 2011;11:1287–95.

46. Faure S, Herrero A, Jung B, et al. Excessive alcohol consumption after liver transplantation impacts on long-term survival, whatever the primary indication. J Hepatol 2012;57:306–12.

47. Rice JP, Eickhoff J, Agni R, et al. Abusive drinking after liver transplantation is associated with allograft loss and advanced allograft fibrosis. Liver Transpl 2013;19:1377–86.

48. Pfitzmann R, Schwenzer J, Rayes N, et al. Long-term survival and predictors of relapse after orthotopic liver transplantation for alcoholic liver disease. Liver Transpl 2007;13:197–205.

49. Patton HM, Yates K, Unalp-Arida A, et al. Association between metabolic syndrome and liver histology among children with nonalcoholic fatty liver disease. Am J Gastroenterol 2010;105:2093–102.

50. Angulo P. Nonalcoholic fatty liver disease. N Engl J Med 2002;346:1221–31.

51. Ong JP, Younossi ZM. Epidemiology and natural history of NAFLD and NASH. Clin Liver Dis 2007;11:1–16, vii.

52. Charlton MR, Burns JM, Pedersen RA, et al. Frequency and outcomes of liver transplantation for nonalcoholic steatohepatitis in the United States. Gastroenterology 2011;141:1249–53.

53. Ong J, Younossi ZM, Reddy V, et al. Cryptogenic cirrhosis and posttransplantation nonalcoholic fatty liver disease. Liver Transpl 2001;7:797–801.

54. Afzali A, Berry K, Ioannou GN. Excellent posttransplant survival for patients with nonalcoholic steatohepatitis in the United States. Liver Transpl 2012;18:29–37.

55. Dureja P, Mellinger J, Agni R, et al. NAFLD recurrence in liver transplant recipients. Transplantation 2011;91:684–9.

56. Wang X, Li J, Riaz DR, et al. Outcomes of liver transplantation for nonalcoholic steatohepatitis: a systematic review and meta-analysis. Clin Gastroenterol Hepatol 2014;12(3):394–402.e1.

57. Burke GW, Cirocco R, Hensley G, et al. Liver transplantation for cirrhosis following jejuno-ileal bypass—regional cytokine differences associated with pathological changes in the transplant liver. Transplantation 1992;54:374–7.

58. El-Masry M, Puig CA, Saab S. Recurrence of non-viral liver disease after orthotopic liver transplantation. Liver Int 2011;31:291–302.

59. Patil DT, Yerian LM. Evolution of nonalcoholic fatty liver disease recurrence after liver transplantation. Liver Transpl 2012;18:1147–53.

60. Valenti L, Al-Serri A, Daly AK, et al. Homozygosity for the patatin-like phospholipase-3/adiponutrin I148M polymorphism influences liver fibrosis in patients with nonalcoholic fatty liver disease. Hepatology 2010;51:1209–17.

61. Kotronen A, Johansson LE, Johansson LM, et al. A common variant in PNPLA3, which encodes adiponutrin, is associated with liver fat content in humans. Diabetologia 2009;52:1056–60.

62. Finkenstedt A, Auer C, Glodny B, et al. Patatin-like phospholipase domain-containing protein 3 rs738409-G in recipients of liver transplants is a risk factor for graft steatosis. Clin Gastroenterol Hepatol 2013;11:1667–72.
63. Watt KD, Dierkhising R, Fan C, et al. Investigation of PNPLA3 and IL28B genotypes on diabetes and obesity after liver transplantation: insight into mechanisms of disease. Am J Transplant 2013;13:2450–7.
64. Heimbach JK, Watt KD, Poterucha JJ, et al. Combined liver transplantation and gastric sleeve resection for patients with medically complicated obesity and end-stage liver disease. Am J Transplant 2013;13:363–8.
65. Kilpe VE, Krakauer H, Wren RE. An analysis of liver transplant experience from 37 transplant centers as reported to Medicare. Transplantation 1993;56:554–61.
66. Brandhagen DJ. Liver transplantation for hereditary hemochromatosis. Liver Transpl 2001;7:663–72.
67. Yu L, Ioannou GN. Survival of liver transplant recipients with hemochromatosis in the United States. Gastroenterology 2007;133:489–95.
68. Dar FS, Faraj W, Zaman MB, et al. Outcome of liver transplantation in hereditary hemochromatosis. Transpl Int 2009;22:717–24.
69. Tung BY, Farrell FJ, McCashland TM, et al. Long-term follow-up after liver transplantation in patients with hepatic iron overload. Liver Transpl Surg 1999;5: 369–74.
70. Powell LW. Does transplantation of the liver cure genetic hemochromatosis? J Hepatol 1992;16:259–61.
71. Stuart KA, Fletcher LM, Clouston AD, et al. Increased hepatic iron and cirrhosis: no evidence for an adverse effect on patient outcome following liver transplantation. Hepatology 2000;32:1200–7.
72. Farrell FJ, Nguyen M, Woodley S, et al. Outcome of liver transplantation in patients with hemochromatosis. Hepatology 1994;20:404–10.
73. Cheng F, Li GQ, Zhang F, et al. Outcomes of living-related liver transplantation for Wilson's disease: a single-center experience in China. Transplantation 2009; 87:751–7.
74. Sevmis S, Karakayali H, Aliosmanoglu I, et al. Liver transplantation for Wilson's disease. Transplant Proc 2008;40:228–30.
75. Beinhardt S, Leiss W, Stattermayer AF, et al. Long-term outcomes of patients with Wilson disease in a large Austrian cohort. Clin Gastroenterol Hepatol 2014;12(4):683–9.

Immunosuppression
Trends and Tolerance?

Paige M. Porrett, MD, PhD[a], Sohaib K. Hashmi, BS[b], Abraham Shaked, MD, PhD[c],*

KEYWORDS

- Immunosuppression • Minimization • Tolerance • Biomarkers

KEY POINTS

- Immunosuppression withdrawal or minimization should reduce the long-term morbidity associated with these drugs, but few studies provide evidence of a long-term benefit.
- Multiple approaches to immunosuppression minimization are practiced, but no optimal strategy has been devised.
- Immune tolerance in liver transplant recipients remains elusive and may be unnecessary.
- Biomarkers indicating a patient's immune responsiveness are desperately needed to guide immune management.

The excellent outcomes of contemporary liver transplantation can be directly attributed to improvements in pharmacologic immunosuppression over the last few decades. However, long-term toxicity of many of these agents remains significant; the transplant community continues to seek ways to minimize or discontinue the use of these drugs in liver transplant recipients, despite their critical and historic contribution to transplantation success. In this clinical update, the authors present an overview of current and evolving immunosuppression management in liver transplantation ("Part 1") with a focus on emerging efforts to minimize ("Part 2") or even eliminate ("Part 3") immunosuppression use.

PART I: CURRENT IMMUNOSUPPRESSION PRACTICES

To improve efficacy and diminish toxicity, most transplant centers in the United States use a combination of agents to prevent allograft rejection in liver recipients (**Fig. 1**).[1]

The authors have nothing to disclose.
No funding support.
[a] Division of Liver Transplantation, Department of Surgery, The University of Pennsylvania, 3400 Spruce Street, One Founders Pavilion, Philadelphia, PA 19104, USA; [b] Department of Surgery, The University of Pennsylvania, 3400 Spruce Street, Two Dulles Pavilion, Philadelphia, PA 19104, USA; [c] Division of Liver Transplantation, Department of Surgery, Penn Transplant Institute, The University of Pennsylvania, 3400 Spruce Street, Two Dulles Pavilion, Philadelphia, PA 19104, USA
* Corresponding author.
E-mail address: abraham.shaked@uphs.upenn.edu

Clin Liver Dis 18 (2014) 687–716
http://dx.doi.org/10.1016/j.cld.2014.05.012
1089-3261/14/$ – see front matter © 2014 Elsevier Inc. All rights reserved.

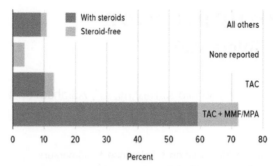

Fig. 1. Initial immunosuppression regimen in adult liver transplant recipients, 2011. Includes all patients transplanted in 2011 and discharged with a functioning graft. MMF/MPA, mycophenolate; TAC, tacrolimus. (*From* Organ Procurement and Transplantation Network (OPTN) and Scientific Registry of Transplant Recipients (SRTR). OPTN/SRTR 2011 Annual Data Report. Rockville, MD: Department of Health and Human Services, Health Resources and Services Administration, Healthcare Systems Bureau, Division of Transplantation; 2012.)

Although the specific mechanism of action of each drug varies widely, the primary goal of all agents currently used in contemporary immunosuppression regimens is to attenuate the allogeneic T-cell response to the donor antigen. This focus on T-cell control stems from decades of immunologic research that has clearly demonstrated the critical role of allogeneic T-cell activation in allograft destruction. Most agents, thus, aim to (1) diminish signaling through the T-cell receptor (TCR) (eg, calcineurin inhibitors), (2) truncate T-cell activation after the TCR has been engaged (eg, costimulatory blockade), or (3) prevent T-cell proliferation by blocking DNA synthesis (eg, antimetabolites) or altering energy metabolism within the cell (mammalian target of rapamycin [mTOR] inhibition). However, as our understanding of alloimmunity evolves and the contribution of additional immune populations to graft destruction is better appreciated (ie, B cells, natural killer [NK] cells), it is likely that additional cell populations will be targeted by immunosuppression agents of the future.

Since the introduction of cyclosporine in the early 1980s, *calcineurin inhibitors* (CNIs) have remained the foundation of immunosuppression in liver transplant recipients (see **Fig. 1**). *Tacrolimus* has replaced *cyclosporine* as the CNI of choice in liver transplant recipients since its introduction in the 1990s, given its improved graft and patient survival and decreased rejection rates.[2] Although tacrolimus is heavily relied on by most centers throughout the country,[1] this agent is rarely used alone early after transplantation. Although 60% of centers use tacrolimus as part of a triple-drug regimen within the first month after transplantation,[1] the number of pharmacologic agents in the regimen of any given recipient is gradually decreased by many centers with increasing time after transplantation. By 1 year after transplantation, more than 30% of centers use tacrolimus alone; this number approaches 50% of centers by 2 years after transplantation.[1]

For many liver recipients, tacrolimus alone may provide adequate immunosuppression given its overall potency and efficacy. However, calcineurin inhibitors are associated with a wide range of serious long-term complications, as discussed in additional detail in the following section of this review ("Part 2"). Arguably, the complications with the greatest impact on long-term patient survival include the development of diabetes mellitus (DM) and nephrotoxicity leading to end-stage renal disease (5% of liver transplant recipients 13 years after transplantation).[3] The avoidance of these complications drives the utilization of multidrug regimens and encourages the development of alternatives for CNI-based immunosuppression.

As shown in **Fig. 2**, 2 additional classes of drugs are frequently used by the transplant community to further improve posttransplant outcomes and decrease CNI use. These classes include corticosteroids and the purine synthesis inhibitors, azathioprine and mycophenolate mofetil.

Corticosteroids have been used in immunosuppression regimens since the first successful solid organ transplant in the 1950s. Despite their extensive use over the last several decades, however, very little is understood about their exact mechanism of action. It is widely assumed that most of their immunosuppressive effect is caused by repression of cytokines and the reduction of inflammation, but the wide tissue distribution of glucocorticoid receptors and their modulation of the promoters of many different genes suggest pleiotropic effects. Although these agents have been widely used to support excellent outcomes in liver transplantation, concern persists that long-term corticosteroid use exacerbates diabetes, hyperlipidemia, and hepatitis C virus (HCV) recurrence in an at-risk posttransplant population. Consequently, several randomized controlled trials (RCTs) have been performed to better delineate the transplant outcome among patients whose immunosuppression regimens do not contain steroids. Unfortunately, the results of many of these trials are difficult to generalize given their heterogeneity; sample sizes in the trials have varied widely, and steroids were replaced in some trials with additional immunosuppressive agents. Nevertheless, a recent meta-analysis of these 19 RCTs of steroid avoidance demonstrated that steroid-free patients enjoyed lower rates of diabetes and hypercholesterolemia. Although steroid-free patients had higher rates of acute rejection, graft loss and patient death were comparable between patients treated with or without steroids.[4]

Twenty years ago, *azathioprine* was used in approximately 50% of recipients at the time of liver transplantation; but most centers rapidly converted to *mycophenolate mofetil* (MMF) in the late 1990s after its approval by the Food and Drug Administration (FDA) in 1995.[1,5] Although MMF is a more potent agent than azathioprine, only 2 randomized controlled trials in liver transplant recipients have been performed comparing the two agents, and neither has shown the superiority of MMF over azathioprine with respect to 1-year patient and graft survival.[6] Although rejection rates were significantly

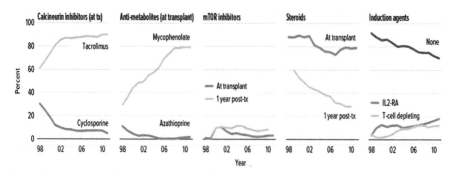

Fig. 2. Trends in immunosuppression use in adult liver transplant recipients, 1998 to 2011. IL2-RA, Interleukin 2-Receptor Alpha; tx, Transplant. (*From* Organ Procurement and Transplantation Network (OPTN) and Scientific Registry of Transplant Recipients (SRTR). OPTN/SRTR 2011 Annual Data Report. Rockville, MD: Department of Health and Human Services, Health Resources and Services Administration, Healthcare Systems Bureau, Division of Transplantation; 2012.)

better in MMF-treated patients (21% [MMF] vs 44% [azathioprine]),[6] it is important to recognize that these studies were conducted in patients treated with cyclosporine instead of tacrolimus. In addition, the follow-up in these studies was very short (approximately 10 months); the dose of MMF was significantly higher than that used in most regimens today (3 g/d vs 2 g/d). In summary, there have been no studies to demonstrate the superiority of MMF over azathioprine in a tacrolimus-based regimen despite the wide adoption of this practice.[1]

Although no single agent or group of drugs has shown adequate efficacy to replace calcineurin inhibitors altogether, the mTOR inhibitors have been the most heavily investigated agents with the potential to supplant CNI-based immunosuppression. Although a variety of single-center and retrospective studies have assessed the ability of *sirolimus* (rapamycin) to replace CNIs and preserve renal function, a recently published multicenter randomized trial has demonstrated that renal function 12 months after liver transplant is no better in patients converted to sirolimus than treated with CNIs alone.[7] In this trial, graft and patient survival were similar after conversion from CNIs to sirolimus, but no appreciable nephron-sparing effect of sirolimus was observed. Moreover, biopsy-proven acute rejection was significantly higher in patients converted to sirolimus; 50% of patients in the study were ultimately removed from the sirolimus arm because of adverse events. The results of this study and others may explain in part the tepid use of sirolimus in contemporary immunosuppression regimens in liver transplant recipients (see **Fig. 2**).

Everolimus is a derivative of sirolimus and the most recent mTOR inhibitor approved by the FDA for use in kidney (2010) as well as liver transplant recipients (2013). Like sirolimus, everolimus has been specifically targeted for use in CNI withdrawal studies. In patients withdrawn from CNIs relatively late after transplant, everolimus has been shown to be safe without an increased incidence of acute rejection episodes; but there was no overall improvement in renal function.[8] However, in a recent study that converted patients to everolimus monotherapy from cyclosporine much earlier after transplantation (<30 days posttransplant), renal function was preserved at a superior level throughout the first posttransplant year; the incidence of stage III chronic kidney disease was significantly diminished.[9] Although everolimus in this trial was associated with complications that may deter its use and have been previously observed in patients treated with mTOR inhibitors (incisional hernia [46.1% vs 27.0% in cyclosporine-treated patients] and limb edema [9.6% vs 0% in cyclosporine-treated patients]), the study highlights the importance of timing in CNI withdrawal. Although the transplant community has generally thought that decreasing the cumulative dose of calcineurin inhibitors will improve renal function, this study and others suggest that permanent CNI-mediated nephrotoxicity may occur much earlier than previously appreciated. Future trials may better incorporate these data and focus on renal preservation by minimizing CNI use very early after transplantation.

The goal of renal preservation in liver transplant recipients has also revived interest in older agents. Antibodies that deplete the T-cell compartment (antithymocyte globulin [ATG] [Thymoglobulin]) or block the interleukin 2 (IL-2) receptor (basiliximab) can be administered to liver recipients at the time of transplantation and may have value in the quest to minimize CNI toxicity. However, 75% of centers in the United States do not report utilization of antibody induction therapy, despite the potency of these agents and their proven track record in kidney transplant recipients.[1] Much of the hesitancy to use these therapies in liver transplant recipients stems from a prevailing concern that excessive immunosuppression in HCV+ liver transplant recipients can lead to aggressive and rapid recurrence of HCV,[10] although no RCTs using T-cell depletion in patients stratified by HCV status have been performed. In the absence of an RCT, only a recently published analysis of the Scientific Registry of Transplant Recipients' database provides the most robust data with respect to outcomes among HCV+ recipients treated with ATG.[11] This study found that 5-year patient and graft survival was improved in liver transplant recipients independent of HCV status, thereby suggesting that antibody induction therapy in liver transplant recipients is not harmful and may even provide a benefit. Although most centers in the United States have yet to embrace these therapies, the utilization of antibody induction therapy has increased consistently in the last 5 years.[1] Whether these agents can be used in an optimum regimen that will allow CNI minimization and improve renal function in liver transplant recipients has not yet been well studied.

The use of other biologic agents in immunosuppression regimens is gaining additional traction within the transplant community as longer follow-up of kidney transplant recipients treated with belatacept has become available.[12] Belatacept is a recombinant fusion protein that prevents T cell costimulation through the CD28 pathway and was approved by the FDA in 2011 for use in kidney transplant recipients in combination with basiliximab induction, MMF, and corticosteroids as part of a CNI-free regimen.[13] When compared with kidney transplant recipients treated with a cyclosporine-based regimen, patients who received belatacept had significantly improved renal function early and late after transplantation. This initial experience in kidney transplant recipients prompted the evaluation of this drug in de novo liver transplant recipients (NCT00555321), but this phase II clinical trial of belatacept as a first-line agent in a CNI-free regimen was terminated early because of high rates of graft loss and patient death during the first year of follow-up.[14] Although these initial results are indeed discouraging, the optimal dose and timing of belatacept in liver transplant recipients is unknown and may be significantly different from that used with success in kidney transplant recipients. Furthermore, belatacept has not yet been studied in liver transplant recipients as a bridge to CNI withdrawal or minimization. In sum, the efficacy of this agent in a highly immunogenic group of kidney transplant recipients suggests great potential for use in other transplant populations; it is, thus, likely that additional trials with belatacept in liver transplant recipients will be performed given the successful preservation of renal function that has been observed.

PART II: MINIMIZATION AS A GOAL FOR TRANSPLANTATION
Overview

It is seldom that the fate of the transplanted liver is determined solely by the immune response against the allograft. Episodes of acute rejection are usually not associated with long-lasting tissue damage, and the incidence of graft loss caused by chronic rejection is low.[15–17] Instead, in many recipients, morbidity and mortality is directly related to the burden of immunosuppression as evidenced by organ system damage that is mediated by their side effects, by compromised immune surveillance resulting in the development of opportunistic infection and malignancies, and by the rapid and severe recurrence of HCV infection.[18–27] Consequently, minimization of this burden should have a direct impact on the long-term well-being of the recipient.

In principle, the minimization of immunosuppression in the setting of organ transplantation is aimed at finding the most effective balance of controlling the alloimmune response while allowing the immune system to regain its surveillance function of harmful processes. As most immunosuppressive drugs have significant toxic side effects, efforts are also directed at reducing injury by designing protocols that include a combination of drugs that will prevent rejection while preserving the best organ system function. Because most injury is apparent in the early postoperative period, the current approach is geared toward using induction and maintenance immunosuppression that would spare the known side effects of drugs, such as CNIs or steroids, yet command a good control of rejection.[9,28–30]

Management of Immunosuppression with the Aim of Decreasing Adverse Effects

Immunosuppression-induced kidney injury

Chronic renal failure is the most well-known complication of CNI-based immunosuppression, the injury is superimposed onto preexisting hepatorenal injury as well as the development of systemic hypertension and worsening posttransplant diabetes. In a study by Ojo and colleagues,[24] the frequency of chronic renal failure was 13.2% at 3 years and climbed to 27.0% at 10 years, and chronic renal failure was associated with a relative risk of death of 4.45. Similar findings of kidney damage were reported in other studies that correlated the initial posttransplant glomerular filtration rate (GFR) with long-term kidney function, demonstrating a continuous decline over the years.[29] Renal morbidity in children is likely even greater than that described in adults, as children have longer posttransplant life spans with greater cumulative exposure to tacrolimus-mediated injury. The Studies in Pediatric Liver Transplantation (SPLIT) database outcomes indicate that at a mean of 5.2 years posttransplantation, 17.6% of pediatric transplant recipients have an estimated GFR (eGFR) less than 90 mL/min/1.73 m^2; multivariate analysis demonstrated that primary immunosuppression was among the independent variables associated with this injury.[31] Longitudinal follow-up of inulin clearance in a smaller cohort demonstrated the cumulative incidence of chronic renal impairment to be 25% (eGFR 60 mL/min/1.73 m^2).[32]

The use of multiple-drug regimens is one way to lessen drug-related organ dysfunction while maintaining adequate alloimmune control. However, the main strategies of CNI reduction, CNI withdrawal, and CNI avoidance do not provide a very good answer as to whether minimization at a late stage after transplantation is associated with an improvement of kidney function. Several studies have explored antibody induction with the aim to delay or reduce the exposure to CNIs in the immediate posttransplant period. The initial outcomes demonstrate higher GFR early on, but the impact on long-term outcomes is yet to be determined. It is still unclear whether the replacement of CNIs with TOR inhibitors is associated with an improvement in GFR.[9,33,34] Replacement immunosuppression, however, has its own toxicities to consider. Sirolimus, for example, has significant metabolic (hyperlipidemia), hematologic (anemia in the presence of renal failure), and growth factor inhibition–related ulceration (impaired wound healing) side effects.[35] The feasibility of reduction or replacement of CNI with mycophenolate mofetil was shown in studies demonstrating improvement in GFR.[36–38] These studies support the hypothesis that the reduction in CNI may halt or ameliorate renal dysfunction without compromising patient and graft survival.

Metabolic syndrome

Metabolic syndrome (MS) is a group of risk factors associated with insulin resistance and an increased risk for the development of DM and cardiovascular disease. According to the Framingham study, MS alone can predict at least 25% of all new-onset cardiovascular diseases.[39–41] MS was defined by the Adult Treatment Panel III as the presence of 3 or more of the following: (1) abdominal obesity, (2) hypertriglyceridemia, (3) low high-density lipoprotein levels, (4) high blood pressure, and (5) high fasting glucose levels. Importantly, most current immunosuppression agents that are used in liver transplant recipients are described to be associated with one or more of the aforementioned risk factors.[42]

New-onset DM after transplantation (NODAT) is reported with an incidence of 10% to 36% in liver transplant recipients.[43–49] The variation in the incidence of NODAT is caused by differences in the diagnostic criteria for NODAT, patient characteristics, duration of the study period, and variation of the immunosuppressive regimens used. A recent study of the United Network for Organ Sharing's database demonstrated that the incidence of NODAT is 12.5%, 3.4%, and 1.9% at 1, 3, and 5 years, respectively, after transplant in those undergoing deceased donor liver transplantation (DDLT) and slightly less for those undergoing living donor transplantation, suggesting the contribution of donor factors in the development of the disease.[50]

In patients followed for at least 1 year after orthotopic liver transplantation (OLT), the incidence of hypertension increased from 19.0% before transplantation to 64.2% posttransplantation.[51] Glucocorticoids are still used in 49% and 33% of liver allograft recipients at the end of the first year and second year, respectively, in North America and are recognized as a cause of hypertension. CNIs were demonstrated to induce sympathetic hyperactivity, stimulate renin release, and induce renal artery vasoconstriction and sodium reabsorption, all of which contribute to the persistence of hypertension.[52] The adjustment of CNI immunosuppression may reduce the incidence of this complication. In the case of steroids, the clinical tendency is to move from withdrawal to steroid avoidance protocols, and most studies show that patient and graft survival are not compromised. Indeed, these protocols demonstrated beneficial findings in relation to the metabolic effects as demonstrated by a reduction in the relative risk of diabetes and hypertension.[4]

A significant increase in cholesterol and triglycerides has been reported in liver transplant recipients, specifically with the use of mTOR inhibitors, leading to the frequent use of statins.[53] It is the authors' experience that the discontinuation of sirolimus reverses these trends.

Malignancy and infections

Meta-analysis studies have demonstrated the increased incidence of cancer in the transplant population. Many cancers that occur at higher rates are those with known or suspected infectious causes, such as Epstein-Barr virus. For most of the common epithelial cancers, including cancer of the colon, rectum, breast, ovary, and prostate, there is little evidence of increased risk in the transplant population.[21] However, the incidence of lung cancer is much higher among kidney transplant recipients than patients undergoing dialysis, suggesting that immune deficiency could have a direct role.[54] Infection and rejection remain major causes of morbidity after a liver transplant. Two-thirds of all infections occurred during the first 100 days after transplantation in this study and were found to be bacterial in 48% of the cases, fungal in 22%, and viral in 12%. The bacterial infection rate peaked during the first month following transplantation.[55] Opportunistic bacterial infections are uncommon after 6 months in patients receiving stable and reduced maintenance doses of immunosuppression with good graft function.[55] In contrast, viral infections, such as the influenza epidemics, constitute a major infectious disease problem for liver transplant recipients early and late after the procedure.[56] In theory, the minimization of immunosuppression should provide improved pathogen immunity, improved vaccination efficacy, and reduced morbidity and mortality.

HCV recurrence

More than 40% of liver transplants are done in patients who are infected with HCV. Reinfection is universal; histologic evidence of hepatitis can be observed in up to

97% of recipients, many of whom also have elevated aminotransferases.[20,57] Chronic inflammation and the development of mild to severe fibrosis are associated with the development of cirrhosis. Posttransplant HCV RNA levels do not correlate with serum transaminase or histologic findings and cannot be used alone to assess the severity of hepatitis or the degree of allograft injury. Nevertheless, viral levels and histologic findings serve as good markers to evaluate new therapeutic modalities aimed at the control of HCV disease before transplantation and may be used in a similar way to assess the impact of minimizing immunosuppression on anti-HCV activity. Continuous suppression of the immune response is thought to contribute to the rapid progression of recurrent HCV (leading to graft failure and decreased survival) and cirrhosis in 20% within 5 years after transplantation.[58,59] The HCV RNA concentration increases rapidly in patients receiving corticosteroid boluses to treat acute rejection; however, the relationship between viral titer and the severity of HCV recurrence is controversial.[60–63]

Clinical Observation of Minimization of CNI Immunosuppression in Liver Transplantation

The strategies that have been used to prevent long-term CNI-related complications were either CNI reduction or complete avoidance, and these have been made possible by the supplementation of non-CNI immunosuppression.

Reduction and/or delayed introduction of CNI are possible in the early posttransplant period with the use of induction with lymphocyte-depleting or neutralizing antibodies. Examples of such regimens include daclizumab or basiliximab induction with a delay of therapeutic dosing of tacrolimus.[30,64] These protocols allowed significant reduction in the target levels of CNI in the critical immediate posttransplant period without an increase in the rate of acute cellular rejection. The results demonstrated preservation and/or improvement in renal function; however, there are no long-term studies to demonstrate whether the initial reduction in CNI translates to a permanent renal-sparing effect.

A similar approach was taken with the introduction of mycophenolate mofetil that allowed a reduction in the CNI dose at an early or late stage after transplantation. Renal function was improved in small groups of pediatric recipients who were placed on MMF.[65,66] In adult recipients, studies have taken the approach of minimizing or complete replacement of CNI with mycophenolate mofetil.[36–38,67] These are mostly nonrandomized studies with a relatively small group of patients. Nevertheless, the important lesson learned is that there is some potential for improving kidney function by the reversal of CNI-induced kidney damage. CNI minimization is associated with a modest improvement in renal function, but it is yet to be determined whether persistent damage is observed on biopsies as long as the CNIs are continued.[29]

It is the authors' impression that the aforementioned studies describe conversion rather than minimization of immunosuppression, with the general approach to replace CNIs with non-CNIs and that the end points were aimed at reducing CNI-induced injury with no attempt to improve systemic immunity.

Long-term Management of Immunosuppression in Adult Transplant Recipients

Although the concept of immunosuppression minimization (IM) intuitively seems to be in transplant patients' best interest, analysis of available data demonstrates that consistent, standardized IM is not currently practiced.

The authors think that most US programs have no standard protocols for long-term management of immunosuppression in OLT recipients, and there are no attempts to decrease immunosuppression over the years. Preliminary analysis of 120 stable recipients at 6 Immune Tolerance Network (ITN) transplant centers demonstrated that LDLT and DDLT patients and patients with HCV and non-HCV patients were kept at twice-daily dosing of tacrolimus at similar trough levels at the end of years 1, 2, and 3 after transplant. To quantify the overall use of immunosuppression, a standardized scoring system was used, whereby a 1-unit score was assigned to certain drugs and doses (1 mg tacrolimus = 100 mg cyclosporine = 1 mg sirolimus = 1000 mg MMF = 5 mg prednisone = 1 unit). This study showed that patients who were HCV+ were receiving less immunosuppression than patients who were HCV− at the end of years 1 and 2, with the difference being less significant at the end of year 3 **(Table 1)**. Additionally, patients who were HCV+ received a lower tacrolimus dose than patients who were HCV− at the end of years 1 and 2 **(Table 2)**. However, the average trough levels (HCV+ 6.95 ng/mL, HCV− 7.2 ng/mL) did not show significant differences ($P = .69$). Even though patients who were HCV+ had lower immunosuppression scores and tacrolimus doses than patients who were HCV−, the similar trough levels between the groups seem to indicate differential tacrolimus pharmacokinetics in patients who are HCV+ and that current strategies are not sufficient to reduce immunosuppression in patients who are HCV+ in the first 3 years after transplant.[68]

The results from studies whereby minimization was used in patients who are HCV+ are important to note. In a 2006 study, Tisone and colleagues[69] attempted immunosuppression withdrawal in 34 patients who were HCV RNA+ under cyclosporine A monotherapy and at least 12 months after transplant who showed normal graft function but had biopsy-proven recurrence. Eight patients achieved complete and permanent immunosuppression withdrawal (23.4%), whereas 14 (41.2%) developed rejection within 8 months, and 12 (35.2%) developed rejection during tapering of immunosuppression. Patients who were successfully weaned entirely from immunosuppression showed stabilization or improvement of fibrosis, reduced necroinflammation, and improved liver function compared with nontolerant patients. Low trough levels of cyclosporine A in the first week after OLT and initial steroid-free immunosuppression were shown to be independent predictors of successful, sustained weaning. Furthermore, an immunosuppression-free state did not influence metabolic, renal, or blood pressure changes. The 3-year survival was also unaffected. There was a statistically significant decrease in HCV RNA levels in weaned patients compared with weaning nontolerant patients. Thus, this study showed that immunosuppression withdrawal led to reconstitution of the immune system and subsequent reduction in fibrosis progression.

A 10-year follow-up of this immunosuppression withdrawal study in HCV liver transplant recipients reported that 6 out of the 8 originally tolerant patients remained off all immunosuppression. Twenty-two of the patients who could not be weaned off were

Table 1
Immunosuppression scores at the end of years 1 to 3

		Year 1	Year 2	Year 3
HCV−	*Mean*	6.99	5.91	5.03
	SD	3.47	3.04	2.48
HCV+	*Mean*	4.61	4.09	4.05
	SD	3.29	3.39	2.84
	P	.0002	.0031	.07

Data from Tchao N, Sayre P, Feng S, et al. Long-term immunosuppression management in OLT recipients. American Transplant Congress. San Francisco, CA, May 5–9, 2007.

Table 2
Tacrolimus usage at the end of years 1 to 3

		Year 1	Year 2	Year 3
HCV−	Mean	6.37	5.39	4.56
	SD	3.38	3.01	2.89
HCV+	Mean	4.42	3.97	3.74
	SD	3.09	3.25	2.79
	P	.0005	.04	.24

Data from Tchao N, Sayre P, Feng S, et al. Long-term immunosuppression management in OLT recipients. American Transplant Congress. San Francisco, CA, May 5–9, 2007.

alive at the time of assessment and showed a significant increase in staging as opposed to the tolerant patients who showed no significant staging increase. Furthermore, 9 nontolerant patients also showed frank cirrhosis, whereas none of the tolerant patients showed evidence of cirrhosis. In addition to this sustained stabilization of cirrhosis progression, the tolerant group was also superior to the nontolerant group with regard to immunosuppression-related morbidity.[70] In summary, these studies show a clear benefit of immunosuppression withdrawal in patients with HCV with not only a reduction in disease progression but also a lower incidence of diseases associated with long-term immunosuppression.

Minimization in the Pediatric Liver Transplant Setting

Although pediatricians, in particular, are acutely aware of the need to minimize the long-term side effects of these powerful immunosuppressive agents, most attempts at minimization remain reactive and/or consist of avoiding dose increases as recipients grow in size and age. Analysis of the SPLIT database demonstrated that at 5 years after transplant, most children from 45 participating North American transplant centers continue CNI suppression (74% tacrolimus, 24% cyclosporine), receive twice-daily dosing, and are maintained at trough levels of 6 ng/mL and 100 ng/mL for tacrolimus and cyclosporine, respectively.[71,72] A review of the Children's Hospital of Philadelphia's (CHOP) outcome data demonstrated similar management (**Table 3**), with minimal changes in drug dosage occurring after the first year. Although somewhat lower tacrolimus trough levels are seen in later years, these, again, likely represent patients outgrowing their doses rather than true proactive attempts at IM. SPLIT data demonstrate that only 64% of OLT recipients receive single-drug therapy at 5 years after transplant, presumably because of pretransplant immune-related hepatitis and/or past history of rejection. CHOP outcome data demonstrate a similar trend (**Table 4**). Although it is common practice to reactively minimize tacrolimus in individual

Table 3
Tacrolimus dosages and troughs after OLT

Time After OLT	Dosage (mg), BID (Mean ± SD)	Trough Level (Mean ± SD)
1 month	3.18 ± 2.84	10.23 ± 4.41
1 y	2.85 ± 2.38	7.60 ± 4.45
2 y	2.46 ± 2.07	6.40 ± 6.79
3 y	2.06 ± 1.88	4.02 ± 3.65
5 y, SPLIT data	3.40 ± 2.6	6.0

Table 4
Number of immunosuppressive drugs by posttransplant year

Time After OLT	1 (%)	2 (%)	3 (%)
1 y (n = 61)	70.5	21.3	8.2
3 y (n = 26)	80.8	19.2	0
5 y, SPLIT data	64.0	25.0	11.0

recipients when drug-related complications such as posttransplant lymphoprolifera-tive disorder (PTLD) develop, proactive minimization is not routine.

Feasibility of Immunosuppression Minimization

A few trials have reported that a small proportion of pediatric and adult liver transplant recipients can be prospectively weaned from immunosuppression without undue detriment to the larger proportion that fail, requiring treatment of rejection and rein-statement of immunosuppression. Published literature suggests that about 20% of liver transplant recipients will develop operational tolerance and that this phenomenon is observed in the setting of nonimmune liver disease causes.[69,73–77] Recipients greater than 8 years from the transplant procedure and those on minimal immunosup-pression before complete withdrawal have better chances at being weaned. Using strict inclusion criteria and consents, Feng and colleagues[78] recently conducted an excellent ITN investigation of stable pediatric liver transplant recipients greater than 4 years after transplantation. In this study, 60% of recipients of parental LDLT were weaned from and remained off of immunosuppression therapy for at least 1 year with normal graft function and stable allograft histology. The total LDLT population eligible for withdrawal in the participating centers greatly exceeded the number that could participate (n = 129). One wonders whether additional recipients could have been minimized, whether any of the participating recipients could have been mini-mized earlier, and whether those failing withdrawal could be maintained on less intense immunosuppression.

Can IM Be Personalized?

At present, there is no induction immunosuppression setting known to enhance the potential for long-term CNI minimization or induction of tolerance; there are no vali-dated biomarkers that can identify tolerant patients. Therefore, current attempts at IM remain guided by clinical judgment and gross indicators of allograft function (eg, alanine transaminase, aspartate transaminase). Ideally, specific markers of im-mune function should guide IM, allowing a more personalized approach to dose reduction. Similarly, immunosuppression-related end-organ injury should be recog-nized early at the molecular level before organs are noticeably and irrevocably damaged.

Data published by the authors' group and others have recently identified biomarkers with the potential to predict operational tolerance in pediatric and adult liver transplant recipients.[75,79,80] These techniques show great promise in their ability to discriminate tolerant from nontolerant individuals and are discussed later in this article. The ultimate goal is to develop practical, yet clinically robust immune assessment profiles and markers of end-organ damage that will allow identification and long-term manage-ment of liver transplant recipients who can safely undergo IM without compromising graft function.

PART III: TOLERANCE

Although the minimization of immunosuppression may indeed limit chronic toxicity and improve patient outcomes, the elimination of immunosuppression dependence entirely would, in theory, be the preferred goal for transplant recipients. If true immunologic tolerance could be induced in patients, it would overcome the 2 major factors contributing to morbidity and limiting allograft survival: chronic rejection and immunosuppression toxicity.[79] Although operational tolerance has been reported in some liver transplant recipients who have stopped their immunosuppression as discussed further later, robust immunologic tolerance has yet to be achieved in human liver transplant recipients in any therapeutically durable or reproducible way.[78,81,82] Operational transplant tolerance is defined as prolonged allograft survival in patients in the absence of immunosuppression, with no evidence of a destructive response and normal responses to immune stimuli, such as infections and tumors.[83]

Conceptual Approach to the Induction of Donor-Specific Tolerance

In principle, tolerance can be achieved in allograft recipients through 2 approaches. First, control of alloreactive recipient T cells can be obtained by promoting endogenous immunoregulatory mechanisms or inducing active deletion (**Table 5**). Alternatively, donor-specific tolerance can be achieved by the creation of a chimeric immunologic state whereby the recipient's immune system is reconstituted with T cells of donor origin. In macrochimerism, donor-derived hematopoietic stem cells (HSCs) engraft within the recipient and produce all blood cell lineages. Chimerism can also be observed on a smaller scale, and varying degrees of microchimerism have been observed when donor passenger leukocytes migrate out of the allograft and produce small numbers of donor-derived cell populations in the recipient.[84] In early studies, microchimerism has been detected in patients more than 10 years after the transplant who were not pharmacologically immunosuppressed.[85,86] This early work suggests that donor-recipient chimerism may be a successful strategy to achieve long-term donor-specific tolerance and has inspired several investigators to use this approach over the last decade, as discussed further later. However, many practical challenges remain with respect to the induction of donor-recipient chimerism, and other experimental strategies have focused instead on the manipulation of only the recipient immune system as outlined in **Table 5**.[79,87]

Clinical and Experimental Approach to the Induction of Donor-Specific Tolerance

Molecular therapeutics

The repertoire of exogenously administered pharmacologic agents that can delete T cells or induce T-cell anergy is currently limited to biologic agents, such as ATG

Table 5	
Mechanisms for inducing tolerance in alloreactive T cells	
Mechanism	**Pathway**
Deletion	Removal of immature T cell in the thymus or mature T cells in the periphery
Anergy	Activated cells are made unresponsive to further stimulation
Immune deviation	Activated cells initiate an alternative cytokine response
Suppression	T cells are activated but are actively restrained from acquiring effector function

Data from Bishop GA, Ierino FL, Sharland AF, et al. Approaching the promise of operational tolerance in clinical transplantation. Transplantation 2011;91(10):1065–74.

and Cytotoxic T-Lymphocyte Antigen 4 immunoglobulin (CTLA-4 Ig) (belatacept). As discussed previously, ATG is a polyclonal antibody formulation produced by the immunization of animals with human T-cell preparations. The administration of ATG to allograft recipients results in nonspecific T-cell lysis and, thus, deletes most T cells transiently from the recipient T-cell repertoire.[88,89] Recipient T-cell anergy can be induced by the blockade of T-cell costimulation through the CD28-B7 pathway or via agonism of CD28 interaction with CTLA-4 (belatacept). Although T-cell anergy has been induced experimentally with these agents in animals to promote donor-specific tolerance, belatacept has not yet been used to induce allograft tolerance in humans.[90–96] Although the importance of regulatory T cells in tolerance to both autoantigen and alloantigen is well established, there are currently no pharmacologic agents that selectively manipulate or expand this T-cell population.

Cellular therapeutics

Infusion of immunoregulatory cell populations or donor HSCs has produced tolerance in both animal models and preliminary clinical investigations in humans. Donor-recipient chimerism achieved by total lymphoid irradiation of the recipient followed by infusion of donor bone marrow or stem cells has resulted in clinical tolerance of kidney transplants as discussed further later.[97,98] However, the toxicity of the conditioning required and the need for donor cells renders this approach difficult and impractical in most patients.[99] Cluster of Differentiation 4$^+$ (CD4$^+$) regulatory T cells (Tregs) have been positively associated with good liver, kidney, and lung graft function,[100–102] and infusion of these cells in animals[103–106] and in humans[107–110] has led to donor-specific tolerance of diverse allograft types. This preliminary work has inspired ongoing attempts to artificially expand human Tregs ex vivo,[111] and clinical trials are currently planned to treat solid organ transplant recipients with these ex vivo–expanded Tregs in the future.[112] In addition to Tregs, certain mesenchymal stem cells (MSCs) have been used to prevent graft-versus-host disease (GVHD) after bone marrow transplant. In vitro studies have demonstrated the immunosuppressive potential of MSCs as they cause inhibition of T-cell proliferation in response to alloantigens, reduce T-cell activation, prevent the maturation of cytotoxic T cells, and decrease the secretion of proinflammatory cytokines by dendritic cells. These cell types are all involved in pathways related to rejection; by regulating them, MSCs may improve allograft tolerance.[113–115]

Experimental Models of Liver Transplant Tolerance in Animals

Several animal models of liver allograft tolerance have been developed. It has been well appreciated for decades that the liver is one of the least immunogenic allografts, and liver tolerance occurs spontaneously in most rat and mouse strain combinations.[83] The mechanisms underlying liver tolerance in rodents have been heavily investigated for many years and are briefly summarized later.

Induction of recipient T-cell apoptosis by the allograft has been implicated as an important mechanism for preventing graft rejection. Chen and colleagues[116] showed in a 2008 study in adult male rats that Kupffer cells (KCs) may induce T-cell deletion through the Fas/FasL pathway, thus leading to allograft tolerance. KCs, which are macrophages in the liver, may cause apoptosis of the recipient T cells entering the allograft from peripheral blood by increasing the expression of Fas ligands on their cell surface. Further evidence of T-cell depletion as a potential tolerance pathway is provided by a 2010 study in rats by Fujiki and colleagues,[117] which used posttransplant total lymphoid irradiation to increase apoptosis of the intragraft T cells and, thereby, allowed an increase in the frequency of Cluster of Differentiation 4$^+$ Cluster of Differentiation 25$^+$ Forkhead Box P3$^+$ (CD4$^+$CD25$^+$FOXP3$^+$) Tregs, which have been implicated in inducing donor-specific tolerance.

CD4$^+$ CD25$^+$FOXP3 Tregs play a key role in promoting immune tolerance. This role was recognized in the pioneering work of Sakaguchi and colleagues[118] who induced a range of autoimmune diseases in mice by depleting CD4$^+$ T cells from the CD4$^+$ CD25$^+$ T-cell subset in 1995. FOXP3 was subsequently identified as the primary regulator of CD4$^+$ CD25$^+$ Tregs in 2003, when FOXP3 deletion caused Tregs to lose their suppressive properties and resulted in lethal autoimmune diseases in mice.[119] Recently, upregulation of Tregs in the periphery and the graft was demonstrated in mice after OLT; treating the mice with Treg-depleting anti-CD25 antibody led to acute rejection.[120] Furthermore, the role of the Treg effector molecule, CTLA-4 has also been outlined as critical to the induction of spontaneous tolerance in mice. Anti-CTLA-4 antibodies protected alloreactive T cells from apoptosis and caused an increase in the activity of donor-specific T cells and NK cells in the liver and spleen.[121] This finding is suggestive of a Treg tolerance induction mechanism that relies on targeting alloreactive T cells in both the periphery and the allograft itself.[117,121] Additionally, Tregs may also be used as biomarkers of tolerance in transplant recipients, although many lines of investigation have found these cells to be numerous in allografts that are also undergoing rejection. In the graft, increased expression of FOXP3 was associated with tolerance in cardiac and liver allografts; increased expression of CD25 was associated with rejection in cardiac allografts.[122]

A variety of experimental rodent models of liver transplantation have also demonstrated the importance of donor-recipient chimerism in liver allograft tolerance. Although recipients can become chimeric when donor-derived cells reconstitute their hematopoietic populations, the allograft can also become chimeric when some of the tissue is replaced by cells derived from the recipient (reverse chimerism). Some of the earliest work in establishing the reverse chimeric state was done by Sanada and colleagues[123] who induced chimerism in rat donor livers by intraportal injection of recipient bone marrow cells followed by intramuscular injection of tacrolimus for 5 days. The livers were then transplanted after 1 to 2 months, and tolerance was induced in the recipients with no immunosuppression required to maintain graft function. Okabayashi and colleagues recently showed that a reverse chimeric state could be attained while undergoing combination therapy with tacrolimus and plerixafor, which leads to increased allograft survival.[124] A low dose of tacrolimus was advantageous for host stem cells, as it permitted low-level rejection and prevented the donor allograft response from dominating. Plerixafor is an HSC mobilizer used to mobilize HSCs into the peripheral blood. It has been approved by the FDA for use in patients with non-Hodgkin lymphoma and multiple myeloma who are being prepared for an autologous stem cell transplant.[125,126] The increase in host stem cells caused by plerixafor enhanced the development and distribution of Tregs, thereby suppressing the graft response. This mobilization of host stem cells by plerixafor combined with the action of tacrolimus was critical to graft survival, with neither tacrolimus nor plerixafor preventing acute rejection on their own. Lastly, chimerism that does not depend on infusion or mobilization of stem cells can also be established in mothers and offspring because of the bidirectional flow of alloantigen across the placenta. Although the importance of this unique type of chimerism is not well established in liver transplantation, Dutta and Burlingham[127] demonstrated in a mouse model of cardiac transplantation that Tregs associated with these nonmaternal antigens led to heart allograft tolerance, whereas mice that did not exhibit maternal microchimerism experienced rejection. However, an unanticipated observation in this study was that tolerance was associated with microchimerism in the heart and lung but not in the liver. Maternal microchimerism in the human liver transplantation setting is discussed in the subsequent section.

Liver transplant tolerance in humans

As mentioned previously, the poor immunogenicity of liver allografts has been appreciated for many years, as liver allografts in humans show lower rejection rates than other organs and operational tolerance has been observed at a higher frequency than in any other transplant scenario.[69,79,128] The authors discuss later the tolerance induction studies performed in the human setting that have used diverse techniques to promote tolerance of the liver allograft with varying degrees of success. In summary, a state of operational tolerance to the liver allograft has been induced through (1) establishment of donor-recipient chimerism, (2) intentional deletion of the alloreactive repertoire or support of endogenous immunoregulatory mechanisms, and (3) progressive withdrawal of immunosuppression. **Table 6** summarizes important tolerance studies performed across multiple centers.

Two types of studies have assessed the role of donor-recipient chimerism in liver allograft tolerance: (1) studies whereby attempts have been made to induce macrochimerism through donor bone marrow transplants and (2) observational studies assessing donor microchimerism in patients who have either been classified as operationally tolerant after weaning off immunosuppression or in patients in whom microchimerism has been naturally established through pregnancy. Patients receiving a donor bone marrow infusion during the transplant were found to have increased chimerism and improved graft survival during withdrawal of CNI-based immunosuppression However, a follow-up analysis suggested that even though tolerant patients displayed 10 times more chimerism (<1%) than nontolerant patients, the establishment of this chimeric state did not lead to long-term operational tolerance, with similar numbers of tolerant and nontolerant patients being donor bone marrow recipients in the long-term.[129,130] In contrast, using regimens based on reduced-intensity preconditioning with cyclophosphamide and fludarabine, 2 patients with cirrhosis and leukemia that were treated with HSC transplantation followed by HLA-matched LDLT went on to achieve an immunosuppression-free, tolerant state for 6 and 7 years, respectively, at the time of the report.[131] Similarly, observational studies have also shown mixed results. Araujo and colleagues[132] found microchimerism in 32 (68.0%), patients with 10 (31.2%) experiencing rejection after immunosuppression withdrawal. This study showed a significant association between microchimerism and the absence of rejection ($P = .02$). On the other hand, Ayala and colleagues[133] observed significantly high donor chimerism in 3 patients on very low immunosuppression but also found that high donor chimerism was associated with an increased incidence of rejection and organ destruction caused by disease recurrence. Pons and colleagues[134] found that endothelial cell chimerism was evident in both tolerant and nontolerant patients and did not play a significant role in inducing tolerance, whereas Aini and colleagues[135] recently showed similar results related to hepatocyte chimerism. Support for a role of maternal microchimerism in liver transplantation tolerance is found in pediatric patients who show lower levels of graft failure and retransplantation when receiving maternal grafts as compared with the paternal grafts.[136] Thus, in the liver transplant setting in humans, there is little conclusive proof that microchimerism is necessary or sufficient to establish operational tolerance; harsh conditioning regimens associated with chimerism induction studies make this approach difficult to broadly implement in transplant recipients.

Table 6
Tolerance studies after liver transplantation in humans

Center	Areas of Investigation	Adult/Pediatric	Total Number of Subjects Enrolled	Tolerant	Nontolerant	Under Weaning
Kyoto[73,137–140,162–164]	LDLT, Tregs, FOXP3, HLA mismatch	Pediatric	190	84 (44.2%)	50 (26.3%)	56 (29.5%)
Miami[129,130]	Donor bone marrow chimerism, sex	Adult	104	23 (22.1%)	81 (77.9%)	—
Ontario[165]	Ursodeoxycholic acid	Adult	26	2 (7.7%)	24 (92.3%)	—
University of California San Francisco[78]	LDLT, time since transplantation, portal inflammation, C4d	Pediatric	20	19 (95%)	1 Patient did not complete the study	
Tor Vergata[69,166]	HCV, cirrhosis, fibrosis, steroid-free immunosuppression	Adult	34	8 (23.5%)	26 (76.5%)	—
King's College[167,168]	Cyclosporine, HLA mismatch, chimerism, non–immune-mediated liver disorders	Adult	18	5 (27.8%)	13 (72.2%)	—
Pittsburgh[151,152,169]	HLA-specific antibodies, cytokine gene polymorphisms, Epstein-Barr Virus, PTLD	Both	95	19	40	34
Oschner[170]	Steroid-free immunosuppression, Liver Function Tests, liver enzymes, tacrolimus monotherapy	Adult	18	1	11	—
Murcia[82,134,141]	Immunosuppression side-effects, endothelial cell chimerism, Tregs, FOXP3	Adult	20	8 (40%)	12 (60%)	—
Barcelona[81]	Time since transplantation, sex, age at transplantation, absence of CNI-inhibition	Adult	102	41 (40.2%)	57 (55.8%)	2 Patients did not complete the study

Other studies of tolerance induction have focused on describing the behavior of the alloreactive repertoire without attempting to induce chimerism. These primarily observational studies have described the state of the recipient's T cells in patients that are either tolerant or are in the midst of tolerance induction or immunosuppression withdrawal. Such studies have included T-cell deletion or inactivation protocols, modulation of cytokine production, and observations of Treg quantity or function.

As seen in animal studies, CD4$^+$ CD25$^+$ Tregs may play an important role in the development of operational tolerance; the groups from Murcia and Kyoto[73,137–139] have shown that Treg induction is one of many graft acceptance pathways. CD4$^+$ T cells from the tolerant recipients on no immunosuppression were hyporesponsive to donor alloantigens but not to third-party antigens, and FOXP3 mRNA expression was found to be greater in tolerant patients as compared with patients on maintenance immunosuppression or in normal liver samples.[140] Additionally, analysis of the Treg profile and FOXP3 mRNA expression in patients being weaned off CNI-based immunosuppression showed evidence of an increase in CD4$^+$ CD25^{high+} cells during withdrawal and a 3.5-fold increase in relative FOXP3 mRNA expression during withdrawal, with a further increase once withdrawal was complete.[141] In an interesting connection to fetomaternal tolerance, IL-10–producing Vδ1γδT cells were found in peripheral blood in tolerant patients and may be responsible for transplant tolerance.[73] Naive Tregs (CD4$^+$CD25^{++}CD45RA$^+$ cells) also play an important role in tolerance, with naive Tregs significantly decreased in nontolerant patients and FOXP3^{high+} cells showing greater expression within the naive Tregs in tolerant patients and those being weaned off immunosuppression.[139]

Progressive immunosuppression withdrawal studies without a definitive focus on tolerance induction have been driven by the earliest cases of transplantation tolerance, which were achieved on minimal immunosuppression and by cases of noncompliant patients. Benitez and colleagues[81] and Feng and colleagues[78] have demonstrated that the development of operational tolerance is significantly more common when immunosuppression is withdrawn after a longer time after transplant. Tolerant patients weaned off immunosuppression show improvements in not only kidney function but also decreases in serum cholesterol (hypercholesterolemia) and uric acid (hyperuricemia), fasting glucose (diabetes), and diastolic arterial pressure (hypertension).[82] They also have a lower incidence of portal inflammation compared with nontolerant patients and lower total C4d (a marker of antibody-mediated rejection) scores as compared with nontolerant patients. Significantly, operational tolerance was found to be independent of HLA mismatch, sensitization status, and the presence of donor-specific antibodies.[78] However, there is evidence of clinically relevant fibrotic lesions in long-term surviving patients, which may be the consequence of chronic underimmunosuppression.[142–144]

Thus, although studies have investigated multiple mechanisms of tolerance induction, there is no agreed on protocol for attempting immunosuppression withdrawal; the lack of tolerance biomarkers limits our ability to both identify tolerant patients and accurately assess tolerance induction during experimental protocols. Given the experimental and clinical data at this time, it remains questionable whether complete immunosuppression withdrawal is even a suitable strategy to induce tolerance, as there are very little long-term data available on the rare patients who maintain operational tolerance.

Lessons from Tolerance in Renal Transplantation and the Quest for Biomarkers

To date, clinical tolerance induction in human allograft recipients has been most successful in recipients of kidney allografts; the lessons learned from these patients may guide future attempts to induce tolerance in liver transplant recipients. Furthermore, cross-platform biomarker studies have identified several potentially important pathways in tolerant kidney patients and is discussed later.

Groups at both the Massachusetts General Hospital (MGH) and Northwestern have conducted seminal work exploring the role of induced donor chimerism in tolerance in kidney transplant recipients. The MGH group has provided key evidence supporting chimerism as a successful strategy to induce tolerance in humans by using a non-myeloablative preconditioning regimen followed by donor bone marrow transplantation to allow complete immunosuppression withdrawal in kidney transplant recipients.[97,145,146] More recently, Leventhal and colleagues[147] have shown that tolerance can be induced using chimerism without the associated negative side effects of GVHD and engraftment syndrome in a phase II clinical trial of dual kidney and hematopoietic transplantation with engraftment, sustainable chimerism, and operational tolerance in 5 out of 8 subjects. These subjects were all successfully weaned from pharmacologic immunosuppression by 1 year post-transplant. This trial was followed by a subsequent study in which chimerism was attempted in 15 HLA-mismatched living donor renal transplant recipients. Complete immunosuppression withdrawal was successful in all patients in whom chimerism was sustained and no GVHD or engraftment syndrome has been observed.[148] Another study on tolerance in HLA-identical sibling renal transplantation used 4 $CD34^+$ donor HSC infusions within the first 9 months after transplantation, and calcineurin-based immunosuppression was replaced over time with sirolimus and eventual complete immunosuppression withdrawal. Peripheral Blood Mononuclear Cell (PBMC) microchimerism was only temporarily observed in year 1 after transplant and was found to be unrelated to tolerance or nontolerance. $CD4^+CD25^{high}CD127^-FOXP3^+$ Tregs and $CD19^+IgD/M^+CD27^-$ B cells were shown to increase through a 5-year period after transplant, regardless of tolerance. Although chimerism was not discretely associated with tolerance in the work of this group, Leventhal and colleagues[149] successfully elucidated a tolerance signature of 783 genes, which suggested that tolerant patients have a type of natural immunosuppression as a consequence of regulatory activity, similar to that of Tregs or regulatory B cells, for which the mechanism is not yet understood. CD25 mRNA and other mRNAs associated with acute cellular rejection were less expressed in tolerant patients, whereas mRNAs for tolerance markers, such as FOXP3, CTLA-4, transforming growth factor (TGF)-β1, IL-10, and CD20, were relatively upregulated in nontolerant patients.

Although both of these groups performed biomarker studies in their studies, the comprehensive analysis to identify a cross-platform biomarker signature for tolerance in renal transplant patients by Sagoo and colleagues[150] is also worth mentioning for its robustness. In their analysis of whole-blood mRNA and PBMCs, Sagoo and colleagues[150] successfully identified a 10-gene signature showing generalized enrichment of B cell–related pathways, T-cell activation–related pathways, and Treg-related pathways in the peripheral blood in tolerant patients. A similar approach may be used in liver transplant recipients to elucidate a tolerance signature. A multicenter analysis using large training and validation cohorts and assessing cross-platform biomarkers and bioassays, such as those considered by Sagoo and colleagues, may be sufficiently powerful to more conclusively identify a liver allograft tolerance signature.

Although the data supporting tolerance studies are less well established in liver transplantation, several tolerance markers, including increased ratio of plasmacytoid to myeloid dendritic cells, an increase in B cells, higher numbers of $CD4^+CD25^+$ T cells, and an increase in $\gamma\delta$ T and NK cells, have been identified. There is also evidence of differential intragraft gene expression between tolerant and nontolerant patients even before immunosuppression minimization, with tolerant patients demonstrating an upregulation of iron homeostasis genes. Lastly, on the onset of rejection, nontolerant patients show a significant overexpression of immune-related genes, including STAT1, IL32, CXCL9, CXCL10, CD83, and CD8A, which were not detectable before immunosuppression minimization.[73,75,79,83,151–154] These results are summarized in **Table 7**.

MicroRNAs (miRNAs) have been assessed as markers of disease, and their differential expression in rejection in both renal and liver transplant settings has been the focus of many studies.[155–160] Recently, B cells from operationally tolerant patients were shown to overexpress miR-142-3p, regardless of immunosuppression. This overexpression of miR-142-3p was found to modulate approximately 1000 genes implicated in the immune response of B cells. There is also evidence of a negative feedback loop involving TGF-β signaling and miR-142-3p expression in B cells playing a role in maintaining the tolerant state. Thus, this study demonstrated a correlation between miR-142-3p and tolerance. However, it remains to be seen whether miR-142-3p is responsible for controlling the inflammatory response leading to tolerance or if it is a product of the tolerant state.[161] In summary, the role of miRNAs in the regulation of alloimmunity is poorly understood and will be an area of robust investigation in future years.

Current Clinical Tolerance Trials

Decades of experimental and observational studies have provided the foundation for ongoing work in clinical tolerance. As summarized in **Table 8**, several current trials

---

Table 7
Summary of biomarkers associated with liver transplant tolerance

First Author,[Ref.] Year	Biomarkers	Regulation	Functional Significance
Martinez-Llordella et al,[79,75] 2007, 2008	TRD@, CD94, NKG2D, NKG7, KLRC2, CD160, KLRB1, KLRC1, KLRF1, SLAMF7, KLRB1, FANCG, GNPTAB, CLIC3, PSMD14, ALG8, CX3CR1, RGS3	Upregulated	Markers of proliferative arrest, γδ T-cell function (transcripts of γδ T cells and NK cells), and non–T-cell mononuclear cells
Martinez-Llordella et al,[79] 2007	CD4⁺CD25⁺ T cells and Vδ1⁺ T cells	Upregulated	Tregs
Martinez-Llordella et al,[79,75] 2007, 2008	SOS-1, BCL-XL, AIOLOS, JAK1, IL2RB	Upregulated	T-cell tolerance (IL-2R signaling)
Martinez-Llordella et al,[79] 2007	RAD21, RAD50, RAD52, PMSL3, UHMK1	Upregulated	Cell cycle control
Martinez-Llordella et al,[79] 2007	RBBP9, APRIN, PML, GCIP-interacting protein p29, I (3)mbtlike, TES, MATK, RASA3, and TUSC1	Upregulated	Suppression of cell proliferation
Martinez-Llordella et al,[79] 2007	F3, DAF, CD83, PLAUR, SDC4, TNFα	Downregulated	Stress response
Martinez-Llordella et al,[79] 2007	CXCL1, CXCL2, TNFAIP6, CCL20, CXCL3, CXCL4	Downregulated	Inflammatory response

Abbreviation: TNF, tumor necrosis factor.
Data from Refs.[75,79,154]

Table 8
Summary of ongoing clinical trials on tolerance after liver or renal transplantation

Primary Center	Study Title	Organ	Summary
Emory University, Harvard Medical School	Associating Renal Transplantation with the ITN Signature of Tolerance (ARTIST)	Kidney	Assess presence and stability of B-cell differentiation tolerance signature, determine other tolerance biomarkers
MGH	Research Study of ATG and Rituximab in Renal Transplantation (RESTARRT)	Kidney	Use ATG (T-cell targeting) and rituximab (B-cell targeting) with maintenance immunosuppression to promote tolerance
MGH	Renal Allograft Tolerance Through Mixed Chimerism	Kidney	Nonmyeloablative conditioning before combined renal and bone marrow transplant
Emory University	Study of Tolerant Kidney Transplant Recipients (FACTOR)	Kidney	Global biorespository to determine biomarkers of renal allograft tolerance
Johns Hopkins Hospital	Posttransplant Cyclophosphamide (ACCEPTOR)	Kidney	Specialized nonmyeloablative conditioning regimen for renal and bone marrow transplant, high-dose post-OLT cyclophosphamide for tolerance induction
University of Pennsylvania	Gradual Withdrawal of Immune System Suppressing Drugs in Patients Receiving a Liver Transplant (AWISH)	Liver	Gradual immunosuppression withdrawal after OLT for HCV+ or nonimmune nonviral causes of liver failure
University of California San Francisco	Withdrawal of Immunosuppression in Pediatric Liver Transplant Recipients (WISP-R)	Liver	Immunosuppression withdrawal in pediatric patients transplanted for nonimmune nonviral causes of liver failure

Data from Immune Tolerance Network. Clinical trials in transplantation. Available at: http://www.immunetolerance.org/researchers/clinical-trials/transplantation. Accessed December 15, 2013.

continue to investigate the role of B cells, donor-recipient chimerism, and progressive immunosuppressive withdrawal on tolerance induction, with a major focus on the identification of tolerance biomarkers.

SUMMARY

Pharmacologic manipulation of the recipient immune system is responsible for the great success of organ transplantation. It has virtually eliminated mortality caused by acute rejection and has resulted in excellent allograft and patient survival. However, significant long-term morbidity caused by off-target effects of these drugs is a major challenge in the field; there is, thus, a great need to develop effective strategies to reduce this morbidity. Although allograft tolerance in the absence of immunosuppression continues to garner great interest, effective and easily reproducible tolerance induction strategies in humans presently elude us; there is an overall lack of data that demonstrates superior long-term outcomes among the few operationally tolerant recipients that are managed off immunosuppression. In conclusion, clinical efforts to define optimal strategies of IM may prove more fruitful in addressing and correcting the long-term morbidity and mortality in liver transplant recipients.

REFERENCES

1. OPTN. 2011 Annual report of the U.S. Organ Procurement and Transplantation Network and the Scientific Registry of Transplant Recipients: Transplant Data 1998-2011. Department of Health and Human Services, Health Resources and Services Administration, Healthcare Systems Bureau, Division of Transplantation, Rockville, MD; United Network for Organ Sharing, Richmond, VA; University of Renal Research and Education Association, Ann Arbor, MI; 13 Dec 2012.
2. McAlister VC, Haddad E, Renouf E, et al. Cyclosporin versus tacrolimus as primary immunosuppressant after liver transplantation: a meta-analysis. Am J Transplant 2006;6(7):1578–85.
3. Gonwa TA, Mai ML, Melton LB, et al. End-stage renal disease (ESRD) after orthotopic liver transplantation (OLTX) using calcineurin-based immunotherapy: risk of development and treatment. Transplantation 2001;72(12):1934–9.
4. Segev DL, Sozio SM, Shin EJ, et al. Steroid avoidance in liver transplantation: meta-analysis and meta-regression of randomized trials. Liver Transpl 2008; 14(4):512–25.
5. Shapiro R, Young JB, Milford EL, et al. Immunosuppression: evolution in practice and trends, 1993-2003. Am J Transplant 2005;5(4 Pt 2):874–86.
6. Germani G, Pleguezuelo M, Villamil F, et al. Azathioprine in liver transplantation: a reevaluation of its use and a comparison with mycophenolate mofetil. Am J Transplant 2009;9(8):1725–31.
7. Abdelmalek MF, Humar A, Stickel F, et al. Sirolimus conversion regimen versus continued calcineurin inhibitors in liver allograft recipients: a randomized trial. Am J Transplant 2012;12(3):694–705.
8. De Simone P, Carrai P, Precisi A, et al. Conversion to everolimus monotherapy in maintenance liver transplantation: feasibility, safety, and impact on renal function. Transpl Int 2009;22(3):279–86.
9. Masetti M, Montalti R, Rompianesi G, et al. Early withdrawal of calcineurin inhibitors and everolimus monotherapy in de novo liver transplant recipients preserves renal function. Am J Transplant 2010;10(10):2252–62.
10. Heimbach JK, Charlton MR. Antibody-based immunosuppression following liver transplantation: the plot thickens. Am J Transplant 2010;10(3):445–6.
11. Moonka DK, Kim D, Kapke A, et al. The influence of induction therapy on graft and patient survival in patients with and without hepatitis C after liver transplantation. Am J Transplant 2010;10(3):590–601.
12. Rostaing L, Vincenti F, Grinyo J, et al. Long-term belatacept exposure maintains efficacy and safety at 5 years: results from the long-term extension of the BENEFIT study. Am J Transplant 2013;13(11):2875–83.
13. Archdeacon P, Dixon C, Belen O, et al. Summary of the US FDA approval of belatacept. Am J Transplant 2012;12(3):554–62.

14. Klintmalm GB. Immunosuppression, generic drugs and the FDA. Am J Transplant 2011;11(9):1765–6.
15. Demetris AJ, Adeyi O, Bellamy CO, et al. Liver biopsy interpretation for causes of late liver allograft dysfunction. Hepatology 2006;44(2):489–501.
16. Jain A, Demetris AJ, Kashyap R, et al. Does tacrolimus offer virtual freedom from chronic rejection after primary liver transplantation? Risk and prognostic factors in 1,048 liver transplantations with a mean follow-up of 6 years. Liver Transpl 2001;7(7):623–30.
17. Shepherd RW, Turmelle Y, Nadler M, et al. Risk factors for rejection and infection in pediatric liver transplantation. Am J Transplant 2008;8(2):396–403.
18. Bianchi G, Marchesini G, Marzocchi R, et al. Metabolic syndrome in liver transplantation: relation to etiology and immunosuppression. Liver Transpl 2008; 14(11):1648–54.
19. Forman LM, Lewis JD, Berlin JA, et al. The association between hepatitis C infection and survival after orthotopic liver transplantation. Gastroenterology 2002;122(4):889–96.
20. Gane EJ. The natural history of recurrent hepatitis C and what influences this. Liver Transpl 2008;14(Suppl 2):S36–44.
21. Grulich AE, van Leeuwen MT, Falster MO, et al. Incidence of cancers in people with HIV/AIDS compared with immunosuppressed transplant recipients: a meta-analysis. Lancet 2007;370(9581):59–67.
22. Guckelberger O. Long-term medical comorbidities and their management: hypertension/cardiovascular disease. Liver Transpl 2009;15(Suppl 2):S75–8.
23. Moon JI, Barbeito R, Faradji RN, et al. Negative impact of new-onset diabetes mellitus on patient and graft survival after liver transplantation: long-term follow up. Transplantation 2006;82(12):1625–8.
24. Ojo AO, Held PJ, Port FK, et al. Chronic renal failure after transplantation of a nonrenal organ. N Engl J Med 2003;349(10):931–40.
25. Watt KD, Charlton MR. Metabolic syndrome and liver transplantation: a review and guide to management. J Hepatol 2010;53(1):199–206.
26. Watt KD, Pedersen RA, Kremers WK, et al. Evolution of causes and risk factors for mortality post-liver transplant: results of the NIDDK long-term follow-up study. Am J Transplant 2010;10(6):1420–7.
27. Watt KD, Pedersen RA, Kremers WK, et al. Long-term probability of and mortality from de novo malignancy after liver transplantation. Gastroenterology 2009; 137(6):2010–7.
28. Becker T, Foltys D, Bilbao I, et al. Patient outcomes in two steroid-free regimens using tacrolimus monotherapy after daclizumab induction and tacrolimus with mycophenolate mofetil in liver transplantation. Transplantation 2008;86(12): 1689–94.
29. Flechner SM, Kobashigawa J, Klintmalm G. Calcineurin inhibitor-sparing regimens in solid organ transplantation: focus on improving renal function and nephrotoxicity. Clin Transplant 2008;22(1):1–15.
30. Neuberger JM, Mamelok RD, Neuhaus P, et al. Delayed introduction of reduced-dose tacrolimus, and renal function in liver transplantation: the 'ReSpECT' study. Am J Transplant 2009;9(2):327–36.
31. Campbell K, Ng V, Martin S, et al. Glomerular filtration rate following pediatric liver transplantation–the SPLIT experience. Am J Transplant 2010;10(12): 2673–82.
32. Harambat J, Ranchin B, Dubourg L, et al. Renal function in pediatric liver transplantation: a long-term follow-up study. Transplantation 2008;86(8):1028–34.

33. Morard I, Dumortier J, Spahr L, et al. Conversion to sirolimus-based immuno-suppression in maintenance liver transplantation patients. Liver Transpl 2007; 13(5):658–64.
34. Watson CJ, Gimson AE, Alexander GJ, et al. A randomized controlled trial of late conversion from calcineurin inhibitor (CNI)-based to sirolimus-based immuno-suppression in liver transplant recipients with impaired renal function. Liver Transpl 2007;13(12):1694–702.
35. Taylor AL, Watson CJ, Bradley JA. Immunosuppressive agents in solid organ transplantation: mechanisms of action and therapeutic efficacy. Crit Rev Oncol Hematol 2005;56(1):23–46.
36. Creput C, Blandin F, Deroure B, et al. Long-term effects of calcineurin inhibitor conversion to mycophenolate mofetil on renal function after liver transplantation. Liver Transpl 2007;13(7):1004–10.
37. Dharancy S, Iannelli A, Hulin A, et al. Mycophenolate mofetil monotherapy for severe side effects of calcineurin inhibitors following liver transplantation. Am J Transplant 2009;9(3):610–3.
38. Reich DJ, Clavien PA, Hodge EE. Mycophenolate mofetil for renal dysfunction in liver transplant recipients on cyclosporine or tacrolimus: randomized, prospective, multicenter pilot study results. Transplantation 2005;80(1):18–25.
39. Franco OH, Massaro JM, Civil J, et al. Trajectories of entering the metabolic syndrome: the Framingham Heart Study. Circulation 2009;120(20):1943–50.
40. Hu G, Qiao Q, Tuomilehto J. The metabolic syndrome and cardiovascular risk. Curr Diabetes Rev 2005;1(2):137–43.
41. Wannamethee SG, Shaper AG, Lennon L, et al. Metabolic syndrome vs Framingham Risk Score for prediction of coronary heart disease, stroke, and type 2 diabetes mellitus. Arch Intern Med 2005;165(22):2644–50.
42. Guize L, Pannier B, Thomas F, et al. Recent advances in metabolic syndrome and cardiovascular disease. Arch Cardiovasc Dis 2008;101(9):577–83.
43. Carey EJ, Aqel BA, Byrne TJ, et al. Pretransplant fasting glucose predicts new-onset diabetes after liver transplantation. J Transplant 2012;2012:614781.
44. Kuo HT, Sampaio MS, Ye X, et al. Risk factors for new-onset diabetes mellitus in adult liver transplant recipients, an analysis of the Organ Procurement and Transplant Network/United Network for Organ Sharing database. Transplantation 2010;89(9):1134–40.
45. Saliba F, Lakehal M, Pageaux GP, et al. Risk factors for new-onset diabetes mellitus following liver transplantation and impact of hepatitis C infection: an observational multicenter study. Liver Transpl 2007;13(1):136–44.
46. Tueche SG. Diabetes mellitus after liver transplant new etiologic clues and cornerstones for understanding. Transplant Proc 2003;35(4):1466–8.
47. Saab S, Shpaner A, Zhao Y, et al. Prevalence and risk factors for diabetes mellitus in moderate term survivors of liver transplantation. Am J Transplant 2006; 6(8):1890–5.
48. Oufroukhi L, Kamar N, Muscari F, et al. Predictive factors for posttransplant diabetes mellitus within one-year of liver transplantation. Transplantation 2008; 85(10):1436–42.
49. Xu X, Ling Q, He ZL, et al. Post-transplant diabetes mellitus in liver transplantation: Hangzhou experience. Hepatobiliary Pancreat Dis Int 2008;7(5): 465–70.
50. Yadav AD, Chang YH, Aqel BA, et al. New onset diabetes mellitus in living donor versus deceased donor liver transplant recipients: analysis of the UNOS/OPTN database. J Transplant 2013;2013:269096.

51. Hanouneh IA, Feldstein AE, McCullough AJ, et al. The significance of metabolic syndrome in the setting of recurrent hepatitis C after liver transplantation. Liver Transpl 2008;14(9):1287–93.

52. Mells G, Neuberger J. Reducing the risks of cardiovascular disease in liver allograft recipients. Transplantation 2007;83(9):1141–50.

53. McKenna GJ, Trotter JF, Klintmalm E, et al. Sirolimus and cardiovascular disease risk in liver transplantation. Transplantation 2013;95(1):215–21.

54. Vajdic CM, McDonald SP, McCredie MR, et al. Cancer incidence before and after kidney transplantation. JAMA 2006;296(23):2823–31.

55. del Pozo JL. Update and actual trends on bacterial infections following liver transplantation. World J Gastroenterol 2008;14(32):4977–83.

56. Vilchez RA, Fung J, Kusne S. The pathogenesis and management of influenza virus infection in organ transplant recipients. Transpl Infect Dis 2002;4(4):177–82.

57. Demetris AJ. Evolution of hepatitis C virus in liver allografts. Liver Transpl 2009; 15(Suppl 2):S35–41.

58. Kuo A, Terrault NA. Management of hepatitis C in liver transplant recipients. Am J Transplant 2006;6(3):449–58.

59. Roche B, Samuel D. Risk factors for hepatitis C recurrence after liver transplantation. J Viral Hepat 2007;14(Suppl 1):89–96.

60. Charlton M. Liver biopsy, viral kinetics, and the impact of viremia on severity of hepatitis C virus recurrence. Liver Transpl 2003;9(11):S58–62.

61. Lake JR. The role of immunosuppression in recurrence of hepatitis C. Liver Transpl 2003;9(11):S63–6.

62. McCaughan GW, Shackel NA, Bertolino P, et al. Molecular and cellular aspects of hepatitis C virus reinfection after liver transplantation: how the early phase impacts on outcomes. Transplantation 2009;87(8):1105–11.

63. Sgourakis G, Radtke A, Fouzas I, et al. Corticosteroid-free immunosuppression in liver transplantation: a meta-analysis and meta-regression of outcomes. Transpl Int 2009;22(9):892–905.

64. Lin CC, Chuang FR, Lee CH, et al. The renal-sparing efficacy of basiliximab in adult living donor liver transplantation. Liver Transpl 2005;11(10):1258–64.

65. Ferraris JR, Duca P, Prigoshin N, et al. Mycophenolate mofetil and reduced doses of cyclosporine in pediatric liver transplantation with chronic renal dysfunction: changes in the immune responses. Pediatr Transplant 2004;8(5):454–9.

66. Tannuri U, Gibelli NE, Maksoud-Filho JG, et al. Mycophenolate mofetil promotes prolonged improvement of renal dysfunction after pediatric liver transplantation: experience of a single center. Pediatr Transplant 2007;11(1):82–6.

67. Kamphues C, Bova R, Rocken C, et al. Safety of mycophenolate mofetil monotherapy in patients after liver transplantation. Ann Transplant 2009;14(4):40–6.

68. Tchao N, Sayre P, Feng S, et al. Long-term immunosuppression management in OLT recipients. San Francisco (CA): American Transplant Congress; 2007.

69. Tisone G, Orlando G, Cardillo A, et al. Complete weaning off immunosuppression in HCV liver transplant recipients is feasible and favourably impacts on the progression of disease recurrence. J Hepatol 2006;44(4):702–9.

70. Manzia TM, Angelico R, Baiocchi L, et al. The Tor Vergata weaning of immunosuppression protocols in stable hepatitis C virus liver transplant patients: the 10-year follow-up. Transpl Int 2013;26(3):259–66.

71. Feng S. Long-term management of immunosuppression after pediatric liver transplantation: is minimization or withdrawal desirable or possible or both? Curr Opin Organ Transplant 2008;13(5):506–12.

72. Ng VL, Fecteau A, Shepherd R, et al. Outcomes of 5-year survivors of pediatric liver transplantation: report on 461 children from a North American multicenter registry. Pediatrics 2008;122(6):e1128–35.
73. Koshiba T, Li Y, Takemura M, et al. Clinical, immunological, and pathological aspects of operational tolerance after pediatric living-donor liver transplantation. Transpl Immunol 2007;17(2):94–7.
74. Lerut J, Sanchez-Fueyo A. An appraisal of tolerance in liver transplantation. Am J Transplant 2006;6(8):1774–80.
75. Martinez-Llordella M, Lozano JJ, Puig-Pey I, et al. Using transcriptional profiling to develop a diagnostic test of operational tolerance in liver transplant recipients. J Clin Invest 2008;118(8):2845–57.
76. Orlando G, Manzia T, Baiocchi L, et al. The Tor Vergata weaning off immunosuppression protocol in stable HCV liver transplant patients: the updated follow up at 78 months. Transpl Immunol 2008;20(1–2):43–7.
77. Yoshitomi M, Koshiba T, Haga H, et al. Requirement of protocol biopsy before and after complete cessation of immunosuppression after liver transplantation. Transplantation 2009;87(4):606–14.
78. Feng S, Ekong UD, Lobritto SJ, et al. Complete immunosuppression withdrawal and subsequent allograft function among pediatric recipients of parental living donor liver transplants. JAMA 2012;307(3):283–93.
79. Martinez-Llordella M, Puig-Pey I, Orlando G, et al. Multiparameter immune profiling of operational tolerance in liver transplantation. Am J Transplant 2007; 7(2):309–19.
80. Li L, Wozniak LJ, Rodder S, et al. A common peripheral blood gene set for diagnosis of operational tolerance in pediatric and adult liver transplantation. Am J Transplant 2012;12(5):1218–28.
81. Benitez C, Londono MC, Miquel R, et al. Prospective multicenter clinical trial of immunosuppressive drug withdrawal in stable adult liver transplant recipients. Hepatology 2013;58(5):1824–35.
82. Pons JA, Ramirez P, Revilla-Nuin B, et al. Immunosuppression withdrawal improves long-term metabolic parameters, cardiovascular risk factors and renal function in liver transplant patients. Clin Transplant 2009;23(3):329–36.
83. Alex Bishop G, Bertolino PD, Bowen DG, et al. Tolerance in liver transplantation. Best practice & research. Clin Gastroenterol 2012;26(1):73–84.
84. Wu SL, Pan CE. Tolerance and chimerism and allogeneic bone marrow/stem cell transplantation in liver transplantation. World J Gastroenterol 2013;19(36): 5981–7.
85. Hundrieser J, Hisanaga M, Boker K, et al. Long-term chimerism in liver transplantation: no evidence for immunological relevance but requirement for graft persistence. Transplant Proc 1995;27(1):216–8.
86. Starzl TE, Zinkernagel RM. Transplantation tolerance from a historical perspective. Nat Rev Immunol 2001;1(3):233–9.
87. Zheng XX, Sanchez-Fueyo A, Domenig C, et al. The balance of deletion and regulation in allograft tolerance. Immunol Rev 2003;196:75–84.
88. Hardinger KL, Schnitzler MA, Miller B, et al. Five-year follow up of thymoglobulin versus ATGAM induction in adult renal transplantation. Transplantation 2004; 78(1):136–41.
89. Hardinger KL, Rhee S, Buchanan P, et al. A prospective, randomized, double-blinded comparison of thymoglobulin versus Atgam for induction immunosuppressive therapy: 10-year results. Transplantation 2008;86(7):947–52.

90. Larsen CP, Elwood ET, Alexander DZ, et al. Long-term acceptance of skin and cardiac allografts after blocking CD40 and CD28 pathways. Nature 1996;381(6581): 434–8.

91. Kawai T, Sogawa H, Boskovic S, et al. CD154 blockade for induction of mixed chimerism and prolonged renal allograft survival in nonhuman primates. Am J Transplant 2004;4(9):1391–8.

92. Kawai T, Cosimi AB, Colvin RB, et al. Mixed allogeneic chimerism and renal allograft tolerance in cynomolgus monkeys. Transplantation 1995;59(2):256–62.

93. Kimikawa M, Kawai T, Sachs DH, et al. Mixed chimerism and transplantation tolerance induced by a nonlethal preparative regimen in cynomolgus monkeys. Transplant Proc 1997;29(1–2):1218.

94. Kimikawa M, Sachs DH, Colvin RB, et al. Modifications of the conditioning regimen for achieving mixed chimerism and donor-specific tolerance in cynomolgus monkeys. Transplantation 1997;64(5):709–16.

95. Xu H, Montgomery SP, Preston EH, et al. Studies investigating pretransplant donor-specific blood transfusion, rapamycin, and the CD154-specific antibody IDEC-131 in a nonhuman primate model of skin allotransplantation. J Immunol 2003;170(5):2776–82.

96. Kirk AD. Transplantation tolerance: a look at the nonhuman primate literature in the light of modern tolerance theories. Crit Rev Immunol 1999;19(5–6): 349–88.

97. Kawai T, Cosimi AB, Spitzer TR, et al. HLA-mismatched renal transplantation without maintenance immunosuppression. N Engl J Med 2008;358(4):353–61.

98. Kawai T, Sachs DH, Sykes M, et al. HLA-mismatched renal transplantation without maintenance immunosuppression. N Engl J Med 2013;368(19): 1850–2.

99. Fändrich F. Tolerance in clinical transplantation: progress, challenge or just a dream? Langenbecks Arch Surg 2011;396(4):475–87.

100. Demirkiran A, Kok A, Kwekkeboom J, et al. Low circulating regulatory T-cell levels after acute rejection in liver transplantation. Liver Transplantation (official publication of the American Association for the Study of Liver Diseases and the International Liver Transplantation Society) 2006;12(2):277–84.

101. Bestard O, Cruzado JM, Rama I, et al. Presence of FoxP3+ regulatory T Cells predicts outcome of subclinical rejection of renal allografts. Journal of the American Society of Nephrology 2008;19(10):2020–6.

102. Meloni F, Vitulo P, Bianco AM, et al. Regulatory CD4+CD25+ T cells in the peripheral blood of lung transplant recipients: correlation with transplant outcome. Transplantation 2004;77(5):762–6.

103. Kim JI, O'Connor MR, Duff PE, et al. Generation of adaptive regulatory T cells by alloantigen is required for some but not all transplant tolerance protocols. Transplantation 2011;91(7):707–13.

104. Sonawane SB, Kim JI, Lee MK, et al. GITR blockade facilitates Treg mediated allograft survival. Transplantation 2009;88(10):1169–77.

105. Yeh H, Moore DJ, Markmann JF, et al. Mechanisms of regulatory T cell counter-regulation by innate immunity. Transplant Rev (Orlando) 2013;27(2):61–4.

106. Issa F, Hester J, Goto R, et al. Ex vivo-expanded human regulatory T cells prevent the rejection of skin allografts in a humanized mouse model. Transplantation 2010;90(12):1321–7.

107. Li L, Godfrey WR, Porter SB, et al. CD4+CD25+ regulatory T-cell lines from human cord blood have functional and molecular properties of T-cell anergy. Blood 2005;106(9):3068–73.

108. Hippen KL, Merkel SC, Schirm DK, et al. Generation and large-scale expansion of human inducible regulatory T cells that suppress graft-versus-host disease. Am J Transplant 2011;11(6):1148–57.
109. Hippen KL, Merkel SC, Schirm DK, et al. Massive ex vivo expansion of human natural regulatory T cells (Tregs) with minimal loss of in vivo functional activity. Sci Transl Med 2011;3(83):83ra41.
110. Sawitzki B, Brunstein C, Meisel C, et al. Prevention of graft-versus-host disease by adoptive T regulatory therapy is associated with active repression of peripheral blood Toll-like receptor 5 mRNA expression. Biol Blood Marrow Transplant 2014;20(2):173–82.
111. June CH, Blazar BR. Clinical application of expanded CD4+25+ cells. Semin Immunol 2006;18(2):78–88.
112. Tang Q, Bluestone JA. Regulatory T-cell therapy in transplantation: moving to the clinic. Cold Spring Harb Perspect Med 2013;3(11). pii:a015552.
113. Le Blanc K, Pittenger M. Mesenchymal stem cells: progress toward promise. Cytotherapy 2005;7(1):36–45.
114. Le Blanc K, Rasmusson I, Sundberg B, et al. Treatment of severe acute graft-versus-host disease with third party haploidentical mesenchymal stem cells. Lancet 2004;363(9419):1439–41.
115. Le Blanc K, Ringden O. Immunomodulation by mesenchymal stem cells and clinical experience. J Intern Med 2007;262(5):509–25.
116. Chen Y, Liu Z, Liang S, et al. Role of Kupffer cells in the induction of tolerance of orthotopic liver transplantation in rats. Liver Transpl 2008;14(6):823–36.
117. Fujiki M, Esquivel CO, Martinez OM, et al. Induced tolerance to rat liver allografts involves the apoptosis of intragraft T cells and the generation of CD4(+)CD25(+)FoxP3(+) T regulatory cells. Liver Transpl 2010;16(2):147–54.
118. Sakaguchi S, Sakaguchi N, Asano M, et al. Immunologic self-tolerance maintained by activated T cells expressing IL-2 receptor alpha-chains (CD25). Breakdown of a single mechanism of self-tolerance causes various autoimmune diseases. J Immunol 1995;155(3):1151–64.
119. Fontenot JD, Gavin MA, Rudensky AY. Foxp3 programs the development and function of CD4+CD25+ regulatory T cells. Nat Immunol 2003;4(4):330–6.
120. Li W, Kuhr CS, Zheng XX, et al. New insights into mechanisms of spontaneous liver transplant tolerance: the role of Foxp3-expressing CD25+CD4+ regulatory T cells. Am J Transplant 2008;8(8):1639–51.
121. Li W, Zheng XX, Kuhr CS, et al. CTLA4 engagement is required for induction of murine liver transplant spontaneous tolerance. Am J Transplant 2005;5(5):978–86.
122. Xie L, Ichimaru N, Morita M, et al. Identification of a novel biomarker gene set with sensitivity and specificity for distinguishing between allograft rejection and tolerance. Liver Transpl 2012;18(4):444–54.
123. Sanada O, Fukuda Y, Sumimoto R, et al. Establishment of chimerism in donor liver with recipient-type bone marrow cells prior to liver transplantation produces marked suppression of allograft rejection in rats. Transpl Int 1998;11(Suppl 1):S174–8.
124. Okabayashi T, Cameron AM, Hisada M, et al. Mobilization of host stem cells enables long-term liver transplant acceptance in a strongly rejecting rat strain combination. Am J Transplant 2011;11(10):2046–56.
125. DiPersio JF, Micallef IN, Stiff PJ, et al. Phase III prospective randomized double-blind placebo-controlled trial of plerixafor plus granulocyte colony-stimulating factor compared with placebo plus granulocyte colony-stimulating factor for

autologous stem-cell mobilization and transplantation for patients with non-Hodgkin's lymphoma. J Clin Oncol 2009;27(28):4767–73.

126. DiPersio JF, Stadtmauer EA, Nademanee A, et al. Plerixafor and G-CSF versus placebo and G-CSF to mobilize hematopoietic stem cells for autologous stem cell transplantation in patients with multiple myeloma. Blood 2009;113(23):5720–6.

127. Dutta P, Burlingham WJ. Correlation between post transplant maternal microchimerism and tolerance across MHC barriers in mice. Chimerism 2011;2(3):78–83.

128. Pons JA, Revilla Nuin B, Ramirez P, et al. What do we know about the clinical impact of complete withdrawal of immunosuppression in liver transplantation? Transplant Proc 2012;44(6):1530–2.

129. Tryphonopoulos P, Ruiz P, Weppler D, et al. Long-term follow-up of 23 operational tolerant liver transplant recipients. Transplantation 2010;90(12):1556–61.

130. Tryphonopoulos P, Tzakis AG, Weppler D, et al. The role of donor bone marrow infusions in withdrawal of immunosuppression in adult liver allotransplantation. Am J Transplant 2005;5(3):608–13.

131. Kim SY, Kim DW, Choi JY, et al. Full donor chimerism using stem-cell transplantation for tolerance induction in the human leukocyte antigen-matched liver transplant setting. Transplantation 2009;88(4):601–3.

132. Araujo MB, Leonardi LS, Leonardi MI, et al. Prospective analysis between the therapy of immunosuppressive medication and allogeneic microchimerism after liver transplantation. Transpl Immunol 2009;20(3):195–8.

133. Ayala R, Grande S, Albizua E, et al. Long-term follow-up of donor chimerism and tolerance after human liver transplantation. Liver Transpl 2009;15(6):581–91.

134. Pons JA, Yelamos J, Ramirez P, et al. Endothelial cell chimerism does not influence allograft tolerance in liver transplant patients after withdrawal of immunosuppression. Transplantation 2003;75(7):1045–7.

135. Aini W, Miyagawa-Hayashino A, Ozeki M, et al. Frequent hepatocyte chimerism in long-term human liver allografts independent of graft outcome. Transpl Immunol 2013;28(2–3):100–5.

136. Nijagal A, Fleck S, MacKenzie TC. Maternal microchimerism in patients with biliary atresia: implications for allograft tolerance. Chimerism 2012;3(2):37–9.

137. Yoshizawa A, Ito A, Li Y, et al. The roles of CD25+CD4+ regulatory T cells in operational tolerance after living donor liver transplantation. Transplant Proc 2005;37(1):37–9.

138. Ohe H, Waki K, Yoshitomi M, et al. Factors affecting operational tolerance after pediatric living-donor liver transplantation: impact of early post-transplant events and HLA match. Transpl Int 2012;25(1):97–106.

139. Nafady-Hego H, Li Y, Ohe H, et al. The generation of donor-specific CD4+CD25++CD45RA+ naive regulatory T cells in operationally tolerant patients after pediatric living-donor liver transplantation. Transplantation 2010;90(12):1547–55.

140. Li Y, Zhao X, Cheng D, et al. The presence of Foxp3 expressing T cells within grafts of tolerant human liver transplant recipients. Transplantation 2008;86(12):1837–43.

141. Pons JA, Revilla-Nuin B, Baroja-Mazo A, et al. FoxP3 in peripheral blood is associated with operational tolerance in liver transplant patients during immunosuppression withdrawal. Transplantation 2008;86(10):1370–8.

142. Evans HM, Kelly DA, McKiernan PJ, et al. Progressive histological damage in liver allografts following pediatric liver transplantation. Hepatology 2006;43(5):1109–17.

143. Abraham SC, Poterucha JJ, Rosen CB, et al. Histologic abnormalities are common in protocol liver allograft biopsies from patients with normal liver function tests. Am J Surg Pathol 2008;32(7):965–73.
144. Sanchez-Fueyo A. Tolerance profiles and immunosuppression. Liver Transpl 2013;19(Suppl 2):S44–8.
145. Buhler LH, Spitzer TR, Sykes M, et al. Induction of kidney allograft tolerance after transient lymphohematopoietic chimerism in patients with multiple myeloma and end-stage renal disease. Transplantation 2002;74(10):1405–9.
146. Fudaba Y, Spitzer TR, Shaffer J, et al. Myeloma responses and tolerance following combined kidney and nonmyeloablative marrow transplantation: in vivo and in vitro analyses. Am J Transplant 2006;6(9):2121–33.
147. Leventhal J, Abecassis M, Miller J, et al. Chimerism and tolerance without GVHD or engraftment syndrome in HLA-mismatched combined kidney and hematopoietic stem cell transplantation. Sci Transl Med 2012;4(124):124ra28.
148. Leventhal J, Abecassis M, Miller J, et al. Tolerance induction in HLA disparate living donor kidney transplantation by donor stem cell infusion: durable chimerism predicts outcome. Transplantation 2013;95(1):169–76.
149. Leventhal JR, Mathew JM, Salomon DR, et al. Genomic biomarkers correlate with HLA-identical renal transplant tolerance. J Am Soc Nephrol 2013;24(9):1376–85.
150. Sagoo P, Perucha E, Sawitzki B, et al. Development of a cross-platform biomarker signature to detect renal transplant tolerance in humans. J Clin Invest 2010;120(6):1848–61.
151. Mazariegos GV, Zahorchak AF, Reyes J, et al. Dendritic cell subset ratio in tolerant, weaning and non-tolerant liver recipients is not affected by extent of immunosuppression. Am J Transplant 2005;5(2):314–22.
152. Mazariegos GV, Sindhi R, Thomson AW, et al. Clinical tolerance following liver transplantation: long term results and future prospects. Transpl Immunol 2007;17(2):114–9.
153. Sanchez-Fueyo A. Identification of tolerant recipients following liver transplantation. Int Immunopharmacol 2010;10(12):1501–4.
154. Bohne F, Martinez-Llordella M, Lozano JJ, et al. Intra-graft expression of genes involved in iron homeostasis predicts the development of operational tolerance in human liver transplantation. J Clin Invest 2012;122(1):368–82.
155. Farid WR, Pan Q, van der Meer AJ, et al. Hepatocyte-derived microRNAs as serum biomarkers of hepatic injury and rejection after liver transplantation. Liver Transpl 2012;18(3):290–7.
156. Anglicheau D, Sharma VK, Ding R, et al. MicroRNA expression profiles predictive of human renal allograft status. Proc Natl Acad Sci U S A 2009;106(13):5330–5.
157. Lorenzen JM, Volkmann I, Fiedler J, et al. Urinary miR-210 as a mediator of acute T-cell mediated rejection in renal allograft recipients. Am J Transplant 2011;11(10):2221–7.
158. Scian MJ, Maluf DG, David KG, et al. MicroRNA profiles in allograft tissues and paired urines associate with chronic allograft dysfunction with IF/TA. Am J Transplant 2011;11(10):2110–22.
159. Wei L, Gong X, Martinez OM, et al. Differential expression and functions of microRNAs in liver transplantation and potential use as non-invasive biomarkers. Transpl Immunol 2013;29(1–4):123–9.
160. Hu J, Wang Z, Tan CJ, et al. Plasma microRNA, a potential biomarker for acute rejection after liver transplantation. Transplantation 2013;95(8):991–9.

161. Danger R, Pallier A, Giral M, et al. Upregulation of miR-142-3p in peripheral blood mononuclear cells of operationally tolerant patients with a renal transplant. J Am Soc Nephrol 2012;23(4):597–606.

162. Li Y, Koshiba T, Yoshizawa A, et al. Analyses of peripheral blood mononuclear cells in operational tolerance after pediatric living donor liver transplantation. Am J Transplant 2004;4(12):2118–25.

163. Yagi H, Nomura T, Nakamura K, et al. Crucial role of FOXP3 in the development and function of human CD25+CD4+ regulatory T cells. Int Immunol 2004; 16(11):1643–56.

164. Zhao X, Li Y, Ohe H, et al. Intragraft Vδ1 γδ T cells with a unique T-cell receptor are closely associated with pediatric semiallogeneic liver transplant tolerance. Transplantation 2013;95(1):192–202.

165. Assy N, Adams PC, Myers P, et al. Randomized controlled trial of total immunosuppression withdrawal in liver transplant recipients: role of ursodeoxycholic acid. Transplantation 2007;83(12):1571–6.

166. Tisone G, Orlando G, Angelico M. Operational tolerance in clinical liver transplantation: emerging developments. Transpl Immunol 2007;17(2):108–13.

167. Devlin J, Doherty D, Thomson L, et al. Defining the outcome of immunosuppression withdrawal after liver transplantation. Hepatology 1998;27(4): 926–33.

168. Girlanda R, Rela M, Williams R, et al. Long-term outcome of immunosuppression withdrawal after liver transplantation. Transplant Proc 2005;37(4):1708–9.

169. Girnita A, Mazariegos GV, Castellaneta A, et al. Liver transplant recipients weaned off immunosuppression lack circulating donor-specific antibodies. Hum Immunol 2010;71(3):274–6.

170. Eason JD, Cohen AJ, Nair S, et al. Tolerance: is it worth the risk? Transplantation 2005;79(9):1157–9.

Improving Long-Term Outcomes After Liver Transplantation

Michael R. Charlton, MBBS, FRCP

KEYWORDS

- Liver transplantation • Metabolic syndrome • Immunosuppression • Graft rejection

KEY POINTS

- About two-thirds of deaths after the first year following liver transplantation are unrelated to graft dysfunction.
- Although chronic rejection is an unusual cause of graft loss and mortality, treated acute cellular rejection is associated with attenuated patient and graft survival for patients with hepatitis C virus infection.
- Obesity and components of the metabolic syndrome are important risk factors for many of the most common causes of mortality following liver transplantation.
- The frequency of malignancies is greatly increased among liver transplant recipients, who are at risk of a distinct spectrum of neoplasia.
- Liver transplant recipients should undergo specific screening and management protocols to screen and treat features of the metabolic syndrome and neoplasia.
- Because of the central role of immunosuppression in common causes of morbidity and mortality following liver transplantation, the minimum degree of immunosuppression needed to achieve excellent allograft function should be sought for recipients.

INTRODUCTION

Professor Thomas Starzl performed 5 human liver transplants (LTs) between March and October of 1963. The longest patient survival was 21 days. Shortly after Starzl's initial procedures, surgeons in Boston and Paris made single, failed attempts at LT. In the wake of these poor results, the medical community agreed to a moratorium on LTs that lasted for 3 years. The subsequent evolution of LT from an experimental procedure to a nearly routine operation, limited only by the number of available donor organs, has been one of the most remarkable achievements in medicine. The Scientific Registry of Transplant Recipients reports that more than 60,000 LT recipients are

Disclosure: None.
Department of Medicine, Intermountain Medical Center, 5169 South Cottonwood Street, Murray, UT 84107, USA
E-mail address: michael.charlton@imail.org

Clin Liver Dis 18 (2014) 717–730
http://dx.doi.org/10.1016/j.cld.2014.05.011
1089-3261/14/$ – see front matter © 2014 Elsevier Inc. All rights reserved.

alive with a functioning graft in the United States alone. Currently, overall 3-year patient survival following LT in the United States is 80%, with a 10-year survival rate of approximately 50% (http://www.unos.org). Patient and graft survival rates continue to improve year to year (**Fig. 1**) despite steady increases in the severity of illness (as measured by model for end-stage liver disease [MELD] score) and increasing recipient and donor age at time of transplantation. The sequential improvement in patient and graft survival following LT have been contributed to by many factors. They also have been inversely related to the frequency of steroid-resistant rejection, which now accounts for less than 4% of long-term graft loss.[1] Specific disease etiologies with recurrence of original liver diseases, such as primary sclerosing cholangitis (PSC) and hepatitis C virus (HCV), are the basis of one-third of late posttransplant deaths.[2] As LT recipients live longer, the impact of long-term side effects of highly effective calcineurin inhibitor (CNI)-based immunosuppression has become more important. Understanding graft and nongraft-related causes of long-term mortality is critical to enhancing long-term outcomes.

CAUSES OF DEATH AFTER LT

The most robust data regarding medium and long-term causes of mortality after LT were generated by the National Institute of Diabetes and Digestive and Kidney Diseases prospective multicenter study.[2] Causes of death beyond the first postoperative year were 28% hepatic, 22% malignancy, 11% cardiovascular, 9% infection, and 6% renal failure (**Fig. 2**).[2] Renal-related death increased dramatically over time. Recurrence of hepatitis C is, by far, the most common cause of late hepatic-related mortality. Risk factors for overall mortality beyond the first postoperative year include male gender, age, pretransplant and posttransplant diabetes, posttransplant hypertension, posttransplant renal insufficiency, retransplantation, pretransplant malignancy, and metabolic liver disease. Optimal management of cardiovascular disease, diabetes, hypertension, malignancy, and renal insufficiency are thus all necessary to reduce long-term mortality for LT recipients. Although considerable attention has been given to center-specific variability in 1-year posttransplant survival, there is much greater center-to-center variation in long-term outcomes, for example, 3 years

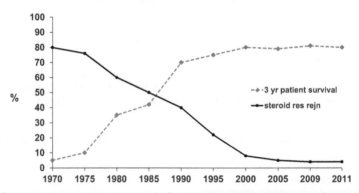

Fig. 1. Changes in 3-year patient survival after LT in the United States are shown. Increased 3-year survival has been mirrored by fall in steroid-resistant rejection, reflecting increasing efficacy of immunosuppression. (*Data from* Scientific Registry of Transplant Recipients. Available at: www.SRTR.org.)

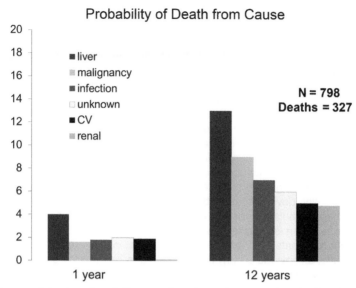

Fig. 2. Causes of death at 1 and 12 years after LT are shown, as described by the NIH Liver Transplant Database Study. Only 4% of late mortality is secondary to chronic rejection. Almost all of the late causes of mortality are contributed to by immunosuppression. CV, cardiovascular disease.

posttransplantation (data source Scientific Registry for Transplant Recipients [SRTR], http://www.srtr.org/). The great majority of variation in long-term outcomes between centers cannot be accounted for recipient or donor-specific parameters, suggesting wide variation and impact of center-specific approaches to the long-term care of LT recipients.

THE IMPACT OF IMMUNOSUPPRESSION AND REJECTION ON OUTCOMES

The development of effective immunosuppressive agents, primarily the advent of CNIs, played a major role in the transformation of posttransplant outcomes. Currently, more than 95% of LT recipients receive immunosuppression with a CNI-based protocol. The decline in the frequency of chronic rejection has closely mirrored the sequential overall improvements in 3-year patient survival (see **Fig. 1**). Contemporary randomized controlled trials of the most widely used immunosuppression combination (tacrolimus and corticosteroids ± mycophenolate) have reported the incidence of treated, biopsy-proven acute cellular rejection (tBPAR) to be 12% to 15% in the first 2 postoperative years.[3,4] The great majority of tBPAR occurs in the first postoperative year (>95%) and the great majority of tBPAR in the first postoperative year occurs in the first 6 postoperative weeks.[3,4,5]

Impact of Acute Cellular Rejection on Overall Patient and Graft Survival Varies with Underlying Liver Disease

The National Institutes of Health (NIH) Liver Transplant Database observed that a single episode of early (first 6 postoperative weeks) tBPAR was associated with superior long-term patient survival when compared with recipients with no episodes of tBPAR ($P = .05$).[5] Graft survival also was superior for patients with a single episode of tBPAR, although the difference was not statistically significant (relative risk [RR] 0.82, $P = .21$). Probably because the highest rates of tBAPR occur among the healthiest recipients (eg, rejection is more common in well-nourished patients with good kidney function), acute rejection was not significantly associated with either patient or graft survival in multivariate analysis, although the RRs were less than 1.0 (patient survival: RR 0.78, $P = .25$; retransplantation-free survival: RR 0.86, $P = .44$). The impact of acute cellular rejection on outcomes appears to vary with etiology of liver disease. In a subsequent analysis of the same cohort of patients (n = 764 adult recipients: 166 HCV-infected and 602 HCV-negative), the NIH Liver Transplant Database study group analyzed the impact of tBPAR according to etiology of liver disease. HCV-infected transplant recipients were seen to experience similar frequencies of acute cellular and steroid-resistant rejection as patients undergoing LT for most other indications. Importantly, the mortality risk was significantly *increased* (RR 2.4; $P = .03$) for HCV-infected transplant recipients who developed early tBPAR compared with HCV-negative transplant recipients. These cumulative observations suggest that, although an episode of early acute cellular rejection is associated with a *lower* risk of mortality among *HCV-negative* transplant recipients, *HCV-infected* transplant recipients are at an *increased* risk for mortality after an episode of early tBPAR. The adverse impact of early acute cellular rejection on patient survival among recipients with HCV infection has been an important consideration in management and development of primary immunosuppression and acute cellular rejection for HCV-infected transplant recipients. The impact, as measured by hazard ratio (HR) for mortality, of events, including acute cellular rejection, is shown in **Fig. 3**. Whether this relationship between tBPAR and mortality for patients with HCV will persist in the era of highly effective antiviral therapy remains to be seen.

The severity of tBPAR is an important factor in long-term patient and graft survival. Patients who experience a severe histologic acute rejection episode have twice the 1-year rate of combined mortality and graft loss as those who experience a mild episode (12% vs 23%).[5]

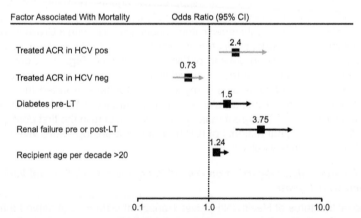

Fig. 3. HRs for causes of mortality associated with rejection (ACR), pretransplantation diabetes, renal failure, and age are shown. The importance of minimizing immunosuppression to avoid renal insufficiency, and diabetes is suggested.

Immunosuppression in Patients with HCV Infection

Corticosteroids

Although treatment of tBPAR has been definitively shown to increase mortality and graft loss in LT recipients with HCV infection, the impact of corticosteroid avoidance and minimization are less clear. By far the best data were generated in a large (n = 312) randomized controlled study, that included a steroid-free arm of immunosuppression. This study, in which steroids were used in modest doses and tapered off in the first postoperative year, found no difference in the rate of recurrence of HCV or in patient or graft survival between steroid-free and steroid-using arms.[6]

Calcineurin inhibitors

The most reliable data concerning the relative impact of cyclosporine and tacrolimus on recurrence of HCV, graft loss, and mortality come from randomized controlled trials and large database analyses. The largest prospective randomized controlled study (n = 495) found no difference in the histologic recurrence rate of hepatitis C at 12 months posttransplantation between patients receiving cyclosporine and tacrolimus.[7] A meta-analysis of studies comparing the 2 CNIs, however, found a patient and graft survival benefit associated with tacrolimus as maintenance immunosuppression (graft loss: HR 0.73, 95% confidence interval [CI] 0.61–0.86).[8] This observation is supported by analyses of the United Network for Organ Sharing (UNOS)/SRTR. In one, risk factors specific for the combined outcomes of death and graft loss among patients with hepatitis C included cyclosporine (increased risk, HR 1.10, CI 0.96–1.27, P = .16), tacrolimus (decreased risk, HR 0.70, CI 0.62–0.79, $P<.0001$), and sirolimus (HR 1.50, CI 1.29–1.74, $P<.0001$).[9] Similar results have been reported in a previous analysis of the SRTR.[10] The lower risk of death and graft loss associated with tacrolimus probably reflects the lower frequency of acute cellular rejection with this agent when compared with cyclosporine. A theoretical case could be made for using tacrolimus as initial (eg, for the first 2 postoperative months) and maintenance immunosuppression for LT recipients, especially those with HCV infection.

Mycophenolate mofetil

Mycophenolate mofetil (MMF) is a potent inosine monophosphate inhibitor (as is ribavirin) that has been shown to have antiviral properties against flaviviruses. Analyses of the UNOS/SRTR database[11] and large randomized controlled trials have found MMF triple therapy is associated with a reduced risk of death (HR 0.77, $P<.001$) and graft loss (HR 0.81, $P<.001$)[11] when compared with MMF-free regimens.

Based on the aggregate of these reports, the impact of MMF on recurrence of HCV appears to be neutral or beneficial to long-term outcomes.

T-cell–depleting therapies

Although the notion of a negative impact of T-cell depletion on posttransplant outcomes in recipients with HCV infection is supported by the potent effect of alemtuzumab (Campath) in exacerbating recurrence of HCV,[12] data concerning the impact of antithymocyte globulin (ATG), an increasingly popular induction agent, are less clear. Outcomes in patients with HCV infection who received induction ATG have been reported to be similar to controls who did not receive ATG, with an analysis of outcomes from 3 centers suggesting that induction with ATG is associated with less-severe fibrosis progression.[13] The interpretability of any of these studies is greatly limited by the lack of protocol biopsies and the use of historical controls.

The results of a prospective randomized study including 93 LT patients suggest that the addition of thymoglobulin to a triple immunosuppressive regimen (tacrolimus, MMF, and steroids) does not modify the incidence of acute rejection episodes or long-term survival and is responsible for increased leukopenia rates.[14] Data from the SRTR suggest a neutral effect of thymoglobulin on patient and graft survival among patients with HCV. Absent data from a large randomized controlled trial, thymoglobulin should probably be used cautiously in LT recipients with HCV infection.

Interleukin-2 receptor inhibition
Large (n = 300) randomized controlled studies of interleukin-2 receptor antibody-based therapy in LT recipients with HCV infection suggest a neutral impact on medium-term outcomes, including allograft histology.[6,15]

Rejection and immunosuppression-related morbidity and mortality in other etiologies of liver disease
The most common causes of death at more than 1 year among LT recipients are 28% hepatic (eg, recurrence of HCV), 22% malignancy, 11% cardiovascular, 9% infection, and 6% renal failure. Renal-related deaths, which are strongly contributed to use of CNIs, increase dramatically over time. Renal failure is *the strongest predictor of late post-LT mortality*. Other important risk factors for death at more than 1 year include post-LT diabetes and hypertension. Each of these predictors of post-LT mortality are associated with immunosuppression. Thus, although acute and chronic rejection may be relatively minor causes of long-term morbidity and mortality, the immunosuppression used to attenuate the impact of rejection has a clear cost. Diligent management of modifiable post-LT factors, including immunosuppression-associated diabetes, hypertension, and renal failure may impact long-term mortality.

Obesity, insulin resistance, and/or diabetes are common metabolic complications in LT recipients and are implicated in increased morbidity and mortality during long-term follow-up.[2] Obesity is generally associated with multiple acquired factors predisposing to insulin resistance, including factors that are associated with LT; for example, sedentary lifestyle, medications (eg, corticosteroids, cyclosporine, tacrolimus, and sirolimus), and hepatic denervation. In addition to the metabolic effects of obesity, LT alters circulating levels of leptin (increased) and adiponectin (decreased), changes that may further contribute to posttransplant obesity and metabolic syndrome (MS). Tumor necrosis factor (alpha), which down-regulates insulin-induced phosphorylation of insulin-receptor substrate-1 and reduces the expression of the insulin-dependent glucose-transport molecule Glut 4, also may be involved in posttransplant insulin resistance.

Corticosteroids decrease beta-cell insulin production in a dose-dependent manner, increase gluconeogenesis, and decrease peripheral glucose utilization.[16] CNIs (cyclosporine and tacrolimus) decrease both insulin synthesis and secretion (pancreatic beta-cell toxicity).[17] Mammalian target of rapamycin (mTOR) inhibitors may block B-cell proliferation, theoretically increasing the risk for diabetes, but mTOR inhibitors also may be insulin sensitizing through their effect on stimulation of GLUT-4.[18] Thus, the effect of sirolimus on posttransplant insulin sensitivity is evolving.

Increased oxidative stress is a hallmark of nonalcoholic steatohepatitis (NASH) with subsequent mitochondrial dysfunction playing an important role in NASH physiology. Almost all LT recipients are maintained on either cyclosporine or tacrolimus, both of which are associated with resultant increased generation of reactive oxygen species, mitochondrial dysfunction, and lipid peroxidation. This may have important implications for the development of insulin resistance and recurrence of NASH after LT.

Whether CNI dosing should be minimized in patients with recurrence of MS and/or NASH is not known, but there exists a reasonable rationale for such an approach.

POSTTRANSPLANT MS AND LONG-TERM MORTALITY AND GRAFT LOSS

The decline in chronic rejection as a cause of long-term mortality after LT has occurred simultaneously with a rise in the impact of posttransplant MS. MS, as defined by the criteria of the National Cholesterol Education Program Adult Treatment Panel III, is a constellation of physiologic consequences of obesity, including increased abdominal girth, hypertension, hyperglycemia, and dyslipidemia. The MS is an important factor for nearly all of the major causes of long-term posttransplant mortality, including cardiovascular disease, renal insufficiency, and neoplasia. Enhancing posttransplant outcomes requires minimizing the impact of posttransplant MS.

The prevalence of MS varies with the etiology of liver disease. Patients with cryptogenic cirrhosis, for example, have a higher reported prevalence of MS (29%) than patients with other etiologies of liver disease (~6%).[19] The lower pretransplant prevalence of MS almost certainly relates, at least in part, to the low systemic vascular resistance with associated systemic hypotension that is a hallmark of portal hypertension, combined with the low lipid levels (with the exception of primary biliary cirrhosis) associated with chronic liver disease and cirrhosis, reducing the frequency of criteria for MS in patients with cirrhosis. As portal hypertension resolves, the prevalence of features of MS increases after LT, with the absolute prevalence of diabetes rising from approximately 15% to more than 30% after transplantation, hypertension rising from approximately 15% to more than 60% after transplantation and hyperlipidemia occurring in more than 50% of LT recipients.[4] Overall, MS is present in approximately 50% of patients after transplantation and is associated with increased cardiovascular and cerebrovascular events.[20]

COMPONENTS OF MS POST-LT
Obesity

Obesity is the physiologic engine of MS. The global increase in the prevalence of obesity has been mirrored by patients undergoing LT. More than a third of patients with end-stage liver disease are obese.[21,22] Between 1990 and 2012, the proportion of LT recipients classified as obese increased from 15% in the early 1990s to just more than 25% since 2002, and 27% in 2012, with an increase in average recipient weight of approximately 1 kg per year.[23] With few exceptions, patients who are overweight or obese before transplantation will remain overweight or obese after, with approximately one-third of patients of normal weight at the time of transplantation becoming obese after transplantation.[23] The potential impact of posttransplant weight gain includes increased risk of diabetes and MS and associated complications, including cardiovascular disease, renal disease, and NASH in the allograft. As in the nontransplant setting, sustained weight reduction is difficult to achieve posttransplantation. The comparative effectiveness of a multidisciplinary protocol for obese patients requiring LT, including a noninvasive pretransplant weight loss program, with and without a combined LT plus sleeve gastrectomy for obese patients who failed to lose weight before LT, has recently been described.[24] In 37 patients who received LT alone, weight gain to body mass index (BMI) greater than 35, posttransplant diabetes, hepatic, deaths, and grafts loss were all less frequent among the 7 patients undergoing the combined LT/sleeve gastrectomy procedure. Although the role of bariatric surgery continues to evolve during and after LT, these preliminary results suggest that combined LT plus sleeve gastrectomy might be considered in selected patients with persistent pretransplant obesity and MS.

Posttransplant Pharmacotherapy of Obesity

The impact of the 2 newly approved therapies for obesity, lorcaserin (a selective 5-HT2C agonist) and phenteramine/topiramate extended-release, have not been reported in the LT population. Because lorcaserin (Belviq) is metabolized by multiple pathways and multiple enzymes, immunosuppressive agents are predicted to have minimal impact on lorcaserin exposure and vice versa. In addition, lorcaserin does not require dose adjusting in mild to moderate renal insufficiency or hepatic impairment, both of which are common following LT. Lorcaserin would appear to have a superior safety profile to phenteramine/topiramate. Ezetimide, an agent that inhibits the enterohepatic recirculation of lipids and has minimal cytochrome P450 metabolism, has been shown to be well tolerated and effective when used in combination with statin drugs in a small retrospective study of LT patients.[25] There is a theoretical concern of hepatotoxicity with ezetimide, particularly when used with statins; thus, caution should be exercised until more data are available in LT recipients. Tetrahydrolipstatin (Orlistat), a reversible inhibitor of pancreatic lipase, has been investigated in the posttransplant setting and appears to be of limited efficacy and may interfere with immunosuppression absorption.[26] Bariatric surgery before transplantation is a difficult proposition in patients with portal hypertension, but may be an option in carefully selected patients.

Diabetes

Glucose intolerance is common in cirrhosis, largely due to peripheral insulin resistance. Although a small minority of patients will experience improved insulin sensitivity after LT, more will either remain diabetic or develop new-onset diabetes (NOD) after LT, with about a third of LT recipients developing diabetes.[27] Most NOD (80%) develops within 1 month of transplantation.[27] Diabetes significantly affects posttransplant outcomes, particularly in patients with hepatitis C who receive a transplant.[28,29] The 5-year occurrence of advanced fibrosis is increased in patients treated for diabetes mellitus (49%) when compared with patients with normal insulin sensitivity (20%) ($P = .01$). Posttransplant diabetes mellitus also is significantly associated with late-onset hepatic artery thrombosis, and acute and chronic rejection.[28] Overall patient morbidity and mortality are greater in patients with both pretransplantation and post-transplantation diabetes, even when posttransplantation diabetes is transient.[29]

Pretransplantation diabetes, elevated BMI, hepatitis C infection (HR 2.5, $P = .001$), and methylprednisolone boluses (HR 1.09 per bolus, $P = .02$) are independent risk factors for the development of NOD.[30] The transplanted liver itself may contribute to the increase in insulin resistance, as denervation/vagotomy of the liver during LT has been associated with increased insulin resistance. Posttransplantation immunosuppression typically impairs insulin sensitivity. As discussed earlier, corticosteroids induce insulin resistance in a dose-dependent manner by decreased beta-cell insulin production, increased gluconeogenesis, and decreased peripheral glucose utilization.[17] CNIs (cyclosporine and tacrolimus) both decrease insulin synthesis and secretion (pancreatic beta-cell toxicity) and induce insulin resistance and hyperinsulinemia.[18] Sirolimus, an mTOR inhibitor, blocks B-cell proliferation, theoretically increasing the risk for diabetes, but also increases GLUT-4 signaling in insulin-responsive cells.[31] The net effect of the mTOR inhibitors everolimus and sirolimus on posttransplant diabetes is not known.

In the nontransplant population, target glycosylated hemoglobin is less than 7%, fasting blood sugar is 70 to 130 mg/dL (3.9–7.2 mmol/L), and peak postprandial glucose is less than 180 mg/dL (10 mmol/L) in diabetic patients. Treatment of early posttransplant diabetes is largely with insulin. As steroids are tapered, lifestyle modifications (diet and physical exercise) should be encouraged and conversion to an oral hypoglycemic agent considered. Most oral hypoglycemic agents have not been formally studied in the posttransplant setting. In the nontransplant setting, weight gain and hypoglycemia are less common with biguanides (metformin) than sulfonylureas or thiazolidinediones. Metformin should be avoided in the setting of renal failure, which is common among LT recipients, because of the increased risk of lactic acidosis. Annual retinal examinations, urinary protein screening, and foot care should be encouraged for LT recipients with diabetes.

Dyslipidemia

Dyslipidemia affects approximately two-thirds of LT recipients[32] and is a major risk factor for posttransplant cardiovascular-related morbidity and mortality.[33] Although tacrolimus may be associated with less severe and lower frequencies of dyslipidemia than cyclosporine, both agents are associated with hyperlipidemia.[34] Sirolimus and everolimus are potent hyperlipidemic agents,[35,36] possibly by affecting the insulin signaling pathway, increasing adipose tissue lipase activity, and decreasing lipoprotein lipase activity. The basis of the relatively dyslipidemic effects of cyclosporine are not known but may involve inhibition of hepatic bile acid 26-hydroxylase, decreasing bile acid synthesis from cholesterol and reducing the subsequent transport of cholesterol into bile and the intestine. Cyclosporine binds to the low-density lipoprotein (LDL)-cholesterol receptor, increasing circulating levels of LDL-cholesterol. Tacrolimus appears less likely to cause hypercholesterolemia than cyclosporine, with conversion of recipients to tacrolimus from cyclosporine for persistent hypercholesterolemia having efficacy in the management of posttransplant dyslipidemia.[37] Posttransplant dyslipidemia is generally resistant to dietary interventions. CNI dosing should probably be minimized in patients with posttransplant MS and dyslipidemia. Corticosteroids are known to produce insulin resistance, truncal fat deposition, hypertension, and dyslipidemia. Only a small minority of patients require maintenance corticosteroids, which typically can be discontinued before the end of the first postoperative year. Pharmacotherapy should be considered in patients with persistent hyperlipidemia. HMG CoA inhibitors (statins), which are well tolerated in solid organ recipients,[38] are an appropriate first-line agent for recipients with both elevations in cholesterol and triglycerides. Statins have been used commonly in solid organ transplant recipients for decades and are well tolerated. Pravastatin is the most studied in transplant recipients and has the theoretical advantage metabolism, in that its metabolism does not require the P450 enzyme system. Other statins (atorvastatin, simvastatin, lovastatin, cerivastatin, and fluvastatin) also are used frequently in transplant patients. A small reduction in cyclosporine and tacrolimus levels during statin therapy has been reported. Simvastatin (40 mg/d), atorvastatin (40 mg/d), or pravastatin (20 mg/d) are reasonable starting doses for posttransplant hypercholesterolemia, in combination with a controlled diet (eg, a Mediterranean diet rich in omega-3 fatty acids, fruits, vegetables, and dietary fiber).

Isolated hypertriglyceridemia also is common following LT and may respond to fish oil (omega-3), which has an excellent safety profile and minimal drug interactions.[39] A starting dosage of 1000 mg twice a day, increasing to a total of 4000 mg daily in divided dosing is reasonable. Fish oil does not affect cyclosporine (a highly lipophilic agent) or tacrolimus levels significantly.[40] Doses higher than 4000 mg can have antiplatelet effects and increased risk of bleeding. Some patients may experience an increase in LDL levels with fish oil. Alternative agents for patients with hypertriglyceridemia include the fibric acid derivatives (gemfibrozil, clofibrate, fenofibrate), which are generally well tolerated but have occasionally been associated with myositis, particularly if used with statins. Fibrates are highly protein bound and cytochrome P450 metabolized with some evidence of a mild effect of increasing CNI levels.[40]

Ezetimide, an agent that inhibits the enterohepatic recirculation of lipids and has minimal cytochrome P450 metabolism, has been shown to be well tolerated and effective when used in combination with statin drugs in a small retrospective study of LT patients.[25] There is a theoretical concern about hepatotoxicity with ezetimide, particularly when used with statins, thus caution should be exercised until more data are available in LT recipients.

Hypertension

Hypertension is unusual before transplantation but occurs in approximately 70% of LT recipients.[20] Steroids contribute to posttransplant hypertension through mineralocorticoid effects and by increasing sustained virologic response and cardiac contractility. Sirolimus increases the risk of hypertension when added to CNIs.[41] CNIs are a major cause of posttransplant hypertension, largely related to renal (and systemic) vasoconstriction, as well as impaired glomerular filtration rate and sodium excretion. Because of the contribution of renal arteriolar vasoconstriction to posttransplant hypertension, calcium channel blockers (amlodipine, isradipine, and felodipine) are excellent first-line agents. Nifedipine is an inhibitor of intestinal cytochrome P450, predictably increasing CNI levels with potential for CNI toxicity, and may cause leg edema. Second-line therapies include specific beta blockers (nonspecific beta blockers may reduce portal blood flow), angiotensin-converting enzyme (ACE) inhibitors, angiotensin receptor blockers, and loop diuretics. ACE inhibitors and angiotensin receptor blockers may exacerbate CNI-induced hyperkalemia, but also may protect against calcineurin-induced renal injury.[42] Thiazides and other diuretics should be used with caution in transplant recipients due to potentiation of electrolyte abnormalities and a mechanism of action that is relatively removed from the physiology of posttransplant hypertension. Up to 30% of LT recipients require 2 or more antihypertensives to achieve blood pressure goals.

Cardiovascular Disease

Cardiovascular disease is a leading cause of morbidity and mortality in LT patients. About a quarter of LT recipients have underlying coronary artery disease.[43] The 10-year probability of a coronary event is higher in LT recipients (11%) than the general population (7%).[44] The RR of ischemic cardiac events is approximately threefold greater in LT recipients when compared with the age-matched and sex-matched general population.[45] Minimization of cardiovascular events after LT revolves around effective pretransplant screening (eg, with stress echocardiography and serum troponin levels[32]) and management of the components of the MS.

MALIGNANCY

The probability of LT recipients developing de novo malignancy at 1, 5, and 10 years posttransplantation is 4%, 12%, and 22%, respectively (**Fig. 4**).[46] This is about twice the risk for matched nontransplant patients. About half of posttransplant malignancies are skin cancers. The probability of developing nonskin malignancy is significantly higher in patients with PSC (22% at 10 years) or alcohol-related liver disease

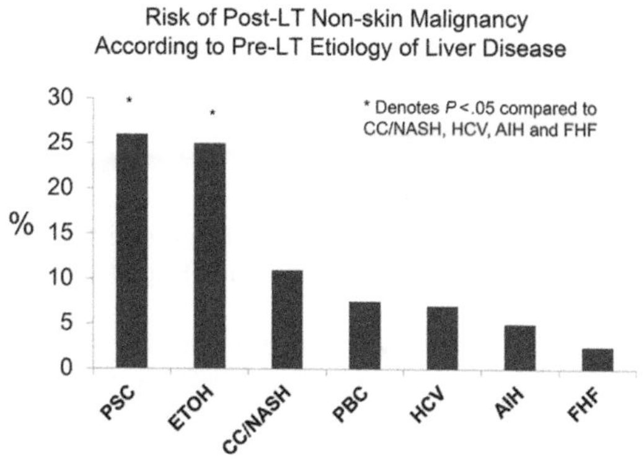

Risk of Post-LT Non-skin Malignancy
According to Pre-LT Etiology of Liver Disease

Fig. 4. Variation in risk of nonskin malignancy with original liver disease is shown, as observed by the NIH Liver Transplant Database Study. Patients with PSC and alcoholic liver disease (ETOH) have significantly greater risk. AIH, autoimmune hepatitis; CC/NASH, cryptogenic/nonalcoholic steatohepatitis; FHF, fulminant hepatic failure; PBC, primary biliary cirrhosis.

(ETOH; 18% at 10 years), when compared with all other diagnoses (10% probability) (see **Fig. 3**). In multivariate analyses, increased age by decade (HR 1.33, $P = .01$) and a history of smoking (HR 1.6, $P = .046$) are associated with increased risk for development of solid malignancies after LT. The development of hematologic and solid organ malignancies greatly affects survival, with probabilities of death after diagnosis of approximately 40% at 1 year. The increased risk for malignancies among LT recipients is multifactorial, with important attributable risks, including exposure to chronic immunosuppression, concomitant viral infection (eg, Epstein-Barr), and sun exposure. Much of the increased risk for skin and nonskin malignancies in LT recipients is on the basis of immunosuppression, with good evidence that reducing immunosuppression reduces risk of malignancy.[47] A summary of recommendations for cancer screening adapted to LT in solid organ recipients is provided in **Table 1**.

Table 1
Interpretive summary of American Society of Transplantation and US Preventive Services Task Force Recommendations for cancer screening in LT recipients

Cancer Type	Recommendation
Breast	Women 50 to 74 y of age: biennial screening; other ages: screening left to the physician and patient
Skin	Monthly self-examination; physician examination annually.
Cervical	Screening for cervical cancer in women ages 21 to 65 y with cytology (Pap smear) every 3 y or, for women ages 30 to 65 y who want to lengthen the screening interval, screening with a combination of cytology and human papillomavirus testing every 5 y
Anogenital	Yearly physical examination of the anogenital area, including pelvic examination and cytological studies for women.
Prostate	Consider annual screening for men $\geq$50 y. If positive family history or African American race, may start annual screening earlier.
Colorectal	Age 50–75: annual fecal occult blood test (FOBT) and colonoscopy every 10 y (or flexible FOBT every 3 y with sigmoidoscopy every 5 y).
Lung	Annual chest radiograph if history of smoking.
Hepatocellular carcinoma	For patients with cirrhosis or active hepatitis C virus or hepatitis B virus infection, serum alpha-fetoprotein and liver ultrasound every 6–12 mo.

Because of the unequivocal role of immunosuppression in posttransplant malignancy risk and MS, consideration should be given to determining the minimal amount of immunosuppression required to maintain excellent graft function.

REFERENCES

1. Adam R, McMaster P, O'Grady JG, et al. Evolution of liver transplantation in Europe: report of the European Liver Transplant Registry. Liver Transpl 2003;9: 1231–43.
2. Watt KD, Pedersen RA, Kremers WK, et al. Evolution of causes and risk factors for mortality post-liver transplant: results of the NIDDK long-term follow-up study. Am J Transplant 2010;10:1420–7.
3. Neuberger JM, Mamelok RD, Neuhaus P, et al. Delayed introduction of reduced-dose tacrolimus, and renal function in liver transplantation: the 'ReSpECT' study. Am J Transplant 2009;9:327–36.
4. De Simone P, Nevens F, De Carlis L, et al. Everolimus with reduced tacrolimus improves renal function in de novo liver transplant recipients: a randomized controlled trial. Am J Transplant 2012;12:3008–20.
5. Wiesner RH, Demetris AJ, Belle S, et al. Acute hepatic allograft rejection: incidence, risk factors and impact on outcome. Hepatology 1998;28:638–45.
6. Klintmalm GB, Davis GL, Teperman L, et al. A randomized, multicenter study comparing steroid-free immunosuppression and standard immunosuppression for liver transplant recipients with chronic hepatitis C. Liver Transpl 2011;17: 1394–403.
7. Levy G, Grazi GL, Sanjuan F, et al. 12-month follow-up analysis of a multicenter, randomized, prospective trial in de novo liver transplant recipients (LIS2T) comparing cyclosporine microemulsion (C2 monitoring) and tacrolimus. Liver Transpl 2006;12:1464–72.
8. McAlister VC, Haddad E, Renouf E, et al. Cyclosporin versus tacrolimus as primary immunosuppressant after liver transplantation: a meta-analysis. Am J Transplant 2006;6:1578–85.
9. Watt KD, Dierkhising R, Heimbach JK, et al. Impact of sirolimus and tacrolimus on mortality and graft loss in liver transplant recipients with or without hepatitis C virus: an analysis of the Scientific Registry of Transplant Recipients Database. Liver Transpl 2012;18:1029–36.
10. Irish W, Arcona S, Bowers D, et al. Cyclosporine versus tacrolimus treated liver transplant recipients with chronic hepatitis C: outcomes analysis of the UNOS/OPTN database. Am J Transplant 2011;11(8):1676–85.
11. Wiesner RH, Shorr JS, Steffen BJ, et al. Mycophenolate mofetil combination therapy improves long-term outcomes after liver transplantation in patients with and without hepatitis C. Liver Transpl 2005;11:750–9.
12. Marcos A, Eghtesad B, Fung JJ, et al. Use of alemtuzumab and tacrolimus monotherapy for cadaveric liver transplantation: with particular reference to hepatitis C virus. Transplantation 2004;78:966–71.
13. Belli LS, Burroughs AK, Burra P, et al. Liver transplantation for HCV cirrhosis: improved survival in recent years and increased severity of recurrent disease in female recipients: results of a long term retrospective study. Liver Transpl 2007;13:733–40.
14. Stevens RL, Fluharty AL, Killgrove AR, et al. Arylsulfatase of human tissue. Studies on a form of arylsulfatase B found predominantly in brain. Biochim Biophys Acta 1977;481:549–60.

15. Filipponi F, Salizzoni M, Grazi G, et al. Study of simulect-based, steroid-free immunosuppressive regimen in HCV+ de novo liver transplant patients: preliminary results. Transplant Proc 2001;33:3211–2.

16. Schacke H, Docke WD, Asadullah K. Mechanisms involved in the side effects of glucocorticoids. Pharmacology Therapeutics 2002;96:23–43.

17. Ozbay LA, Moller N, Juhl C, et al. Calcineurin inhibitors acutely improve insulin sensitivity without affecting insulin secretion in healthy human volunteers. Br J Clin Pharmacol 2011;73:536–45.

18. Newgard CB, An J, Bain JR, et al. A branched-chain amino acid-related metabolic signature that differentiates obese and lean humans and contributes to insulin resistance. Cell Metab 2009;9:311–26.

19. Tellez-Avila F, Sanchez-Avila F, García-Saenz-de-Sicilia M, et al. Prevalence of metabolic syndrome, obesity and diabetes type 2 in cryptogenic cirrhosis. World J Gastroenterol 2008;14:4771–5.

20. Laryea M, Watt KD, Molinari M, et al. Metabolic syndrome in liver transplant recipients: prevalence and association with cardiovascular events. Liver Transpl 2007; 13:1109–14.

21. Bianchi G, Marchesini G, Marzocchi R, et al. Metabolic syndrome in liver transplantation: relation to etiology and immunosuppression. Liver Transpl 2008;4: 1648–54.

22. Poonawala A, Nair S, Thuluvath P. Prevalence of obesity and diabetes in patients with cryptogenic cirrhosis: a case-control study. Hepatology 2000;32:689–92.

23. Everhart JE, Lombardero M, Lake JR, et al. Weight change and obesity after liver transplantation: incidence and risk factors. Liver Transpl Surgery 1998;4: 285–96.

24. Heimbach JK, Watt KD, Poterucha J, et al. Combined liver transplantation and gastric sleeve resection for patients with medically complicated obesity and end-stage liver disease. Am J Transplant 2013;13(2):363–8.

25. Almutairi F, Peterson T, Molinari M, et al. Safety and effectiveness of ezetimibe in liver transplant recipients with hypercholesterolemia. Liver Transpl 2009;15: 504–8.

26. Cassiman D, Roelants M, Vandenplas G, et al. Orlistat treatment is safe in overweight and obese liver transplant recipients: a prospective, open label trial. Transpl Int 2006;19:1000–5.

27. Moon J, Barbeito R, Faradji R, et al. Negative impact of new-onset diabetes mellitus on patient and graft survival after liver transplantation: long-term follow up. Transplantation 2006;82:1625–8.

28. John P, Thuluvath P. Outcome of patients with new-onset diabetes mellitus after liver transplantation compared with those without diabetes mellitus. Liver Transpl 2002;8:708–13.

29. Baid S, Cosimi A, Farrell M, et al. Posttransplant diabetes mellitus in liver transplant recipients: risk factors, temporal relationship with hepatitis C virus allograft hepatitis, and impact on mortality. Transplantation 2001;72:1066–72.

30. Vodenik B, Rovira J, Campistol JM. Mammalian target of rapamycin and diabetes: what does the current evidence tell us? Transplant Proc 2009;41:S31–8.

31. Gisbert C, Prieto M, Berenguer M, et al. Hyperlipidemia in liver transplant recipients: prevalence and risk factors [see comments]. Liver Transpl Surg 1997;3: 416–22.

32. Watt KD, Coss E, Pedersen RA, et al. Pretransplant serum troponin levels are highly predictive of patient and graft survival following liver transplantation. Liver Transpl 2010;16:990–8.

33. Canzanello VJ, Schwartz L, Taler SJ, et al. Evolution of cardiovascular risk after liver transplantation: a comparison of cyclosporine A and tacrolimus (FK506). Liver Transpl Surg 1997;3:1–9.

34. Sanchez EQ, Martin AP, Ikegami T, et al. Sirolimus conversion after liver transplantation: improvement in measured glomerular filtration rate after 2 years. Transplant Proc 2005;37:4416–23.

35. Saliba F, De Simone P, Nevens F, et al. Renal function at two years in liver transplant patients receiving everolimus: results of a randomized, multicenter study. Am J Transplant 2013;13(7):1734–45.

36. Roy A, Kneteman N, Lilly L, et al. Tacrolimus as intervention in the treatment of hyperlipidemia after liver transplant. Transplantation 2006;82:494–500.

37. Martin J, Cavanaugh T, Trumbull L, et al. Incidence of adverse events with HMG-CoA reductase inhibitors in liver transplant patients. Clin Transplant 2008;22:113–9.

38. McKenney J, Sica D. Role of prescription omega-3 fatty acids in the treatment of hypertriglyceridemia. Pharmacotherapy 2007;27:715–28.

39. Asberg A. Interactions between cyclosporin and lipid-lowering drugs: implications for organ transplant recipients. Drugs 2003;63:367–78.

40. Gonwa T, Mendez R, Yang H, et al. Randomized trial of tacrolimus in combination with sirolimus or mycophenolate mofetil in kidney transplantation: results at 6 months. Transplantation 2003;75:1213–20.

41. Lubel J, Herath C, Burrell L, et al. Liver disease and the renin-angiotensin system: recent discoveries and clinical implications. J Gastroenterol Hepatol 2008;23:1327–38.

42. Tiukinhoy-Laing SD, Rossi JS, Bayram M, et al. Cardiac hemodynamic and coronary angiographic characteristics of patients being evaluated for liver transplantation. Am J Cardiol 2006;98:178–81.

43. Neal D, Tom B, Luan J, et al. Is there disparity between risk and incidence of cardiovascular disease after liver transplant? Transplantation 2004;77:93–9.

44. Johnston S, Morris J, Cramb R, et al. Cardiovascular morbidity and mortality after orthotopic liver transplantation. Transplantation 2002;73:901–6.

45. Watt KD, Pedersen RA, Kremers WK, et al. Long-term probability of and mortality from de novo malignancy after liver transplantation. Gastroenterology 2009;137:2010–7.

46. Dantal J, Hourmant M, Cantarovich D, et al. Effect of long-term immunosuppression in kidney-graft recipients on cancer incidence: randomised comparison of two cyclosporin regimens. Lancet 1998;351:623–8.

47. Kasiske BL, Vazquez MA, Harmon WE, et al. Recommendations for the outpatient surveillance of renal transplant recipients. American Society of Transplantation. J Am Soc Nephrol 2000;11(Suppl 15):S1–86.

Hepatic Retransplant
What Have We Learned?

William H. Kitchens, MD, PhD[a], Heidi Yeh, MD[b], James F. Markmann, MD, PhD[b],*

KEYWORDS

- Liver transplant • Retransplant • Risk prediction models • Hepatitis C virus
- MELD scores

KEY POINTS

- Hepatic retransplant accounts for 5% to 15% of liver transplants in most series.
- Liver retransplants are associated with significantly increased hospital costs and inferior patient survival when compared with primary liver transplants.
- The indications for hepatic retransplant vary depending on the time interval between prior transplant and retransplant. Early retransplants (within the first few days or weeks) are usually due to primary graft nonfunction (PNF) or vascular thrombosis, whereas later retransplants are most commonly necessitated by chronic rejection or recurrent primary liver disease.
- A variety of recipient and donor characteristics predict poor survival after hepatic retransplant, including history of multiple prior liver transplants, need for retransplant 7 to 30 days after prior transplant, high Model for End-stage Liver Disease (MELD) score at the time of retransplant, need for preoperative mechanical ventilation, cold ischemia times greater than 12 hours, advanced donor age, and use of split liver grafts or grafts from donors after cardiac death.
- Several risk prediction models have been developed to characterize high-risk candidates for hepatic retransplant, allowing futile retransplants to be avoided. Better stratification of retransplant candidates has improved the outcomes of retransplant in the contemporary era.

Advances in surgical technique, immunosuppression, and perioperative care have significantly improved the outcomes of liver transplantation over the past 30 years, offering new hope to patients with end-stage liver disease. These clinical innovations have underpinned a dramatic prolongation in graft survival. Indeed, the most recent

Conflicts of interest: the authors disclose no conflicts.
Funding: the authors disclose no funding.
[a] Department of Surgery, Massachusetts General Hospital, 55 Fruit Street, Boston, MA 02114, USA; [b] Division of Transplantation, Department of Surgery, Massachusetts General Hospital, 55 Fruit Street, Boston, MA 02114, USA
* Corresponding author. Massachusetts General Hospital, White 517A, 55 Fruit Street, Boston, MA 02114.
E-mail address: jmarkmann@partners.org

Clin Liver Dis 18 (2014) 731–751
http://dx.doi.org/10.1016/j.cld.2014.05.010
1089-3261/14/$ – see front matter © 2014 Elsevier Inc. All rights reserved.

liver.theclinics.com

Organ Procurement and Transplantation Network (OPTN) annual report indicated that at the end of 2011, only 2.8% of patients on the liver transplant waiting list had undergone a prior liver transplant and only 6.2% of the actual transplants performed in 2011 were retransplants, a significant decline from the 1980s when retransplants comprised up to one-third of liver transplants.[1–3] For the patients whose grafts do fail, however, retransplant remains the only life-saving option.

Hepatic retransplant remains a formidable technical challenge, and it also raises critical ethical concerns given the current organ shortage. At present, 1 of every 12 donor livers is allocated for a hepatic retransplant, underscoring the role played by retransplant in exacerbating donor organ scarcity.[4] It is well-documented that the outcomes of hepatic retransplant are inferior to those of primary liver transplant (**Fig. 1**).[5–12] For example, in a large series of liver retransplants from University of California Los Angeles (UCLA), the 1-, 5-, and 10-year patient survival rates for liver retransplant recipients (62%, 47%, and 45%, respectively) were significantly worse than those of primary liver transplant recipients (83%, 74%, and 68%, respectively).[7] In addition, hepatic retransplant often consumes far more health care resources than primary liver transplant.[7,13] Indeed, one series demonstrated that hepatic retransplants were associated with almost double the inpatient hospital stay and over twice the immediate hospital cost ($122,358 vs $289,302) when compared with primary liver transplants.[11]

Given the inferior outcomes of hepatic retransplants, some clinicians and ethicists have argued that hepatic retransplant should be abandoned. Back in the early 1990s, for example, Powelson and colleagues[14] used an elegant model of hepatic retransplants in the New England organ procurement region. Given the relatively poor 1-year survival rates of retransplants in their series (48%) compared with the survival rates of primary liver transplants (70%), the investigators found that permitting hepatic retransplant improved the predicted 1-year survival of liver transplant recipients, but at the cost of decreasing the overall survival of patients on the liver transplant waiting list, because organs allocated for repeat transplants obviously deny the opportunity of primary transplant for someone else on the waiting list.

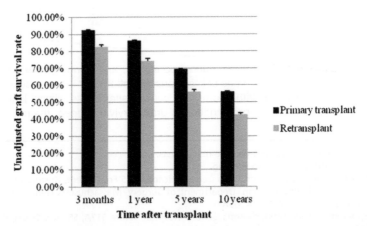

Fig. 1. Hepatic retransplant has inferior graft survival compared with initial primary liver transplants. Error bars show standard error. (*Adapted from* Organ Procurement and Transplantation Network (OPTN) and Scientific Registry of Transplant Recipients (SRTR). OPTN/SRTR 2010 Annual Data Report. Rockville (MD): Department of Health and Human Services HRSA, Healthcare Systems Bureau, Division of Transplantation; 2011.)

Although this article makes a persuasive case for restricting hepatic retransplant, it must be noted that this analysis preceded the adoption of the MELD system of organ allocation and that it also does not take into account changes in physician behavior that might result from a blanket policy of denying retransplant. A refusal to permit retransplant would provide perverse incentives for transplant surgeons to accept only the most ideal hepatic grafts and restrict them for the least sick patients. This incentive would undermine current efforts to transplant more patients through the use of marginal grafts, because there would no longer be the option of replacing grafts with primary nonfunction, vascular and nonanastomotic biliary complications, or recurrent disease. A moratorium on hepatic retransplant, therefore, could paradoxically decrease patient access to liver transplant.

Yet, although a blanket policy may be unwise, some hepatic retransplant candidates are likely so sick that any new hepatic transplant would almost certainly fail. Indeed, up to 75% of deaths after hepatic retransplant over the course of some case series occur within the first 6 months of retransplant[15,16]; many of these early deaths likely occurred in patients who were poor candidates for retransplant in the first place. It is critical to find a means to identify those patients for whom retransplant is likely futile, because performing transplant in these patients would only serve to deny the procedure to other patients on the waiting list, with no real benefit to the retransplant candidate. Identification of those patients in whom liver retransplant is futile requires a thorough understanding of the causes and epidemiology of hepatic graft failure.

WHY DO LIVER TRANSPLANTS FAIL?

Patients require hepatic retransplant for a multitude of different clinical indications. These causes of prior allograft failure tend to vary markedly depending on how soon after this prior transplant another liver is required. Broadly speaking, one can consider indications for retransplant that manifest in the early postoperative period (typically, within the first month), and then consider the late indications for retransplant (**Table 1**). The vast majority of early retransplants are due either to PNF of the first graft or to vascular complication (usually hepatic artery or portal vein thrombosis).[17] One recent review found that PNF and vascular thrombosis accounted for 40% and 19%, respectively, of hepatic graft failure requiring retransplant and that approximately 80% of the patients requiring new livers for these indications underwent retransplant within 7 months of their last transplant.[18]

Increasing reliance on marginal grafts over the past 2 decades has increased the rates of PNF in many transplant series. The development of PNF can be attributed to multiple causes, including issues with the donor graft (ie, steatosis, grafts from donors >50 years of age, and use of split livers), recipient variables (ie, preoperative renal failure), and perioperative factors (cold ischemic time >12 hours, prolonged warm ischemic time).[19,20] The other major driver of early hepatic retransplant is early hepatic artery thrombosis (HAT), which is a devastating technical complication of liver transplant. Early HAT occurs in approximately 2.9% of adult liver transplants and up to 8.3% of pediatric transplants, and it is associated with an almost 33% mortality rate.[21] Although some patients have a favorable clinical course with either close observation or attempted revascularization, almost 50% ultimately proceed to hepatic retransplant.[21]

Acute rejection is another indication for retransplant, which typically happens relatively early, although the incidence of acute rejection causing graft loss has grown vanishingly rare in the modern era of tacrolimus-based immunosuppression. For

Table 1
Early versus late indications for hepatic retransplant

Cause of Graft Failure	Time from Primary Transplant to Retransplant			
	0–14 d	15–222 d	223–1307 d	>1308 d
Primary graft nonfunction (%)	64.1	21.1	10.1	8.9
Hepatic artery/portal vein thrombosis (%)	27.8	32.9	11.5	5.3
Biliary tract complication (%)	1.4	14.7	14.7	5.3
De novo hepatitis (%)	0	0.1	0.1	1.0
Recurrent hepatitis (%)	0.5	5.3	5.3	20.2
Recurrent disease (%)	0.1	1.2	1.2	17.6
Acute rejection (%)	4.1	6.9	6.9	2.2
Chronic rejection (%)	0.1	3.5	3.5	20.6
Infection (%)	1.5	8.6	8.6	2.5
Patient noncompliance (%)	0	0	0	0.6
Unknown (%)	12.4	27.4	27.4	37.0

Primary graft nonfunction and vascular complications account for the overwhelming majority of early hepatic retransplants, whereas chronic rejection and recurrent primary liver disease dominate as the interval between primary transplant and retransplant lengthens.

Data from Thuluvath PJ, Guidinger MK, Fung JJ, et al. Liver Transplantation in the United States, 1999–2008. Am J Transplant 2010;10(4p2):1015.

example, in the University of Pittsburgh experience, acute rejection as a reason for retransplant declined from 13.2% of patients in the early 1980s to 1% in the 1990s.[3] Very rarely, a perfectly functioning donor graft is explanted in the immediate perioperative period because of a delayed finding that the liver donor had unrecognized cancer, thereby placing the recipient at risk of developing a donor-derived malignancy.[22–24]

Among patients requiring late hepatic retransplant, the indications for retransplant tend to be more diverse. Chronic rejection (usually a result of recurrent or smoldering episodes of acute rejection) remains a major indication for retransplant, accounting for almost 18% of total retransplants in one review.[18] Similar to acute rejection, the incidence of chronic rejection seems to be diminishing in the contemporary era. Complex biliary strictures, often a result of either earlier HAT or prolonged warm or cold ischemic times before implantation, are another common reason to pursue retransplant in the months after initial transplant. The incidence of these strictures is estimated between 5% and 15% in many liver transplant series, and although some can be successfully treated endoscopically, other ischemic biliary strictures result in chronic cholangitis and eventual graft loss (or development of multidrug-resistant organisms that can only be treated by graft removal).[18]

An increasingly common cause of late liver retransplant is recurrent primary liver disease. Although de novo autoimmune disease of the liver is an uncommon cause of liver transplant, up to 20% to 40% of liver transplant recipients with prior autoimmune hepatitis, primary biliary cirrhosis, or sclerosing cholangitis develop recurrent disease in their allografts within 5 years of transplant. More concerning, between 5% and 10% of these patients eventually develop recurrent liver failure that may lead to retransplant.[25–27]

Alcoholic liver disease is now the second leading indication for liver transplant in Western countries, accounting for 20% of recipients in the United States and up to 40% of those in Europe.[28] Recidivism of alcohol abuse is common after liver transplant in alcoholics, and studies have demonstrated that between 20% and 50% of patients who undergo transplant for end-stage alcoholic liver disease endorse some alcohol use within the first 5 years after transplant and up to 10% to 15% resume heavy drinking.[29–31] Despite these high rates of relapse, however, the incidence of recurrent alcoholic cirrhosis in transplant recipients is rare. Indeed, only 0% to 5% of deaths in patients who undergo transplant for alcoholic liver disease can be attributed to recurrent cirrhosis and graft failure due to recurrent alcohol abuse.[32,33]

Similarly, nonalcoholic steatohepatitis (now representing the fourth leading cause of primary liver transplant in the United States) has a high rate of recurrence but rarely leads to retransplant. Rates of recurrent steatohepatitis after liver transplant vary widely in the literature, ranging from 0% to 33% in follow-up periods extending from 4 months to 10 years.[34,35] However, despite this high rate of recurrent steatosis posttransplant, only 5% and 10% of patients with recurrent steatosis ultimately develop advanced fibrosis at 5 and 10 years posttransplant, respectively.[36] The relatively benign clinical course of recurrent steatohepatitis after liver transplant is also demonstrated by the finding that patients with recurrent disease have identical survival to those patients transplanted initially for steatohepatitis who do not develop recurrent disease.[35] Furthermore, at least one case report suggests that the rare cases of recurrent nonalcoholic steatohepatitis that do result in graft dysfunction can successfully be treated by a posttransplant Roux-en-Y gastric bypass.[37]

Finally, recurrent hepatitis viral infections are another leading cause of retransplant. Recurrent hepatitis B virus was formerly so ubiquitous and severe that infection was once on the verge of being considered a contraindication to liver transplant.[38] However, the advent of effective antiviral treatment with hepatitis B immune globulin and nucleoside analogs such as lamivudine, tenofovir, and entecavir have rendered hepatitis B virus an increasingly rare indication for either primary liver transplant or hepatic retransplant.[39]

SHOULD HEPATITIS C RECURRENCE PRECLUDE RETRANSPLANT?

Although hepatitis B has largely receded as an indication for retransplant, the most prominent (and likely most controversial) recurrent primary liver disease necessitating late liver retransplant is recurrent infection of the allograft with hepatitis C virus (HCV).[18] This fact is perhaps unsurprising, given that the leading indication for orthotopic liver transplant is now HCV-induced cirrhosis.[40] Recurrent primary disease has become an increasingly common indication for hepatic retransplant, and many of these patients undergo retransplant for recurrent HCV. These recurrent HCV infections of the allograft liver are ubiquitous among transplant recipients with confirmed HCV infection,[41,42] although not all patients proceed to develop recurrent liver fibrosis and cirrhosis. However, the recurrent fibrosis in HCV-positive liver transplant recipients tends to follow a much more virulent and rapidly progressive course than it does in patients who have not undergone transplant.[43,44] Cirrhosis develops in approximately 20% of HCV-positive liver transplant recipients within 5 years of transplant, and up to 10% of these infected recipients die or lose their allografts secondary to recurrent HCV.[45] This more virulent course perhaps explains why several early reports found markedly worse survival outcomes in patients who received a hepatic retransplant for recurrent HCV infection compared with those retransplanted for other indications.[6,46–52] An analysis of all United Network for Organ Sharing (UNOS) database cases from 1987 to 2001 found that transplant recipients infected with HCV were 20% more likely to lose their grafts than non-HCV-infected recipients at 1 year and 30% more likely at 3 years.[6] In one case series of hepatic retransplant for recurrent HCV, for example, almost 50% of the patients were dead within 6 months of retransplant, mostly due to overwhelming sepsis.[53]

Even among HCV-positive transplant recipients, some are more likely to have inferior survival after retransplant. For example, compared with HCV-positive transplant recipients who require retransplant for other indications, those HCV-positive patients whose indication for retransplant is recurrent HCV infection have markedly worse 5-year graft survival rates (45% vs 80%).[54] Survival after retransplant is particularly poor for HCV-positive patients who are also coinfected with human immunodeficiency virus (HIV); in one series, the 3-year survival of HCV-positive patients undergoing retransplant was 22% and 65% for HIV-positive and HIV-negative patients, respectively.[55] All these factors led several investigators to argue that recurrent HCV should be a contraindication for hepatic retransplant, except in a handful of carefully selected low-risk patients, such as those with late HCV recurrence and well-preserved renal function.[56,57]

Efforts to improve the inferior clinical outcomes of hepatic retransplant for recurrent HCV have focused on better recipient and donor selection. For example, older hepatic donors (>60 years of age) were associated with worse outcomes in HCV-positive patients undergoing liver retransplant.[53] Many centers exclude HCV-positive liver recipients who develop early HCV recurrence,[58] but some studies have found that the interval to clinical HCV recurrence after a first liver transplant could not predict the HCV recurrence course after retransplant.[53] Other investigators argued that the worse outcomes of hepatic retransplant for recurrent HCV-associated graft failure could be avoided if these patients underwent retransplant at lower MELD scores.[48,59] Going a step further, Andres and colleagues[60] developed a risk score model specifically designed to predict survival after hepatic retransplant in HCV-positive patients. This model incorporates variables such as donor and recipient age, the interval between transplant, as well as the recipient international normalized ratio and albumin and creatinine levels at the time of retransplant. At 3 years postretransplant, the survival of HCV-positive patients was 71% in the low-risk category versus 37% in the high-risk category.[60]

Several more recent studies have found no difference in liver retransplant outcome between HCV-positive and HCV-negative patients (**Fig. 2**).[15,61–67] Indeed, at least one series found improved patient and graft survival 3 years after initial retransplant in HCV-positive recipients compared with HCV-negative recipients, a finding attributed to the younger donor age and better patient selection in HCV-positive recipients undergoing retransplant.[68] In this case series, for example, the average donor age was 31.8 years for patient undergoing retransplant due to recurrent HCV, versus 42.8 years for those with a non-HCV indication for retransplant. The advent of a new generation of antiviral drugs such as simeprevir and sofosbuvir (which target the HCV protease and RNA polymerase, respectively) offers a new potential means to treat recurrent HCV in allograft recipients and may further obviate the argument that recurrent HCV should contraindicate hepatic retransplant.[69]

LIVER ALLOCATION FOR HEPATIC RETRANSPLANT: THE STATUS QUO

At present, livers are allocated to patients being considered for hepatic retransplant based purely on their laboratory MELD score, just as they are allocated for primary transplant. Exceptions to the use of MELD scores are patients who require urgent retransplant within the first week of transplant for PNF or early HAT (who are awarded UNOS Status 1A) or patients who develop HAT within 8 to 14 days of transplant, who are granted an exceptional MELD score of 40.[70] However, accumulating evidence

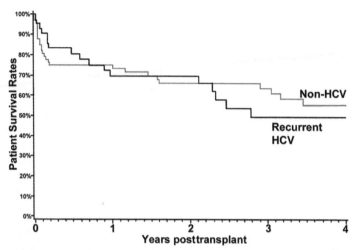

Fig. 2. Hepatic retransplant for recurrent HCV. In a multicenter US study, patients receiving hepatic retransplants for biopsy-proven recurrent HCV had no statistically significant differences in overall survival compared with those receiving hepatic retransplants for other indications. (*Adapted from* McCashland T, Watt K, Lyden E, et al. Retransplantation for hepatitis C: results of a U.S. multicenter retransplant study. Liver Transpl 2007;13(9):1250; with permission.)

suggests that MELD scores may not be as accurate for risk stratification of retransplant candidates as they are for patients considered for primary liver transplant.[71] For example, Edwards and Harper[72] demonstrated that MELD scores systemically underestimate the risk of death on transplant waiting lists for patients awaiting a hepatic retransplant compared with those waiting for a first liver graft (**Fig. 3**). Another study found that compared with primary transplant candidates, patients awaiting liver retransplant had particularly high waiting list mortality at lower MELD scores (MELD

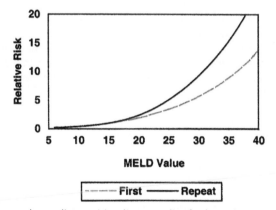

Fig. 3. MELD score underpredicts waiting list mortality for hepatic retransplant. Compared with patients on waiting list for primary liver transplant, those waiting for a retransplant have a higher relative risk of dying on the waiting list at equivalent MELD score levels. (*From* Edwards E, Harper A. Does MELD work for relisted candidates? Liver Transpl 2004;10(10 Suppl 2):S12; with permission.)

<25) but a lower waiting list mortality at higher MELD scores (25–40).[73] Many of these studies demonstrate that candidates for hepatic retransplant tend to have higher MELD scores at the time of their retransplant compared with the average MELD score of recipients of primary liver grafts, bolstering the common consensus that patients who undergo retransplant tend to be sicker at the time of their new transplant.[71,72,74,75]

Given the limitations of the current MELD system, improving the outcomes of hepatic retransplant almost certainly requires development of improved risk stratification models that prevent wasteful allocation of another liver allograft to high-risk patients with failing prior grafts, preventing retransplant when this is likely to be a futile maneuver. The definition of futility when considering liver allocation has been a matter of great controversy for both transplant clinicians and medical ethicists.[76] As gatekeepers and stewards of a scarce societal resource such as donor livers, transplant clinicians must perform a delicate moral calculus, balancing their duties to current transplant recipients (and their duty not to abandon these patients) against the needs and interests of other patients on the transplant waiting list who may die before receiving a first liver transplant. In an effort to define a fair definition of futile transplantation, a national UK panel in 1998 determined that with few exceptions, patients should be denied either primary liver transplant or hepatic retransplant if their expected 5-year survival would be less than 50%,[77] and a subsequent US consensus report validated this 50% survival benchmark, although it elided whether this should be 1-year or 5-year survival rate.[78]

Careful analysis of several large case series of hepatic retransplant have offered several important variables that might better predict outcomes after liver retransplant, identifying clinical situations where retransplant is likely to lead to a poor or futile outcome. These factors include both the timing of retransplant (specifically, the interval between the prior transplant and the retransplant) and several different recipient and donor characteristics.

CAN THE TIMING OF RETRANSPLANT PREDICT PATIENT SURVIVAL?

The time interval between hepatic retransplant and prior transplant is often quite broad; UNOS data show that in the United States from 1999 to 2008, the mean interval to retransplant was 962 ± 1453 days and the median time was 222 days.[4] Although some liver retransplants are not performed until years after the first transplant, most hepatic retransplants occur relatively early after the primary graft. For example, 25% of retransplants in the United States are performed within the first 2 weeks,[4] and in one recent case series from Spain, 12.2% were done within 3 days of the first transplant, 34.7% were performed between 4 to 30 days after the first transplant, and another 18.4% were performed within the first year thereafter.[17]

Amassing evidence strongly suggests that the timing of hepatic retransplant may significantly affect the ultimate success or failure of the procedure. Several studies have shown that urgent early retransplants (within 3–7 days of prior liver transplant) and late retransplants (>365 days after prior liver transplant) are associated with improved patient survival compared with retransplant on a semiurgent basis (7–30 days after prior transplant).[14,17,63,79–82] The inferior survival encountered with semiurgent transplant is likely a reflection of the indications for retransplant that would be most commonly encountered during this time interval. Patients requiring retransplant between 7 and 30 days are unlikely to have developed recurrent disease or chronic rejection, because this is too early a time frame. Instead, most of these semiurgent retransplant candidates are extremely sick and have multiorgan failure either after developing primary nonfunction of their first graft or having a vascular complication that was managed expectantly. Many of these patients likely share the same indication for retransplant as those who undergo retransplant within the first week, but their retransplants occur later because of either a delay in obtaining a replacement graft or failure of their physicians to recognize their need for retransplant in a timely manner; as a consequence of this delay, they are usually sicker at the time of retransplant, explaining their inferior outcomes compared with those undergoing retransplant within the first week. In addition, in contrast to the relatively easy graft explant encountered in patients who undergo retransplant within a few days of their first transplant, patients undergoing retransplant several weeks after prior transplant would have formed dense adhesions that increase the complexity and potential dangers posed by reoperation. While liver transplant recipients requiring semiurgent retransplant rarely have the luxury of time to postpone their transplant until it is likely to have a more favorable outcome, these findings do help risk-stratify patients undergoing retransplant, identifying those more likely to have a poor result.

WHICH RECIPIENT CHARACTERISTICS ARE ASSOCIATED WITH WORSE PROGNOSIS?

Analysis of various case series has highlighted several recipient variables that are independently associated with worse survival after liver retransplant. As might be expected, sicker patients at the time of retransplant tend to have inferior outcomes. Specifically, preoperative mechanical ventilation,[80,83] increased recipient creatinine levels, increased recipient bilirubin levels,[49,63,83] and MELD scores greater than 25[82,84–87] have all been independently linked to worse survival rates after retransplant. Consistent with the hypothesis that sicker patients fare worse after retransplant, patients requiring emergent liver retransplant (eg, UNOS Status 1) have also been claimed to have inferior outcomes according to some case series.[7,10] However, other groups failed to demonstrate a difference in patient survival for urgent versus elective retransplant.[17] Increasing recipient age is another variable linked to worse retransplant outcomes.[15,49,80,88–90] However, beyond the age of 60 years, there is no further augmentation in recipient risk, suggesting that advanced age alone should not be a disqualification for hepatic retransplant.[91]

In addition to older and sicker patients, retransplant should also be approached with caution for patients requiring more than 2 liver transplants, because they have markedly inferior outcomes compared with those undergoing a first hepatic retransplant.[82] Perioperative mortality within the first month of transplant increased to 17%, 25%, 20%, and 50% for recipients of a second, third, fourth, or fifth liver transplant, respectively.[92] In contrast, immediate perioperative death occurred in only 6% of recipients of primary grafts. Another case series of multiple retransplants validated these findings, determining that 10-year patient survival was 52% for recipients of a first liver transplant versus 32% for a second transplant, 25% for a third, and 13% for 4 or more transplants.[3] Transplant of more than 2 liver allografts is not an unusual occurrence. Indeed, UNOS data from 1987 to 2001 showed that more than 23% of patients receiving a second liver transplant would ultimately require a third transplant (compared with only 7.4% of primary liver transplant recipients who would eventually require retransplant).[6]

Several other recipient factors affect the outcome after retransplant. Patients infected with HIV undergoing liver transplant were found to have inferior outcomes after retransplant, although patient survival was significantly better for the subset of HIV-infected patients who were not coinfected with HCV and who did not require retransplant within 30 days of their prior transplant.[55] Finally, one intriguing study highlighted the impact of recipient preformed anti-HLA class I antibodies on survival after hepatic retransplant. This study retrospectively examined sera from 139 patients undergoing hepatic retransplant on a Luminex platform to determine anti-HLA antibodies. The presence of anti-HLA class I antibodies was associated with an absolute 20% reduction in patient survival at 1, 3 and 5 years in adult patients.[93] There was no specific association of donor-specific antibody with worse outcome after retransplant in this study. Although needing verification, this study suggests a potential role for determining panel-reactive antibody in candidates being considered for retransplant.

BETTER DONOR GRAFTS, BETTER OUTCOMES

Improving the outcome of hepatic retransplant likely requires better matching of donor grafts to recipients. Although important recipient factors governing survival after hepatic retransplant have already been discussed, several groups have also focused on donor graft characteristics that may predict more favorable (or unfavorable) outcomes. Many have hypothesized that given the higher risks and inferior clinical outcomes associated with hepatic retransplant, only the best quality donor grafts should be used for this purpose. Indeed, an analysis of the Scientific Registry of Transplant Recipients examining liver transplants in the United States from 1999 to 2008 found that the quality of donor grafts (as measured by the donor risk index, DRI) used in hepatic retransplant increased markedly over time, including a 36% decrease in use of grafts from donors with DRI greater than 1.8.[4] This finding is in sharp contrast to the trend of donors used in primary liver transplant, where the average donor DRI has marched steadily upward. In the setting of urgent retransplant (such as primary nonfunction or HAT), there is rarely the luxury of being able to carefully match donor to recipient, because usually the first available liver must be accepted to save the patient's life. However, in the setting of elective liver retransplant for recurrent disease or chronic rejection, there is generally more time available to carefully select an optimal donor graft.

Analyses of case series by several investigators have found that use of grafts from older donors (usually defined as >60 years of age) adversely affects hepatic retransplant recipient survival.[60,67,80,82,86,94] By similar logic, it could be argued that use of grafts from extended criteria donors (ECD) should also be discouraged for retransplant. However, investigators from the University of Barcelona found that in their series of patients undergoing liver retransplant, ECD liver grafts functioned as well as non-ECD livers.[94] Even in HCV-positive patients requiring retransplant, equivalent patient survival is achieved using ECD versus non-ECD donors.[95] In contrast, retransplant using liver grafts obtained after cardiac death had more unfavorable outcomes, especially for candidates with higher MELD scores at the time of retransplant.[96]

Extended cold ischemia times are also associated with inferior patient and graft survival after retransplant, especially if these cold ischemia times extend beyond 12 hours.[83,86] Finally, use of split liver grafts rather than whole liver grafts for retransplant was found to be an independent variable predicting worse survival in several case series, especially in pediatric recipients of hepatic retransplants.[86,97]

ACHIEVING OPTIMAL OUTCOMES AFTER RETRANSPLANT: THE UTILITY OF RISK PREDICTION MODELS

Many groups have attempted to develop prognostic scores that take into account preoperative patient and donor variables to predict outcomes of hepatic retransplant, with the goal of screening out patients who are unlikely to benefit from the procedure (**Table 2**).[49,62,83,85] Several of these models indicate that MELD scores may

Table 2
Prediction models for hepatic retransplant

Author	Retransplant Prediction Model	Risk Categories	1-y Survival
Markmann et al,[83] 1999	Give 1 point for: total bilirubin level$\geq$13 mg/dL, Cre$\geq$1.6 mg/dL, preoperative ventilator requirement, cold ischemia$\geq$12 h, transplant into adult recipient	Very low risk (score = 1) Low risk (score = 2) Medium risk (score = 3) High risk (score = 4) Very high risk (score = 5)	83% 67%–72% 43%–53% 20%–27% 6%
Rosen et al,[49] 1999	RS = 0.024* (recipient age) + 0.112*$\sqrt{}$(bilirubin in mg/dL) + 0.230*($\log_e$ Cre in mg/dL) – 0.974*(cause of graft failure) + UNOS coefficient Cause of graft failure: 1 if PNF, 0 for non-PNF UNOS coefficient: Status 1 = –0.261, Status 2 = –0.463, Status 3 = –1.07	Low risk: R<0.75 Medium risk: R = 0.75–1.46 High risk: $R\geq$1.47	70%–76% 49%–59% 28%–40%
Azoulay et al,[90] 2002	R = 0.04*(recipient age) + 0.89*($\log_e$ Cre in μmol/L) – 1.28*(1 if PNF is indication, 0 if non-PNF) + 1.38*(1 if emergent, 0 if nonemergent) + 1.27*(1 if urgent, 0 if nonurgent) – 0.23*$\sqrt{}$(total bilirubin in μmol/L) – 1.38*($\log_e$ factor II level) + 0.05*($\sqrt{}$(total bilirubin) * $\log_e$(factor II level))	Low risk: R = –0.6 Medium risk: R = 0.42 High risk: R = 1.7	88% 70% 26%
Rosen et al,[62] 2003	R = 10 * [0.0236*(recipient age) + 0.125*$\sqrt{}$(bilirubin in mg/dL) + 0.438*($\log_e$ Cre in mg/dL) – 0.234 (interval to retransplant, 0 for 15–60 d, 1 for >60 d)]	Low risk: R<16 Medium risk: R = 16–20 High risk: R>20	75% 58% 42%
Ravaioli et al,[84] 2004	MELD score$\geq$25 is valid cutoff to predict poor outcome after retransplant		
Linhares et al,[63] 2006	Give 14 points for urgent/emergent retransplant Give 4 points for every 10-year increment in recipient age Give 4 points for every 100 μmol/L increment in Cre Subtract 10 points if retransplant required within 7 d	Low risk: <24 points Medium risk: 24–32 points High risk: >32 points	85% 69% 21%
Maggi et al,[86] 2008	log (odds of death in 1 y) = –4.81 + 2.23*(recipient sex, 1 for male, 0 for female) + 1.86*(donor age, 0 for <40 y, 1 for 40–59 y, 2 for$\geq$60 y) + 1.60*(MELD score, 0 for <26, 1 for$\geq$26)		

(continued on next page)

Table 2
(continued)

Author	Retransplant Prediction Model	Risk Categories	1-y Survival
Davis et al,[97] 2009	Pediatric retransplant RS: Assign 1 point for: neonatal cholestasis/paucity of bile ducts, being on life support at time of retransplant, receiving a split liver graft Subtract 1 point for: age 5–18 y at time of retransplant, acute rejection as indication for retransplant	Low risk: <0 points Medium risk: 0 points High risk: 1–3 points	82% 62% 49%
Hong et al,[67] 2011	Assign 2 RS points for: intraoperative pRBC >30 units, more than 1 prior liver transplant, mechanical ventilation before retransplant, or interval from prior transplant to retransplant of 15–30 d. Assign 1 RS point for: interval from prior transplant to retransplant of 31–180 d, donor age >45 y, MELD score >27, serum albumin level <2.5 g/dL at time of retransplant, recipient age >55 y	PIC I: RS = 0 Category II: RS = 1–2 Category III: RS = 3–4 Category IV: RS = 5–12	84% 75% 63% 33%
Andres et al,[60] 2012	Specifically for HCV-positive retransplant candidates: RS = 0.23*(donor age) + 4.86*log (Cre) – 2.45*log (interval between transplants in days) + 2.69*INR + 0.1*(recipient age) – 3.27*(serum albumin) + 40	Low risk: RS <30 Medium risk: RS 30–40 High risk: RS >40	72.2%–87.3% 62.5%–71.7% 50%

Abbreviations: Cre, creatinine; INR, international normalized ratio; PIC, predictive index category; pRBC, packed red blood cells; RS, risk score.

underrepresent the degree of illness experienced by patients with a failing liver allograft. Thus, use of the MELD system may delay allocation of new livers to retransplant candidates, perhaps explaining their inferior outcomes compared with primary graft recipients. In an effort to provide an opportunity for retransplant when patients are less sick and might stand to benefit more from the retransplant, some centers have turned to living donor donation, which allows patients to sidestep MELD requirements.[98] This approach may prove problematic, however, in the complex retransplant cases in which vascular conduits are needed to reconstruct the hepatic artery or portal vein, because unlike deceased donor organs that bring with them iliac artery and vein, donor vessel conduits are typically not available from live donors.

One of the earliest prognostic models for retransplant emerged from the UCLA group based on their large cohort of more than 350 hepatic retransplants. The investigators found that poor clinical outcomes after hepatic retransplant could be predicted based on several preoperative variables, including levels of serum creatinine and bilirubin, recipient age range, and the need for preoperative mechanical ventilation.[7] A similar risk score was developed by Linhares and colleagues[63] based on an international patient data set. Multivariate analysis of these patients flagged recipient age, serum creatinine levels, urgency of retransplant, and early failure of the first graft as clinical variables that independently predicted mortality after retransplant.

Perhaps the most commonly used risk score for retransplant is the Rosen score, based on recipient age, serum bilirubin and creatinine levels, cause of graft failure of prior transplant, and UNOS status.[49] This prognostic scoring system was subsequently validated in an international case series data set.[62] However, the criticism raised about this scoring system is that it was formulated in the pre-MELD era of liver allocation. Modern liver allocation practices may therefore render the Rosen score less prognostic of actual clinical outcomes. The UCLA group recently published a new risk stratification scoring system based on more contemporary clinical data (**Fig. 4**).[67] This system assigns points for high-risk clinical variables, including recipient age greater than 55 years, MELD scores greater than 27, history of a prior retransplant, serum albumin levels less than 2.5 g/dL, donor age greater than 45 years, performance of retransplant between 15 to 180 days after prior transplant, and intraoperative red blood cell transfusion requirement greater than 30 units during retransplant. All variables except for the last can be used preoperatively to assign a cumulative risk score, allowing retransplant candidates to be placed into one of 4 predictive index categories (PICs). The most high-risk retransplant recipients (ie, those in PIC IV) had a 5-year patient survival of only 22%, versus a survival rate of 79% for patients undergoing retransplant in PIC I (the most low-risk group). The investigators recommended that retransplant should be denied to candidates who would fall in this high-risk PIC IV.

TECHNICAL CHALLENGES OF HEPATIC RETRANSPLANT

Hepatic retransplant poses some unique technical challenges, but some of the recent improvements in liver retransplant outcomes can likely be attributed to advances in operative technique. The timing of the retransplant (and specifically the interval between prior transplant and retransplant) plays a major role in dictating the complexity

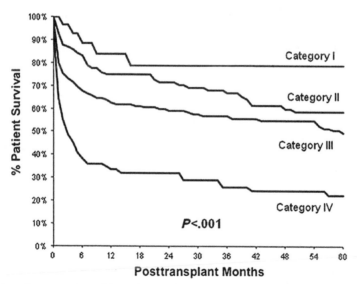

Fig. 4. Hepatic retransplant risk prediction model can stratify patients likely to have poor outcomes from retransplant. In the risk model developed by Hong and colleagues,[67] preoperative variables can assign retransplant candidates into 4 different predictive index categories, which correlate with different postretransplant survival rates. (*From* Hong JC, Kaldas FM, Kositamongkol P, et al. Predictive index for long-term survival after retransplantation of the liver in adult recipients. Ann Surg 2011;254(3):446; with permission.)

of the operation. If retransplant is required within the first few days after a prior trans-plant, the recipient hepatectomy portion of the operation might be considerably easier than for a primary liver transplant, because most of the dissection would already have been performed and portal hypertension often diminished compared with primary transplant.

However, retransplant at later timepoints often poses an extreme technical chal-lenge. The formation of dense adhesions greatly complicates dissection and identifi-cation of key vascular and biliary structures and arterial neovascularization of the graft capsule raises the risk of significant intraoperative bleeding.[99] Before approaching a liver retransplant, it is imperative to fully define the anatomy of vascular and biliary anastomoses via careful review of prior operative notes and cross-sectional imaging. Specifically, it must be determined whether the reconstruction was performed with a piggyback versus caval interposition venous anastomosis and whether the patient's biliary system was reconstructed with a hepaticojejunostomy versus a primary com-mon bile duct anastomosis.

Several techniques have been described to address the unique technical burdens imposed by repeat liver transplant. Zarrinpar and Hong[18] emphasized the importance of venovenous bypass as a means of decompressing the portomesenteric venous system and thereby minimizing bleeding from raw surfaces. As an alternative to tradi-tional venovenous bypass, some groups have also described using a CellSaver (Haemonetics, Braintree, MA) circuit to decompress the portomesenteric system via the recipient inferior mesenteric vein and then return blood through a cannula placed in the internal jugular vein.[100] Also as a means of minimizing bleeding, Akpinar and col-leagues[92] at the University of Miami describe very early mass clamping of the liver hi-lum during recipient hepatectomy, especially when dense scarring precluded the safe dissection or prior anastomoses. Before applying the clamp, a test clamping was per-formed to determine if hemodynamic changes would mandate venous bypass. Once the hilar structures are clamped, the structures can be transected en masse and then subsequently each structure can be dissected out and reanastomosed.

If a bicaval technique was used during the prior liver transplant, the retransplant may be performed using either another bicaval reconstruction or a piggyback technique, in which the anastomosis is performed between suprahepatic vena cava of the new graft and the recipient's conjoined hepatic venous orifices in an end-to-side manner. The benefit of using a piggyback technique in this situation is that the plane between the liver and hepatic cava provides unviolated territory for dissection. If a bicaval implantation is planned for the retransplant, it is often necessary to preserve the previous caval anastomoses to permit sufficient venous length to perform the new suprahepatic and infrahepatic caval anastomoses. Similarly, a segment of the portal vein anastomosis from the prior graft may also be preserved to provide extra length.

In contrast to the veins, the hepatic artery of the prior liver allograft should never be preserved during retransplant. Reuse of these prior graft hepatic arteries is a perilous decision, because these vessels may be prone to thrombosis or rupture after retrans-plant.[2,18] Because of this, arterial reconstruction of hepatic retransplants is greatly aided by having ready access to donor vascular grafts (especially the donor iliac arteries). If retransplant is necessitated by HAT of the prior graft, then anastomosis to the supraceliac or infrarenal aorta may be required. The recipient supraceliac aorta can often be reached when the new donor hepatic artery is harvested along with the donor celiac trunk, but reaching the infrarenal aorta usually requires use of conduit formed from donor iliac arteries. This iliac conduit can be brought through the trans-verse mesocolon in a retrogastric plane, but some investigators have described inter-nal hernias of jejunum through this potential space, leading some to recommend passing the conduit posterior to the mobilized duodenum in a retroperitoneal plane along its entire course to the liver.[101]

Similar to the arteries, none of the bile ducts from the prior graft should be used during biliary reconstruction of the retransplanted graft. To minimize the risk of ischemic cholangiopathy, most investigators recommend use of a Roux-en-Y choledochojejunostomy for biliary reconstruction, because this ensures a tension-free anastomosis.[92] If a Roux-en-Y reconstruction was used during the prior transplant, the blind end of the prior Roux limb should be resected (including the site of the first anastomosis) and a new choledochojejunostomy should be constructed. This dogma that Roux-en-Y biliary reconstructions should always be used for hepatic retransplant was recently challenged by a group at the Mayo Clinic in Florida, who published their retrospective case series showing no difference in biliary complications after retransplant if the biliary reconstruction was performed as a Roux-en-Y versus a primary duct-to-duct anastomosis.[102]

Given the complexity of hepatic retransplant, some have argued that it should be limited to high-volume centers of excellence. However, an analysis of OPTN registry data found no difference in survival after retransplant performed at low-, intermediate-, or high-volume transplant centers.[103]

SUMMARY

Although the incidence of hepatic retransplant is decreasing, it still remains a controversial issue that poses unique technical, medical, and ethical challenges to the transplant physician attempting to balance the interests of current liver transplant recipients against those of patients still waiting for the opportunity of primary transplant. Recent innovations, however, offer much room for optimism. As recent case series have indicated, the indications and outcomes of hepatic retransplant have changed markedly over the past 30 years. Rejection (either acute or chronic) has become a less common

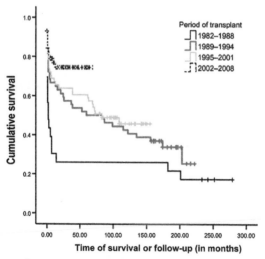

Fig. 5. Hepatic retransplant survival by epoch. Patient survival after hepatic retransplant has improved in the contemporary era compared with that in the 1980s, as shown in this 25-year experience from a single institution (University Hospital of Birmingham, UK). (*Adapted from* Marudanayagam R, Shanmugam V, Sandhu B, et al. Liver retransplantation in adults: a single-centre, 25-year experience. HPB (Oxford) 2010;12(3):222; with permission.)

indication for hepatic retransplant in the contemporary era, but recurrence of primary disease (especially hepatitis C) has increasingly driven hepatic retransplant volume.[65]

Early reports indicated markedly inferior clinical outcomes associated with hepatic retransplants, but more recent case series have shown some improvement (**Fig. 5**).[65,82] On a nationwide level, the Scientific Registry of Transplant Recipients' annual report from 2010 demonstrated that the gap in graft survival between primary liver transplant recipients and retransplant recipients has narrowed considerably in the contemporary era. For example, the 1-year graft survival of deceased donor liver transplants is 86.1% for primary graft recipients versus 74.2% for retransplants; the 10-year survival is similarly 56% and 42.6%, respectively.[104] Much of this improvement can likely be attributed to the more widespread utilization of risk models that reduce the number of patients undergoing futile retransplant.

While consensus guidelines remain elusive, the brunt of evidence identifies several recipient and donor characteristics that should spur hesitancy to offer retransplant. Extremely sick patients (including those with MELD scores >25 or who are mechanically intubated), patients requiring more than one retransplant, and those needing retransplant within 8 to 30 days after their prior transplant are all likely to have high rates of early postoperative mortality after retransplant. However, recipient age and their HCV seropositivity should not preclude being considered for retransplant. Transplant physicians should also be reluctant to offer retransplant using either split liver grafts, grafts from donors older than 60 years, or grafts from donors after cardiac death. Grafts from ECD, an increasingly vital portion of the national organ supply, can be used with confidence in retransplant, however.

Hepatic retransplant remains the sole option for survival in many patients facing allograft failure after liver transplant. With improved techniques to match retransplant candidates with appropriate donor grafts, it is hoped that the outcomes of retransplant will continue to improve in future years.

REFERENCES

1. Organ Procurement and Transplantation Network (OPTN) and Scientific Registry of Transplant Recipients (SRTR). OPTN/SRTR 2011 Annual Data Report. In: Department of Health and Human Services HRaSA, Healthcare Systems Bureau, Division of Transplantation, editors. Rockville (MD): 2012.
2. Shaw BW, Gordon RD, Iwatsuki S, et al. Hepatic retransplantation. Transplant Proc 1985;17(1):264–71.
3. Jain A, Reyes J, Kashyap R, et al. Long-term survival after liver transplantation in 4,000 consecutive patients at a single center. Ann Surg 2000;232(4):490–500.
4. Thuluvath PJ, Guidinger MK, Fung JJ, et al. Liver transplantation in the United States, 1999-2008. Am J Transplant 2010;10(4p2):1003–19.
5. Pfitzmann R, Benscheidt B, Langrehr JM, et al. Trends and experiences in liver retransplantation over 15 years. Liver Transpl 2007;13(2):248–57.
6. Yoo H, Maheshwari A, Thuluvath PJ. Retransplantation of liver: primary graft nonfunction and hepatitis C virus are associated with worse outcome. Liver Transpl 2003;9(9):897–904.
7. Markmann JF, Markowitz JS, Yersiz H, et al. Long-term survival after retransplantation of the liver. Ann Surg 1997;226(4):408–18 [discussion: 418–20].
8. Lang H, Sotiropoulos GC, Beckebaum S, et al. Incidence of liver retransplantation and its effect on patient survival. Transplant Proc 2008;40(9):3201–3.
9. Magee JC, Barr ML, Basadonna GP, et al. Repeat organ transplantation in the United States, 1996-2005. Am J Transplant 2007;7(s1):1424–33.

10. Remiszewski P, Kalinowski P, Dudek K, et al. Influence of selected factors on survival after liver retransplantation. Transplant Proc 2011;43(8):3025–8.
11. D'Alessandro AM, Ploeg RJ, Knechtle SJ, et al. Retransplantation of the liver–a seven-year experience. Transplantation 1993;55(5):1083–7.
12. Yoong KF, Gunson BK, Buckels JA, et al. Repeat orthotopic liver transplantation in the 1990s: is it justified? Transpl Int 1998;11(Suppl 1):S221–3.
13. Reed A, Howard RJ, Fujita S, et al. Liver retransplantation: a single-center outcome and financial analysis. Transplant Proc 2005;37(2):1161–3.
14. Powelson JA, Cosimi AB, Lewis WD, et al. Hepatic retransplantation in New England–a regional experience and survival model. Transplantation 1993;55(4):802–6.
15. Maggi U, Andorno E, Rossi G, et al. Liver retransplantation in adults: the largest multicenter Italian study. PLoS One 2012;7(10):e46643.
16. Crivellin C, De Martin E, Germani G, et al. Risk factors in liver retransplantation: a single-center experience. Transplant Proc 2011;43(4):1110–3.
17. Pérez-Saborido B, Menéu-Díaz JC, de los Galanes SJ, et al. Short- and long-term overall results of liver retransplantation: "Doce de Octubre" Hospital Experience. Transplant Proc 2014;41(6):2441–3.
18. Zarrinpar A, Hong JC. What is the prognosis after retransplantation of the liver? Adv Surg 2012;46(1):87–100.
19. Strasberg SM, Howard TK, Molmenti EP, et al. Selecting the donor liver: risk factors for poor function after orthotopic liver transplantation. Hepatology 1994;20(4 Pt 1):829–38.
20. Ploeg RJ, D'Alessandro AM, Knechtle SJ, et al. Risk factors for primary dysfunction after liver transplantation–a multivariate analysis. Transplantation 1993;55(4):807–13.
21. Bekker J, Ploem S, de Jong KP. Early hepatic artery thrombosis after liver transplantation: a systematic review of the incidence, outcome and risk factors. Am J Transplant 2009;9(4):746–57.
22. Begum R, Harnois D, Satyanarayana R, et al. Retransplantation for donor-derived neuroendocrine tumor. Liver Transpl 2011;17(1):83–7.
23. Lipshutz G. Death from donor-transmitted malignancy despite emergency liver retransplantation. Liver Transpl 2003;9(10):1102–7.
24. Florman S, Bowne W, Kim-Schluger L, et al. Unresectable squamous cell carcinoma of donor origin treated with immunosuppression withdrawal and liver retransplantation. Am J Transplant 2004;4(2):278–82.
25. Mendes F, Couto CA, Levy C. Recurrent and de novo autoimmune liver diseases. Clin Liver Dis 2011;15(4):859–78.
26. Montano-Loza AJ, Mason AL, Ma M, et al. Risk factors for recurrence of autoimmune hepatitis after liver transplantation. Liver Transpl 2009;15(10):1254–61.
27. Molmenti EP, Netto GJ, Murray NG, et al. Incidence and recurrence of autoimmune/alloimmune hepatitis in liver transplant recipients. Liver Transpl 2002;8(6):519–26.
28. Iruzubieta P, Crespo J, Fabrega E. Long-term survival after liver transplantation for alcoholic liver disease. World J Gastroenterol 2013;19(48):9198–208.
29. Mackie J, Groves K, Hoyle A, et al. Orthotopic liver transplantation for alcoholic liver disease: a retrospective analysis of survival, recidivism, and risk factors predisposing to recidivism. Liver Transpl 2001;7(5):418–27.
30. Tome S, Lucey MR. Timing of liver transplantation in alcoholic cirrhosis. J Hepatol 2003;39(3):302–7.

31. Lucey MR. Liver transplantation in the alcoholic patient. In: Maddrey WC, Schiff ER, Sorrel MF, editors. Transplantation of the Liver. Philadelphia: Lipincott Williams and Wilkins; 2001. p. 319–26.

32. Pageaux GP, Bismuth M, Perney P, et al. Alcohol relapse after liver transplantation for alcoholic liver disease: does it matter? J Hepatol 2003;38(5):629–34.

33. Conjeevaram HS, Hart J, Lissoos TW, et al. Rapidly progressive liver injury and fatal alcoholic hepatitis occurring after liver transplantation in alcoholic patients. Transplantation 1999;67(12):1562–8.

34. Patil DT, Yerian LM. Evolution of nonalcoholic fatty liver disease recurrence after liver transplantation. Liver Transpl 2012;18(10):1147–53.

35. Dureja P, Mellinger J, Agni R, et al. NAFLD recurrence in liver transplant recipients. Transplantation 2011;91(6):684–9.

36. Yalamanchili K, Saadeh S, Klintmalm GB, et al. Nonalcoholic fatty liver disease after liver transplantation for cryptogenic cirrhosis or nonalcoholic fatty liver disease. Liver Transpl 2010;16(4):431–9.

37. Duchini A, Brunson ME. Roux-en-Y gastric bypass for recurrent nonalcoholic steatohepatitis in liver transplant recipients with morbid obesity. Transplantation 2001;72(1):156–9.

38. Eason JD, Freeman RB Jr, Rohrer RJ, et al. Should liver transplantation be performed for patients with hepatitis B? Transplantation 1994;57(11):1588–93.

39. Crespo G, Marino Z, Navasa M, et al. Viral hepatitis in liver transplantation. Gastroenterology 2012;142(6):1373–83.e1.

40. Verna EC, Brown RS Jr. Hepatitis C and liver transplantation: enhancing outcomes and should patients be retransplanted. Clin Liver Dis 2008;12(3):637–59, ix–x.

41. Gane E. The natural history and outcome of liver transplantation in hepatitis C virus-infected recipients. Liver Transpl 2003;9(11):S28–34.

42. Garcia-Retortillo M, Forns X, Feliu A, et al. Hepatitis C virus kinetics during and immediately after liver transplantation. Hepatology 2002;35(3):680–7.

43. Berenguer M, Prieto M, Rayon JM, et al. Natural history of clinically compensated hepatitis C virus-related graft cirrhosis after liver transplantation. Hepatology 2000;32(4 Pt 1):852–8.

44. Berenguer M, Ferrell L, Watson J, et al. HCV-related fibrosis progression following liver transplantation: increase in recent years. J Hepatol 2000;32(4):673–84.

45. Charlton M. Natural history of hepatitis C and outcomes following liver transplantation. Clin Liver Dis 2003;7(3):585–602.

46. Carrión JA, Navasa M, Forns X. Retransplantation in patients with hepatitis C recurrence after liver transplantation. J Hepatol 2010;53(5):962–70.

47. Neff GW, O'Brien CB, Nery J, et al. Factors that identify survival after liver retransplantation for allograft failure caused by recurrent hepatitis C infection. Liver Transpl 2004;10(12):1497–503.

48. Sheiner PA, Schluger LK, Emre S, et al. Retransplantation for recurrent hepatitis C. Liver Transpl Surg 1997;3(2):130–6.

49. Rosen HR, Madden JP, Martin P. A model to predict survival following liver retransplantation. Hepatology 1999;29(2):365–70.

50. Chan SE, Rosen HR. Outcome and management of hepatitis C in liver transplant recipients. Clin Infect Dis 2003;37(6):807–12.

51. Biggins SW, Terrault NA. Should HCV-related cirrhosis be a contraindication for retransplantation? Liver Transpl 2003;9(3):236–8.

52. Berenguer M, Prieto M, Palau A, et al. Severe recurrent hepatitis C after liver retransplantation for hepatitis C virus-related graft cirrhosis. Liver Transpl 2003; 9(3):228–35.
53. Roayaie S, Schiano TD, Thung SN, et al. Results of retransplantation for recurrent hepatitis C. Hepatology 2003;38(6):1428–36.
54. Rowe IA. Retransplantation for graft failure in chronic hepatitis C infection: a good use of a scarce resource? World J Gastroenterol 2010;16(40):5070.
55. Gastaca M, Aguero F, Rimola A, et al. Liver retransplantation in HIV-infected patients: a prospective cohort study. Am J Transplant 2012;12(9):2465–76.
56. Llado L, Castellote J, Figueras J. Is retransplantation an option for recurrent hepatitis C cirrhosis after liver transplantation? J Hepatol 2005;42(4):468–72.
57. Wall WJ, Khakhar A. Retransplantation for recurrent hepatitis C: the argument against. Liver Transpl 2003;9(11):S73–8.
58. Wiesner RH, Sorrell M, Villamil F, et al. Report of the first International Liver Transplantation Society expert panel consensus conference on liver transplantation and hepatitis C. Liver Transpl 2003;9(11):S1–9.
59. Burton JR, Sonnenberg A, Rosen HR. Retransplantation for recurrent hepatitis C in the MELD era: maximizing utility. Liver Transpl 2004;10(S10):S59–64.
60. Andres A, Gerstel E, Combescure C, et al. A score predicting survival after liver retransplantation for hepatitis C virus cirrhosis. Transplantation 2012;93(7): 717–22.
61. Ghabril M, Dickson RC, Machicao VI, et al. Liver retransplantation of patients with hepatitis C infection is associated with acceptable patient and graft survival. Liver Transpl 2007;13(12):1717–27.
62. Rosen H. Validation and refinement of survival models for liver retransplantation. Hepatology 2003;38(2):460–9.
63. Linhares MM, Azoulay D, Matos DL, et al. Liver retransplantation: a model for determining long-term survival. Transplantation 2006;81(7):1016–21.
64. Bellido CB, Martínez JM, Artacho GS, et al. Have we changed the liver retransplantation survival? Transplant Proc 2012;44(6):1526–9.
65. Marti J, Charco R, Ferrer J, et al. Optimization of liver grafts in liver retransplantation: a European single-center experience. Surgery 2008;144(5):762–9.
66. McCashland T, Watt K, Lyden E, et al. Retransplantation for hepatitis C: results of a U.S. multicenter retransplant study. Liver Transpl 2007;13(9):1246–53.
67. Hong JC, Kaldas FM, Kositamongkol P, et al. Predictive index for long-term survival after retransplantation of the liver in adult recipients. Ann Surg 2011;254(3): 444–9.
68. Jain A, Orloff M, Abt P, et al. Survival outcome after hepatic retransplantation for hepatitis C virus–positive and –negative recipients. Transplant Proc 2005;37(7): 3159–61.
69. Coilly A, Roche B, Samuel D. Current management and perspectives for HCV recurrence after liver transplantation. Liver Int 2013;33:56–62.
70. Organ distribution: allocation of livers. Available at: http://optn.transplant.hrsa.gov/PoliciesandBylaws2/policies/pdfs/policy_8.pdf. Accessed February 9, 2014.
71. Onaca N, Levy MF, Ueno T, et al. An outcome comparison between primary liver transplantation and retransplantation based on the pretransplant MELD score. Transpl Int 2006;19(4):282–7.
72. Edwards E, Harper A. Does MELD work for relisted candidates? Liver Transpl 2004;10(10 Suppl 2):S10–6.
73. Kim HJ, Larson JJ, Lim YS, et al. Impact of MELD on waitlist outcome of retransplant candidates. Am J Transplant 2010;10(12):2652–7.

74. Watt KDS, Menke T, Lyden E, et al. Mortality while awaiting liver retransplantation: predictability of MELD scores. Transplant Proc 2005;37(5):2172–3.

75. Yan J-Q, Peng C-H, Li H-W, et al. Preliminary clinical experience in liver retransplantation. Hepatobiliary Pancreat Dis Int 2007;6(2):152–6.

76. Biggins SW. Futility and rationing in liver retransplantation: when and how can we say no? J Hepatol 2012;56(6):1404–11.

77. Neuberger J, James O. Guidelines for selection of patients for liver transplantation in the era of donor-organ shortage. Lancet 1999;354(9190):1636–9.

78. Olthoff KM, Brown RS Jr, Delmonico FL, et al. Summary report of a national conference: evolving concepts in liver allocation in the MELD and PELD era. December 8, 2003, Washington, DC, USA. Liver Transpl 2004;10(10 Suppl 2): A6–22.

79. Kim WR, Wiesner RH, Poterucha JJ, et al. Hepatic retransplantation in cholestatic liver disease: impact of the interval to retransplantation on survival and resource utilization. Hepatology 1999;30(2):395–400.

80. Doyle HR, Morelli F, McMichael J, et al. Hepatic retransplantation–an analysis of risk factors associated with outcome. Transplantation 1996;61(10):1499–505.

81. Busuttil RW, Farmer DG, Yersiz H, et al. Analysis of long-term outcomes of 3200 liver transplantations over two decades: a single-center experience. Ann Surg 2005;241(6):905–16 [discussion: 916–8].

82. Marudanayagam R, Shanmugam V, Sandhu B, et al. Liver retransplantation in adults: a single-centre, 25-year experience. HPB (Oxford) 2010;12(3):217–24.

83. Markmann JF, Gornbein J, Markowitz JS, et al. A simple model to estimate survival after retransplantation of the liver. Transplantation 1999;67(3):422–30.

84. Ravaioli M, Grazi GL, Ercolani G, et al. Efficacy of MELD score in predicting survival after liver retransplantation. Transplant Proc 2004;36(9):2748–9.

85. Yao FY, Saab S, Bass NM, et al. Prediction of survival after liver retransplantation for late graft failure based on preoperative prognostic scores. Hepatology 2004; 39(1):230–8.

86. Maggi U, Consonni D, Bertoli P, et al. A risk score and a flowchart for liver retransplantation. Transplant Proc 2008;40(6):1956–60.

87. Ghabril M, Dickson R, Wiesner R. Improving outcomes of liver retransplantation: an analysis of trends and the impact of hepatitis C infection. Am J Transplant 2008;8(2):404–11.

88. Facciuto M, Heidt D, Guarrera J, et al. Retransplantation for late liver graft failure: predictors of mortality. Liver Transpl 2000;6(2):174–9.

89. Wong T, Devlin J, Rolando N, et al. Clinical characteristics affecting the outcome of liver retransplantation. Transplantation 1997;64(6):878–82.

90. Azoulay D, Linhares MM, Huguet E, et al. Decision for retransplantation of the liver: an experience- and cost-based analysis. Ann Surg 2002;236(6):713–21 [discussion: 721].

91. Schmitt TM, Kumer SC, Pruett TL, et al. Advanced recipient age (>60 years) alone should not be a contraindication to liver retransplantation. Transpl Int 2009;22(6):601–5.

92. Akpinar E, Selvaggi G, Levi D, et al. Liver retransplantation of more than two grafts for recurrent failure. Transplantation 2009;88(7):884–90.

93. Goh A, Scalamogna M, De Feo T, et al. Human leukocyte antigen crossmatch testing is important for liver retransplantation. Liver Transpl 2010;16(3):308–13.

94. Marti J, Fuster J, Navasa M, et al. Effects of graft quality on non-urgent liver retransplantation survival: should we avoid high-risk donors? World J Surg 2012; 36(12):2914–22.

95. Northup PG, Pruett TL, Kashmer DM, et al. Donor factors predicting recipient survival after liver retransplantation: the retransplant donor risk index. Am J Transplant 2007;7(8):1984–8.
96. Perry DK, Willingham DL, Sibulesky L, et al. Should donation after cardiac death liver grafts be used for retransplantation? Ann Hepatol 2011;10(4):482–5.
97. Davis A, Rosenthal P, Glidden D. Pediatric liver retransplantation: outcomes and a prognostic scoring tool. Liver Transpl 2009;15(2):199–207.
98. Yoo PS, Umman V, Rodriguez-Davalos MI, et al. Retransplantation of the liver: review of current literature for decision making and technical considerations. Transplant Proc 2013;45(3):854–9.
99. Herrmann J, Herden U, Ganschow R, et al. Transcapsular arterial neovascularization of liver transplants increases the risk of intraoperative bleeding during retransplantation. Transpl Int 2013;26(4):419–27.
100. Sibulesky L, Shine TS, Nguyen JH. A surgical technique for portal vein decompression in retransplantation. J Gastrointest Surg 2011;15(11):2098–100.
101. Maguire D, Hart R, Heaton N, et al. A complication of infrarenal arterial conduit following orthotopic liver transplant. HPB (Oxford) 2001;3(4):275–7.
102. Sibulesky L, Heckman MG, Perry DK, et al. A single-center experience with biliary reconstruction in retransplantation: duct-to-duct or Roux-en-Y choledochojejunostomy. Liver Transpl 2011;17(6):710–6.
103. Reese PP, Yeh H, Thomasson AM, et al. Transplant center volume and outcomes after liver retransplantation. Am J Transplant 2009;9(2):309–17.
104. Organ Procurement and Transplantation Network (OPTN) and Scientific Registry of Transplant Recipients (SRTR). OPTN/SRTR 2010 Annual Data Report. In: Department of Health and Human Services HRSA, Healthcare Systems Bureau, Division of Transplantation, editors. Rockville (MD): 2011.

Index

Note: Page numbers of article titles are in **boldface** type.

Moving?

Make sure your subscription moves with you!

To notify us of your new address, find your **Clinics Account Number** (located on your mailing label above your name), and contact customer service at:

Email: journalscustomerservice-usa@elsevier.com

800-654-2452 (subscribers in the U.S. & Canada)
314-447-8871 (subscribers outside of the U.S. & Canada)

Fax number: 314-447-8029

Elsevier Health Sciences Division
Subscription Customer Service
3251 Riverport Lane
Maryland Heights, MO 63043

*To ensure uninterrupted delivery of your subscription, please notify us at least 4 weeks in advance of move.

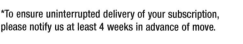
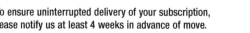

Printed and bound by CPI Group (UK) Ltd, Croydon, CR0 4YY

03/10/2024

01040491-0006